Principles of Pediatric Neurosurgery

Series Editor: Anthony J. Raimondi

Principles of Pediatric Neurosurgery

Head Injuries in the Newborn and Infant

The Pediatric Spine I: Development and the Dysraphic State
The Pediatric Spine II: Developmental Anomalies
The Pediatric Spine III: Cysts, Tumors, and Infections

Edited by Anthony J. Raimondi, Maurice Choux,
and Concezio Di Rocco

The Pediatric Spine II
Developmental Anomalies

Edited by Anthony J. Raimondi,
Maurice Choux, and Concezio Di Rocco

With 151 Figures

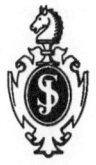

Springer Science+Business Media, LLC

ANTHONY J. RAIMONDI, M.D., 37020 Gargagnago (Verona), Italy

MAURICE CHOUX, M.D., Hôpital des Enfants de la Timone, Rue Saint Pierre, 13005 Marseille, France

CONCEZIO DI ROCCO, M.D., Istituto di Neurochirurgia, Università Cattolica del Sacro Cuore, Largo Gemelli 8, 00168 Rome, Italy

Library of Congress Cataloging-in-Publication Data
The Pediatric spine.
  (Principles of pediatric neurosurgery)
  Includes bibliographies and index.
  Contents: 1. Development and the dysraphic state —
v. 2. Developmental anomalies.
  1. Spine — Diseases. 2. Spine — Abnormalities.
3. Spine — Surgery. 4. Pediatric neurology. I. Raimondi,
Anthony J., 1928-   . II. Choux, M. (Maurice)
III. Di Rocco, C. (Concezio) IV. Series. [DNLM:
1. Spinal Diseases — in infancy and childhood. 2. Spine —
growth & development. WE 725 P3711]
RD768.P36 1989   618.92′73   88-24822

Printed on acid-free paper.

Typeset by Caliber Design Planning, Inc., New York, New York.

9 8 7 6 5 4 3 2 1

ISBN 978-1-4613-8831-9   ISBN 978-1-4613-8829-6 (eBook)
DOI 10.1007/978-1-4613-8829-6

Series Preface

It is estimated that the functionally significant body of knowledge for a given medical specialty changes radically every 8 years. New specialties and "subspecialization" are occurring at approximately an equal rate. Historically, established journals have not been able either to absorb this increase in publishable material or to extend their readership to the new specialists. International and national meetings, symposia and seminars, workshops, and newsletters successfully bring to the attention of physicians within developing specialties what is occurring, but generally only in demonstration form without providing historical perspective, pathoanatomical correlates, or extensive discussion. Page and time limitations oblige the authors to present only the essence of their material.

Pediatric neurosurgery is an example of a specialty that has developed during the past 15 years. Over this period, neurosurgeons have obtained special training in pediatric neurosurgery, and then dedicated themselves primarily to its practice. Centers, Chairs, and educational programs have been established as groups of neurosurgeons in different countries throughout the world organized themselves respectively into national and international societies for pediatric neurosurgery. These events were both preceded and followed by specialized courses, national and international journals, and ever-increasing clinical and investigative studies into all aspects of surgically treatable diseases of the child's nervous system.

Principles of Pediatric Neurosurgery is an ongoing series of publications, each dedicated exclusively to a particular subject, a subject which is currently timely either because of an extensive amount of work occurring in it, or because it has been neglected. The two first subjects, "Head Injuries in the Newborn and Infant" and "The Pediatric Spine," are expressive of those extremes.

Volumes will be published continuously, as the subjects are dealt with, rather than on an annual basis, since our goal is to make this information available to the specialist when it is new and informative. If a volume becomes obsolete because of newer methods of treatment and concepts, we shall publish a new edition.

The chapters are selected and arranged to provide the reader, in each instance, with embryological, developmental, epidemiological, clinical, therapeutic, and psychosocial aspects of each subject, thus permitting each specialist to learn what is current in his field and to familiarize himself with sister fields of the same subject. Each chapter is organized along classical lines, progressing from introduction through symptoms and treatment, to prognosis, for clinical material; and introduction through history and data, to results and discussion, for experimental material.

Contents

Series Preface   v
Contributors   ix

Chapter 1 Malformations of the Vertebrae
           SHIZUO OI   1

Chapter 2 The Normal and Abnormal Aspects of the
           Cranio-Vertebral Junction
           A. WACKENHEIM, J.L. DUTREIX, and G. ZÖLLNER   19

Chapter 3 Chiari Malformations
           CONCEZIO DI ROCCO and MARIO RENDE   57

Chapter 4 Diastematomyelia and Diplomyelia
           P. BRET, J.D. PATET, and C. LAPRAS   91

Chapter 5 Spondylolisthesis
           L. AULISA and F. SERRA   113

Chapter 6 Neurenteric Cysts
           JEAN-FRANÇOIS HIRSCH and ELIZABETH HOPPE-HIRSCH   134

Chapter 7 Sacral and Lumbo-Sacral Agenesis
           GÉRARD BOLLINI   144

Chapter 8 Teratomas
           J.G. RAFFENSPERGER   167

Chapter 9 The Tethered Spinal Cord
           HAROLD J. HOFFMAN   177

Chapter 10   Neuromuscular Scoliosis
             LAWRENCE A. RINSKY and EUGENE E. BLECK 189

Chapter 11   Current Concepts in Long-Term Care of the Deformed Spine
             WILLIAM J. KANE 221

Chapter 12   Congenital Malformations of the Spine in Children:
             Neuro-Imaging
             H.S. CHUANG 251

Index 291

Contributors

LORENZO AULISA
Associate Professor, Department of Orthopaedic Surgery, Catholic University School of Medicine, Rome, Italy

EUGENE E. BLECK
Professor and Chief, Orthopaedic Division, Stanford University School of Medicine, Stanford, California, USA

GÉRARD BOLLINI
Professeur de Chirurgie Infantile, Hôpital Enfants Timone, Marseille, France

PHILIPPE BRET
Professor of Neurosurgery, Université Claude Bernard, U.F.R. Lyon-Nord, France

H.S. CHUANG
Associate Professor, University of Toronto and Head, Division of Special Procedures, Department of Radiology, The Hospital for Sick Children, Toronto, Ontario, Canada

CONCEZIO DI ROCCO
Associate Professor, Pediatric Neurosurgery, Catholic University Medical School, Rome, Italy

J.L. DUTREIX
Centre Hospitalier Universitaire, Tours, France

JEAN-FRANÇOIS HIRSCH
Professeur de Neurochirurgie, Hôpital Necker Enfants Malades, Service de Neurochirurgie Pédiatrique, Paris, France

HAROLD J. HOFFMAN
Professor of Neurosurgery, Division of Neurosurgery, University of Toronto and Chief, Division of Neurosurgery, The Hospital for Sick Children, Toronto, Canada

ELIZABETH HOPPE-HIRSCH
Service de Neuro-Chirurgie, Groupe Hospitalier Necker-Enfants Malades, Paris, France

WILLIAM J. KANE
Professor of Orthopaedic Surgery, Northwestern University Medical School, Chicago, Illinois, USA

CLAUDE LAPRAS
Professor of Neurosurgery, Hôpital Neurologique, Lyon, France

SHIZUO OI
Assistant Professor of Neurosurgery, Department of Neurosurgery, Kobe University, School of Medicine, Kobe, Japan

J.D. PATET
Assistant Neurosurgeon, Hôpital Neurologique, Lyon, France

JOHN G. RAFFENSPERGER
Professor of Surgery, Northwestern University and Surgeon-in-Chief, Children's Memorial Hospital, Chicago, Illinois, USA

MARIO RENDE
Assistant Professor of Human Anatomy, Institute of Normal Human Anatomy, Catholic University School of Medicine, Rome, Italy

LAWRENCE A. RINSKY
Associate Professor, Orthopaedic Division, Stanford University School of Medicine, Stanford, California, USA

FABRIZIO SERRA
Assistant, Department of Orthopaedic Surgery, Catholic University School of Medicine, Rome, Italy

AUGUSTE WACKENHEIM
Professor and Chairman of Radiology, Medical School, University of Strasbourg, Strasbourg, France

GEORG ZÖLLNER
Associate Professor of Radiology, Strasbourg, France

CHAPTER 1

Malformations of the Vertebrae

Shizuo Oi

Embryologic Concepts

Development of the vertebrae and spinal column begins in the third embryonic week and is completed at around 20 years of age. Development occurs by the processes of membrane formation, chondrification (both in the embryonal period), and ossification (in the fetal and postnatal periods). Teratologically speaking, because the embryonic cellular and tissue organization proceed in an exact sequential manner, a congenital malformation is induced in the upper (cephalic site of) vertebrae with early exposure to teratogenic factors, and in the lower (caudal) parts in late exposure (cephalocaudal sequence).[1] Exposure to an effective teratogenic factor causes predictable types of spinal anomalies specific to each temporal period: (1) disorders of the notochord, (2) disorders of the unsegmented paraxial mesoderm, (3) disorders of segmentation, and (4) disorders of sclerotome differentiation.

Classification and Incidence

Classification of congenital vertebral anomalies is based on either roentgenographic/pathoanatomic morphology or embryopathogenesis. Tsou et al.[2] proposed an inclusive classification based on classic embryogenesis and prenatal developmental pattern of the vertebra (Table 1.1). They evaluated congenital vertebral anomalies in 144 patients and revealed the incidence of each specific type of anomaly as shown in the table. It is said that approximately 5% of fetuses have congenital vertebral anomalies.[3]

Vertebral anomalies are classified according to anatomic location in Tables 1.2 to 1.5.

Table 1.1. Classification and incidence of congenital vertebral anomalies from the aspect of embryopathogenesis

Period	Incidence in clinical series
Embryonic (first 56 days postovum fertilization)	
I. Germinal layers midline adhesions (sagittal vertebral cleft)	
A. Neuroendodermal adhesion, mild; irregular or eccentric centrum cleft	
1. Posterior migration of adhesion−intraspinal enteric diverticulum	1[a]
2. Anterior migration of adhesion−anterior myelomeningocoele	0
B. Neuroectoendodermal adhesion, severe; combined centrum and neural arch cleft with diastematomyelia secondary to enterocutaneous fistula/cyst	0
II. Notochordal substance sequestration	
A. In neuroectoendodermal layer; diastematomyelia secondary to midline mesenchymal septum	1[a]
B. In centrum; centrum bifided by smooth hourglass axial channel	4
III. Asynchronous development of hemimetamer pairs−pairing defect anomalies	
A. Solitary hemivertebral−contralateral hemimetameric column shifts one segment caudad	
B. Double hemivertebrae	28
1. Balanced−lower contralateral hemivertebra end caudad shift	20
2. Unbalanced hemivertebrae, nonconsecutive	2
C. Multiple pairing defects; more than two asynchronous pairs complete or partial shifts	8
IV. Hemimetamer hypoplasia and aplasia	
A. Hypoplasia	
1. Mild; ipsilateral diminution of centrum and neural arch; no disturbance of functional segmentation	3
2. Moderate; neural arch elements intersegmental coalition	
a. Apophyseal process bar	2
b. Combined apophyseal process and pedicle bar	2
3. Severe; conjoined neural arch and centrum intersegmental coalition	25
B. Aplasia, unilateral only	
1. Solitary hemivertebra	2
2. Multiple hemivertebrae	3
V. Ventral and lateral processes coalition (rib and transverse process)	1
	101
Fetal (57th day postovum fertilization to birth)	
I. Vertebral amphiarthrodial and arthrodial joints failure of segmentation	
A. Annulus fibrosis osseous metaplasia	
1. Complete-block vertebrae	5
2. Partial-lateral (5), anterior (2), or posterior (1) osseous bar	8
B. Neural arch apophyseal joint failure of segmentation	
1. Unilateral	1
2. Bilateral	0

Table 1.1. *Continued*

Period	Incidence in clinical series
C. Costovertebral joint failure of segmentation (2nd–9th ribs interarticular)	
1. Unilateral	1
2. Bilateral	0
II. Centrum hypoplasia and aplasia	
A. Wedge	6
B. Posterior hemicentrum	6
C. Lateral hemicentrum	3
D. Posterior quadrant centrum	9
E. Centrum aplasia	3
	43

From: Tsou et al[2] with permission.

[a] The same patient had these two anomalies.

Major Anomalies of the Vertebrae

Malformations of the Atlas (Table 1.2)

Arch Defect of the Atlas

As ossification of the atlas proceeds dorsally from the two centers forming the lateral masses, the various types of ossification defects vary from unilateral to total aplasia (Fig. 1.1).[4] A posterior arch defect, or cleft, is seen in 4% and an anterior one in 0.1% of autopsy cases.[5] This rare anomaly is an incidental observation noted at the time of radiologic investigations for other reasons. The patients are essentially symptom-free because the posterior element of the atlas

Table 1.2. Malformations of the atlas

Dysraphism–aplasia–hypoplasia
   Anterior arch defect
   Posterior arch defect
   Hypoplasia of C1

Dysplasia
   Lateral ponticle
   Posterior ponticle
   Epitransverse processes
   Malformations of the transverse process
   Malformations of the lateral masses

Fusion
   Assimilation of the atlas (occipitalization)
   Atlanto-axial fusion

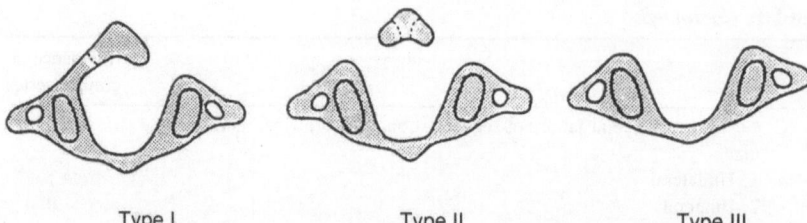

Type I   Type II   Type III

Figure 1.1. Ossification defects of the posterior arch of the atlas.[4] Type I: unilateral aplasia of the posterior arch, with or without complete posterior midline ossification. Type II: bilateral aplasia of the posterior arch, with single midline or paramedian posterior ossicle(s). Type III: total aplasia of the posterior arch. From: Page et al[4] with permission.

contributes negligibly to cervical stability. Hypoplasia of the anterior arch of the atlas is often associated with atlanto-axial fusion and sometimes causes neurologic symptoms. Otherwise, no surgical intervention is indicated even if the posterior arch defect is complete.

Dysplasia of the Atlas

The majority of individuals with this anomaly are asymptomatic. Lateral ponticle is the condition in which a bony spicule extends from the lateral edge of the superior facet of C1 to the transverse process, whereas in posterior ponticle the spicule extends over the posterior margin. Other malformations in this category include epitransverse process, and malformations of the transverse process and the lateral masses.

Fusion

Fusion of the atlas may occur either to the occipital bone (failure of segmentation of the first cervical vertebra from the skull, i.e., assimilation of the atlas,

Table 1.3. Malformations of the axis

Dysplasia–dysgenesis of odontoid process
  Os odontoideum
  Ossiculum terminale
  Agenesis of odontoid base
  Agenesis of apical segment
  Agensis of odontoid

Dysraphism–aplasia–hypoplasia
  Posterior arch defect
  Pedicle defect

Fusion
  Atlanto-axial fusion
  Klippel–Feil syndrome

occipitalization), or to the axis (atlanto-axial fusion). The former anomaly is seen in about 0.1 to 3% of the general population and the latter is extremely rare. Atlanto-axial fusion may cause limitation of rotatory neck motion but is essentially asymptomatic neurologically. Assimilation of the atlas is sometimes associated with basilar impression, protoatlas, and other cervical spine anomalies. Atlanto-axial dislocation may develop and progressively worsen, occurring in approximately half the patients with this anomaly. Various neurologic symptoms occur secondary either to the associated basilar impression or the instability. Nuchal pain/rigidity, motor deficits with or without ataxia, and pain/paresthesia of the extremities are common and often become prominent with episodes of head and neck injury. These conditions require surgical intervention.

Malformations of the Axis (Table 1.3)

Dysplasia–Dysgenesis of Odontoid Process

Greenberg[6] described five variations of odontoid anomalies (Fig. 1.2). These include os odontoideum (joint-like articulation between the odontoid and the body of the axis), ossiculum terminale (failure of fusion of the apical segment of the dens to its base), agenesis of the odontoid base (defect of base of odontoid process), agenesis of apical segment (short odontoid with defect of the apical segment), and agenesis of the odontoid (complete absence of the odontoid process). The embryopathogenesis of this anomaly has been considered, and two theories have been advanced[7]: (1) failure of fusion of the apex or ossiculum terminale to the odontoid and (2) failure of fusion of the odontoid to the axis. No definite explanation has yet been established. The incidence of this anomaly is unclear because so few cases become symptomatic.

The symptomatology depends on whether atlanto-axial dislocation exists. Rowland[8] classified the symptoms of atlanto-axial dislocation into four groups:

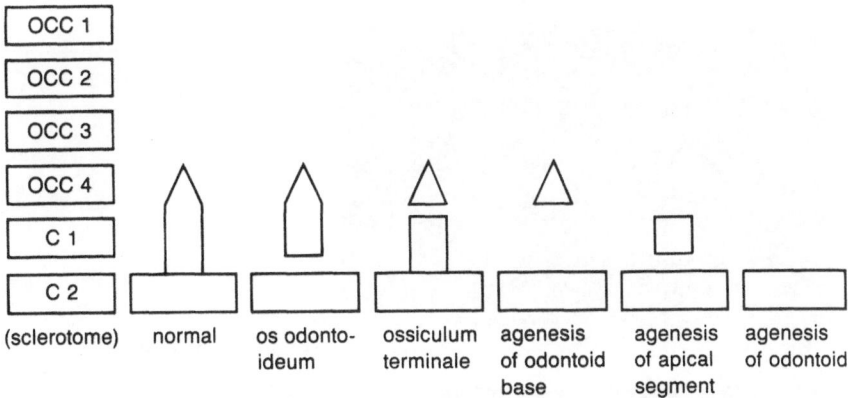

Figure 1.2. Variations of odontoid anomalies. (Modified from Greenberg AD[6]).

group 1, severe cervical pain and marked torticollis, following immediately some kind of trauma, but no neurologic abnormality; group 2, trauma followed by transient weakness of extremities and dysesthesia, torticollis, and permanent neurologic deficit; group 3, slowly progressing or permanent cervical myelopathy without torticollis or neck pain, in the absence of a history of trauma; group 4, cerebral symptoms such as seizures, mental deterioration, unconsciousness, vertigo, and visual disturbances; no cervical myelopathy or nerve root compression. Nagashima[9] ascribed the symptomatology of this condition to the following factors: (1) mechanical neural compression by C1 segment, (2) vertebral circulatory disturbances, and (3) hypertrophic meningopathy. The diagnosis of odontoid anomalies is based on radiologic findings so that the classification and identification of the specific type of anomaly require lateral laminographic studies (Fig. 1.3). The examination must be performed in flexion and extension to rule out instability of the atlanto-axial articulation (Fig. 1.4A–F). Now, magnetic resonance (MR) imaging is available and has the most diagnostic value in detection of the cord compression with the postural changes (Fig. 1.4G–I). Vertebral angiography may be required in cases with symptoms suggestive of vertebral circulatory disturbances. In cases of atlanto-axial dislocation, further diagnostic

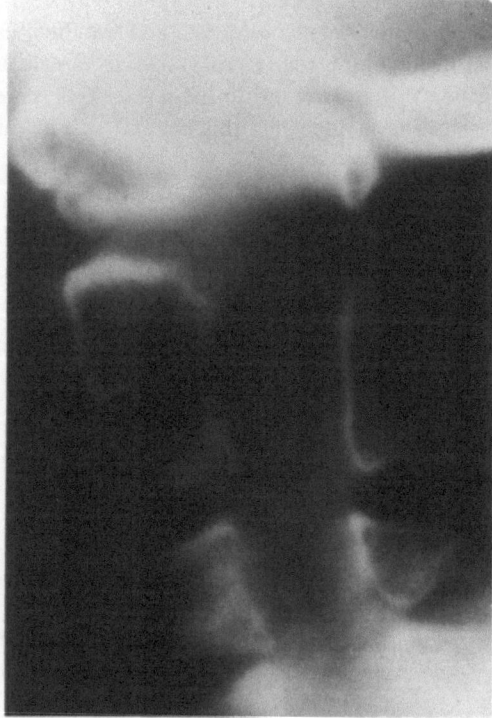

Figure 1.3. Lateral view of laminogram in a patient with os odontoideum.

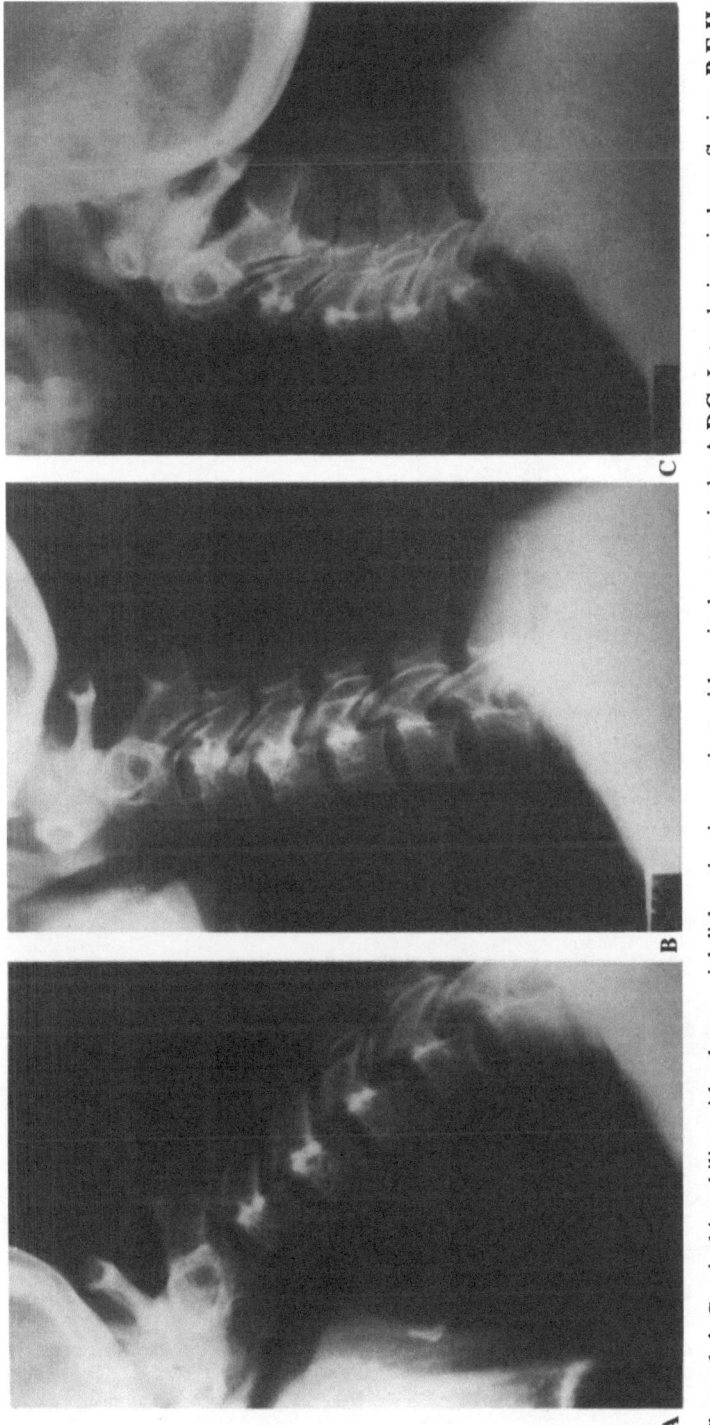

Figure 1.4. Cervical instability with atlanto-axial dislocation in a patient with ossiculum terminale. **A,D,G:** Lateral views in hyperflexion. **B,E,H:** Lateral views in neutral position. **C,F,I:** Lateral views in hyperextension. **A–C:** Plain cervical spine x-ray films. **D–F:** Laminograms. **G–I:** MR images.

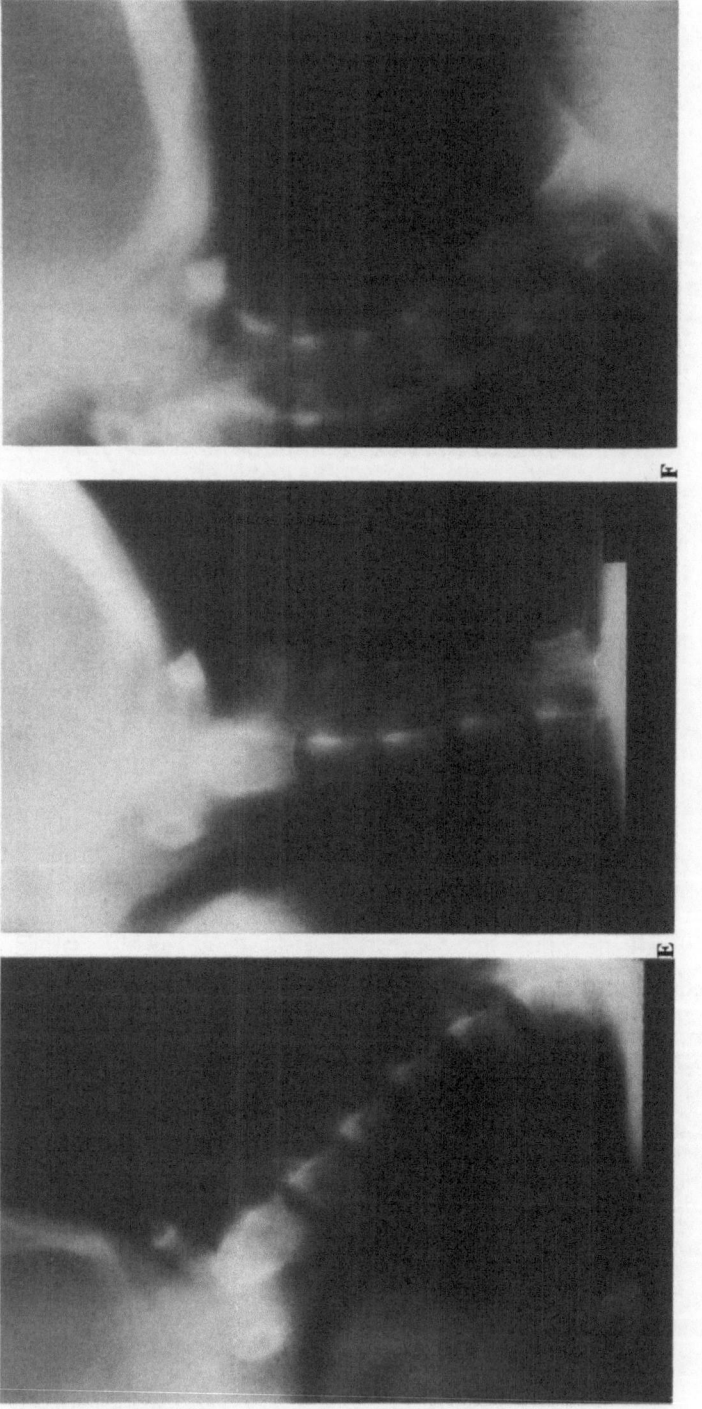

Figure 1.4. *Continued.*

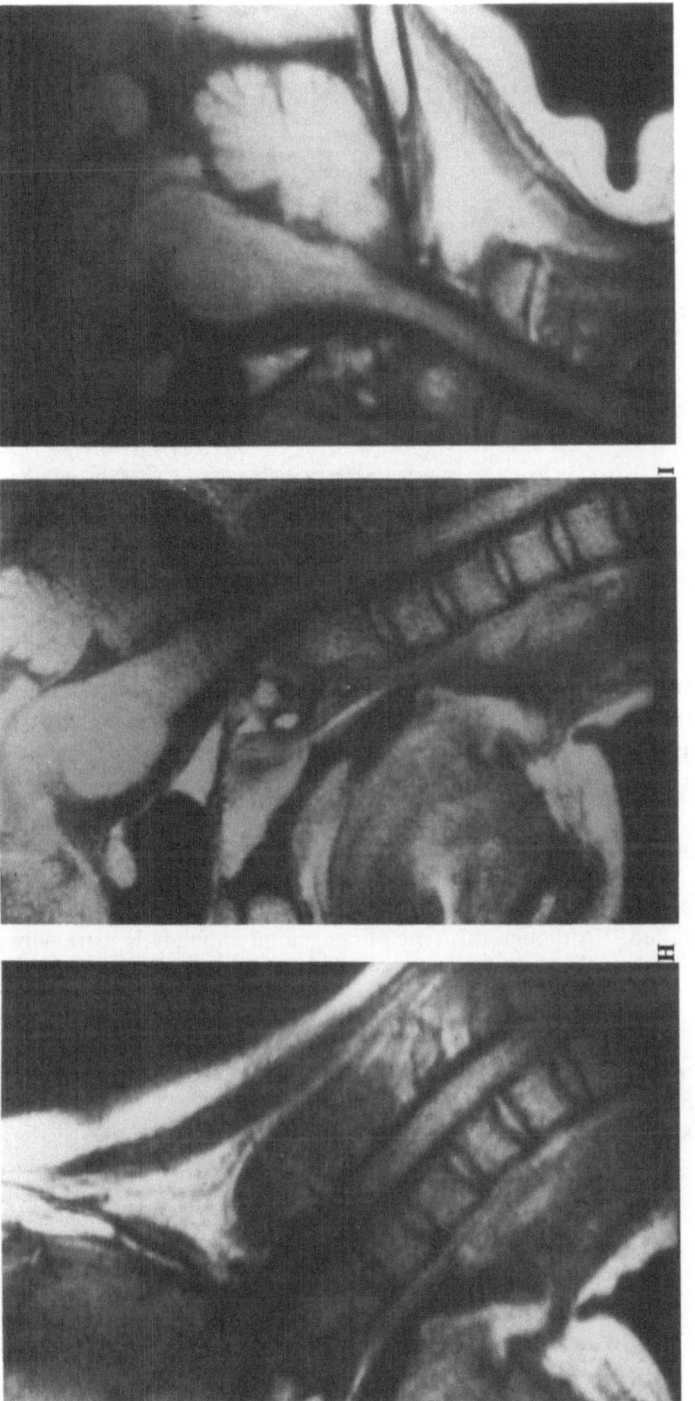

Figure 1.4. *Continued.*

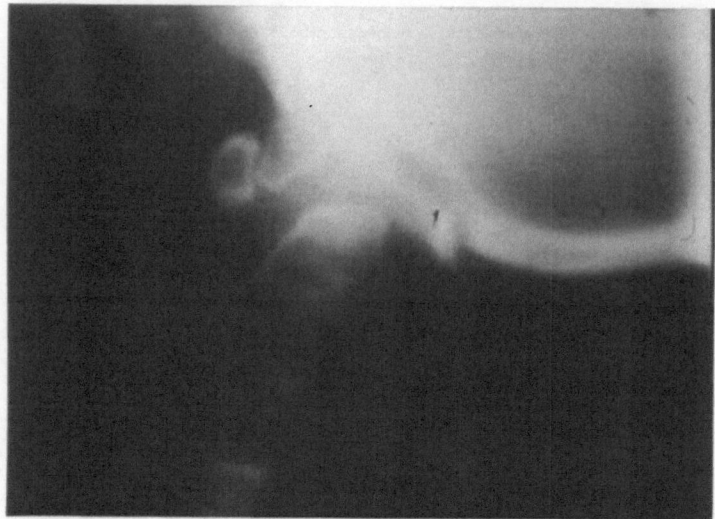

Figure 1.5. Lateral view of laminogram indicates atlanto-axial dislocation with ossiculum terminale in a patient with Down's syndrome.

procedures or informations may be necessary to exclude the possibilities of rheumatoid arthritis, trauma, infection, Down's syndrome[10] (Fig. 1.5), etc. Operative intervention must be considered, especially in symptomatic cases; however, the choice of operative approach, either anterior or posterior, remains controversial.

Dysraphism–Aplasia–Hypoplasia of Arch or Pedicle of C2 (Fig. 1.6)

Only a few cases of absence of the C2 pedicle with or without spondylolysis have been reported.[11] Although this type of congenital anomaly is extremely rare in

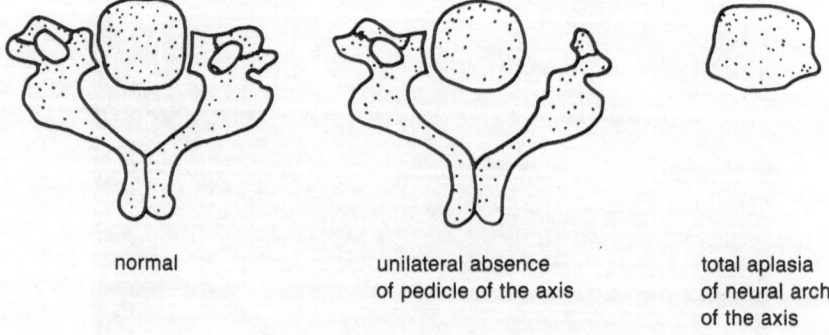

Figure 1.6. Variations of neural arch defects of the axis.

Figure 1.7. Complete neural arch defects of the axis. **A**: Lateral view of laminogram reveals instability and deformity of the cervical spine with complete absence of the neural arch of the axis. **B**: Metrizamid myelographic CT shows the spinal cord without bony covering laterally or posteriorly.

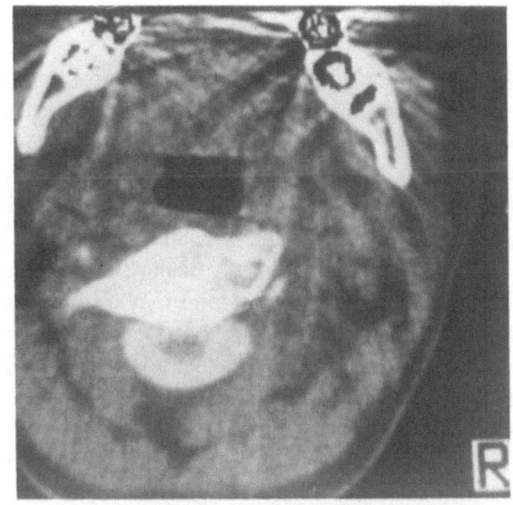

A

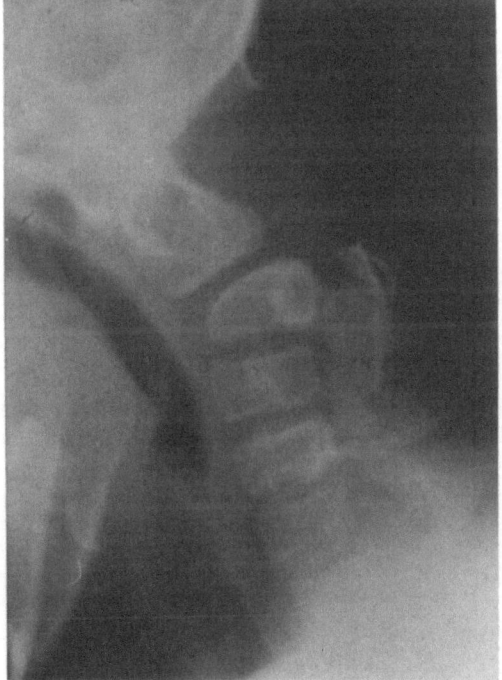

B

the cervical spine, C6 is the most common site for pedicle defects.[12] The author has an experience of familial cases with complete absence of the pedicle and posterior arch of the axis (Fig. 1.7). Cervical instability may occur with spondylolysis. Anterior fusion is the procedure of choice.[13]

Fusion of the Axis

Klippel–Feil syndrome is one of the most common congenital spine anomalies and represents fused vertebra (Fig. 1.8). From the point of view of genetics, there is an obvious inheritance factor. Autosomal dominant inheritance is active in this type of spine anomaly at C2–3, whereas the autosomal recessive form is causative for the ones at C5–6.[14] The triad of this syndrome includes brevicollis (short neck), low posterior hair line, and limited neck motion. Neurologic manifestations such as long tract signs, ocular findings, and pain are occasionally present. These same signs and symptoms may be due to associated malformation anomalies such as basilar impression, Duane–Stilling–Türk syndrome, Turner's syndrome, and cervico-oculo-acoustic dysplasia (Wildervanck's syndrome).[15,16] The Klippen–Feil syndrome is also associated with spina bifida in 45% of cases, spine deformities such as scoliosis and kyphosis in 65%, Sprengel's deformity in 30%, and rib deformities in 33%.[11] Clinical management of these associated problems may be necessary.

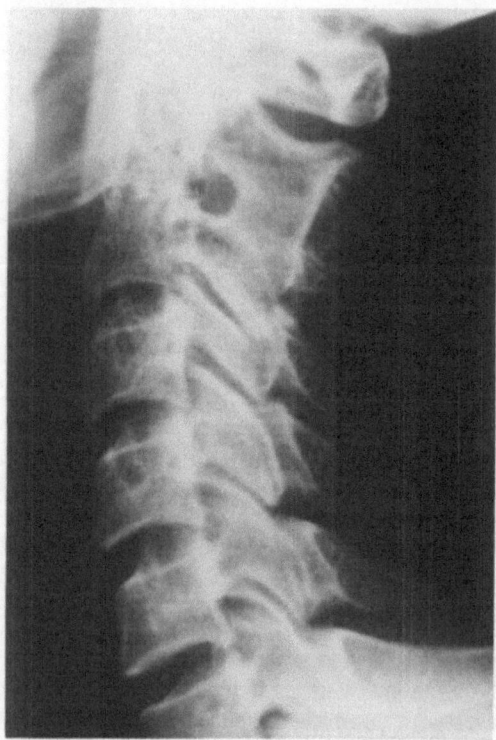

Figure 1.8. Lateral view of cervical spine x-ray film in a patient with Klippel–Feil syndrome.

Malformations Commonly Affecting the Thoracic Vertebrae (Table 1.4)

Hemivertebra and Other Hypoplastic Vertebral Anomalies

Hemivertebra is one of the most common anomalies affecting the thoracic spine. Tsou et al.[2] proposed that this anomaly is the result of pairing defect of sclerotomic cells with asynchronous development of the hemimetameric pair. The most common mechanism of hemivertebra formation is believed by them to consist of paired somite derivatives which are not in the same developmental phase by the time midline fusion occurs. The tardy side may shift one segment caudad (solitary hemivertebra). Also, if two asynchronous pairs deploy tardy hemimetamers on contralateral sides, double-balanced hemivertebrae will develop. The etiopathogenesis of hemivertebrae and other hypoplastic vertebral anomalies is still obscure, though some authors suggest hereditary factors, such as considered in a report of monozygomatic twins,[17] or familial episodes in several generations.[18] Others report chromosomal anomaly[19] (see Spondylothoracic Dysplasia). Spine x-ray films shown in Fig. 1.9 indicate a case of a neonate with unbalanced multiple hemivertebrae and fusion of ribs or transverse processes on contralateral sides. Congenital scoliosis is, of course, the major clinical problem in wedge or hemivertebra.

The conditions of failure of segmentation such as unilateral bar or fused vertebrae may be the cause of congenital scoliosis.[20] This anomaly is more commonly observed in the cervical or lumbar spines (Fig. 1.10). In cases with a scoliotic spine, wedged vertebra does not necessarily indicate congenital asynchronous development. One must be careful to remember that such a deformity of the vertebra may be seen as a complication of severe scoliosis resulting from such other

Table 1.4. Malformations commonly affecting the thoracic vertebra

---

Dysraphism–aplasia–hypoplasia
  Failure of formation
    Wedge
    Hemivertebra
  Sagittal vertebral cleft
    Intraspinal enteric diverticulum
    Anterior myelomeningocele
    Centrum

Dysplasia–dysgenesis
  Spondylocostal dysplasia

Mesenchymal septum
  Diastematomyelia

Fusion–failure of segmentation
  Unilateral bur
  Bilateral ("fusion")

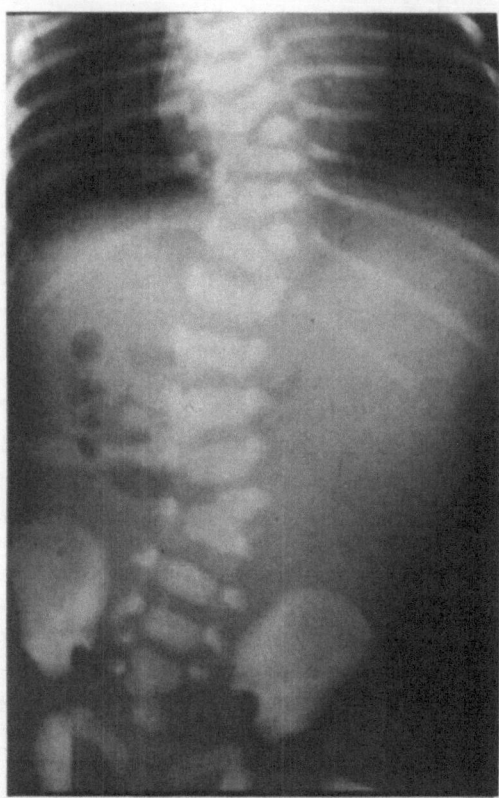

Figure 1.9. Anterior view of spine x-ray film in a newborn reveals unbalanced multiple hemivertebrae and fusion of ribs or transverse processes on the contralateral side. Note complicated scoliotic curvature.

causative pathologies as neuromuscular, tumoral, mesenchymal, traumatic, infectious, metabolic, etc. conditions.

Spondylothoracic Dysplasia

In addition to hereditary factors for congenital scoliosis just described, spondylothoracic dysplasia[21,22] should be considered. This is an autosomal recessive condition which results in lordosis rather than scoliotic spine deformity due to fusion of facets and transverse processes, lateral bar of adjacent ribs, and fusion/wedge deformity of vertebral bodies.

Sagittal Vertebral Cleft/Mesenchymal Septum

See the chapter, "Diastematomyelia" by Lapras in Vol. III.

Fusion–Failure of Segmentation

See page 16.

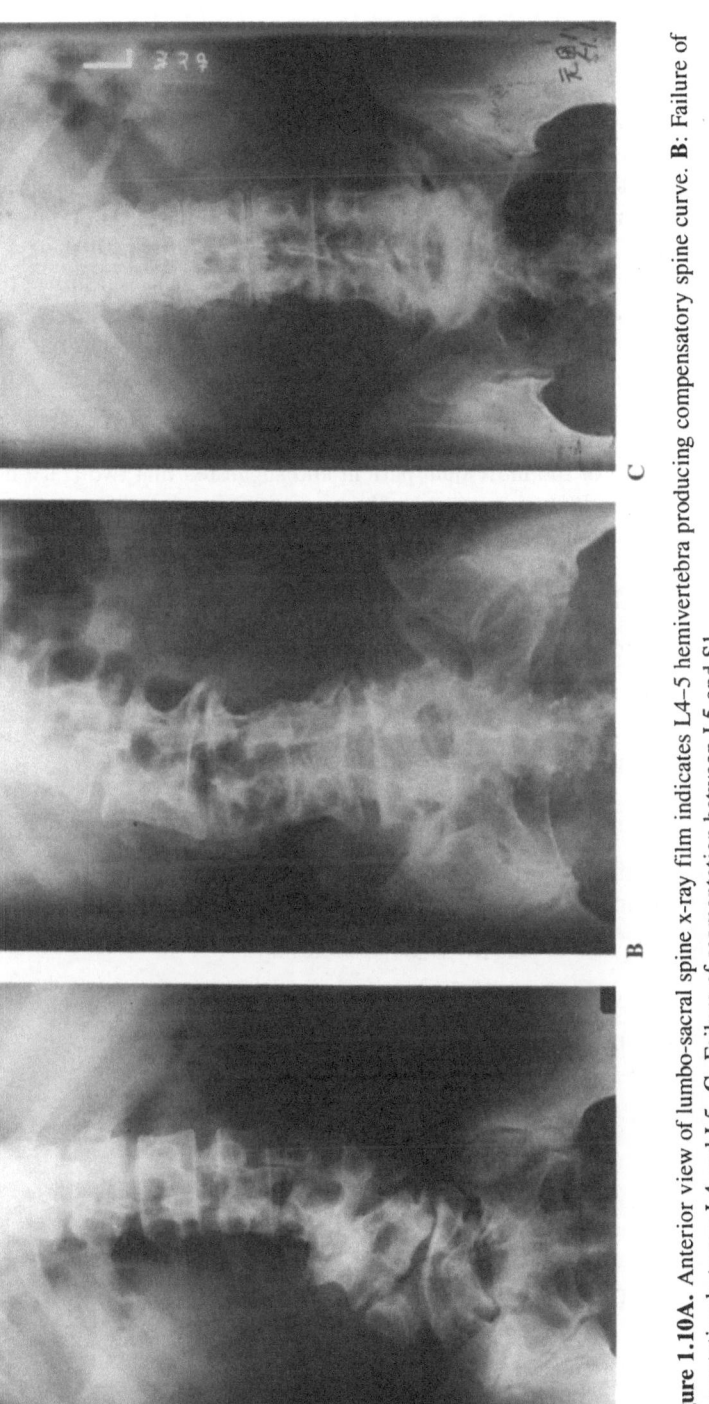

Figure 1.10A. Anterior view of lumbo-sacral spine x-ray film indicates L4–5 hemivertebra producing compensatory spine curve. **B**: Failure of segmentation between L4 and L5. **C**: Failure of segmentation between L5 and S1.

Malformations of Lumbo-sacral Vertebra (Table 1.5)

Lumbo-sacral Hemivertebrae

The anterior view of lumbo-sacral spine x-ray film in Fig. 1.10A indicates L4–5 hemivertebrae producing compensatory spine curve. According to Slabaugh et al.,[23] females are predominantly affected (male/female ratio, 5:9). The hemivertebra occurred at the first sacral level in 11 patients, at L5 in 6, and at L4 in 5. Also, they described two cases of ipsilateral hemivertebra at the L4 and L5 levels. The major clinical problem consists of progressive lateral shift of the trunk with growth, due to lack of a mobile spine and the development of a compensatory spine curve. This latter is, however, necessary to maintain the structural position of the back. The operative approach to correct this unique problem is still controversial because the conventional management, fusion or brace, is not satisfactory. Slabaugh et al.[23] proposed the future management depending on the natural history of the individual patient and suggested that two-stage hemivertebral excision with fusion may give the best results in selected patients who have significant deformity.

Congenital Absence of Lumbo-sacral Spine–Sacral Agenesis

See the chapter, "Sacral Agenesis" by Bollini, this volume.

Dysraphism

See the chapters "The Dysraphic State".

Fusion–Failure of Segmentation

Failure of segmentation between the L5 transverse processes and lateral mass of the S1 segment result in sacralization. Plain x-ray films of lumbo-sacral spine in

Table 1.5. Malformations of lumbo-sacral vertebra

Dysraphism–aplasia–hypoplasia
  Failure of formation
    Wedge
    Hemivertebra
    Congenital absence of lumbo-sacral spine
    Sacral agenesis
  Dysraphism
    Spina bifida
    Anterior myelomeningocele

Dysplasia–dysgenesis
  Dysplasic spondylolisthesis

Fusion–failure of segmentation
  Fusion of lumbar spine
  Sacralization

Fig. 1.10 reveal the failure of segmentation between L4–5 and L5–S1 (sacralization), respectively. These forms of congenital anomaly rarely cause regional signs or symptoms but occasionally associate with developmental narrowing of the lumbo-sacral canal.[24] This category of congenital anomaly of the spine may sometimes be a part of clinical features of certain syndromes involving systemic bony structures such as Turner's syndrome, Stanesco's dysostosis syndrome, etc., suggesting that hereditary or chromosome anomaly factors may be active in the etiopathogenesis.

Acknowledgments. The author acknowledges the permission of Dr. Yasuo Yamanouchi, Assistant Professor of Neurosurgery, Kansai Medical College; Dr. Akira Kimura, Chief of Pediatric Neurosurgery Section, Department of Neurosurgery, Ishikawa Central Prefectural Hospital; and Dr. Akihiro Doi, Chairman of Neurosurgery, Kagawa Central Prefectural Hospital to cite their valuable cases in this chapter. The author also express his sincerest appreciation to Professor Satoshi Matsumoto and Professor Anthony J. Raimondi for kindly reviewing this manuscript.

References

1. Tanimura T: Relationship of dosage and time of administration to teratogenic effects of thio-TEPA in mice. Okajimas Fol Anat Jpn 44:203–253, 1968.
2. Tsou PM, Yau A, Hodgson AR: Embryogenesis and prenatal development of congenital vertebral anomalies and their classification. In: Urist MR (ed): Clinical Orthopedics and Related Research, Vol. 152, Section II. Lippincott, Philadelphia, 1980, pp 211–231.
3. Furukawa C: Clinicopathoanatomical study of congenital vertebral anomalies. Nisseikaishi 37:485–510, 1963.
4. Page GT, Yock DH Jr: Total aplasia of the posterior arch of the atlas. Minn Med: 666–668, 1981.
5. Geipel P: Zur Kenntnis der Spaltbildung des Atlas und Epistropheus. Fortschr Pontgenstr 52:533–570, 1935.
6. Greenberg AD: Atlanto-axial dislocations. Brain 91:655–684, 1968.
7. Hensinger RN, Fielding JW, Hawkins RJ: Congenital anomalies of the odontoid process. Orthop Clin North Am 9:901–912, 1978.
8. Rowland LP, Shapiro JH, Jacobson HG: Neurological syndromes associated with congenital absence of the odontoid process. Arch Neurol Psychiatry 80:286–291, 1958.
9. Nagashima C: Atlanto-axial dislocation due to the os odontoideum and the odontoid agenesis. Report of five cases with comments on pathophysiology and the occipitovertebral fixation with acrylic plastic (N. Dott) as a surgical treatment. No to Shinkei (JPN) 20:881–896, 1968.
10. Nordt JC, Stauffer ES: Sequelae of atlantoaxial stabilization in two patients with Down's syndrome. Spine 6:437–440, 1981.
11. Hensinger RN, MacEwen GD: Congenital Abnormalities of the spine. In: Rathman RH, Simeone FA (eds): The Spine. WB Saunders, Philadelphia, 1982, pp 216–233.

12. Fardon DF, Fielding JW: Defects of the pedicle and spondylolysthesis of the second cervical vertebra. J Bone Joint Surg 63:526–528, 1981.
13. Prioleau GR, Wilson CB: Cervical spondylolysis with spondylolisthesis. J Neurosurg 43:750–753, 1975.
14. Gunderson CH, Greenspan RH, Glaser GH, Lubs HA: The Klippel–Feil syndrome: genetic and clinical reevaluation of cervical fusion. Medicine 46:491–522, .
15. Eisemann ML, Sharma GK: The Wildervanck syndrome: cervico-oculo-acoustic dysplasia. Otolaryngol Head Neck Surg 87:892–897, 1979.
16. Wildervanck LS, Hoekseman PE, Pennings L: Radiological examination of the inner ear of deafmutes presenting the cervico-oculo-acousticus syndrome. Acta Otolaryngol 61:445–453, 1966.
17. Adam MS, and Niswander JD: Health of the American Indian: congenital defects. Eugen Quart 15:227–234, 1968.
18. Carter CO, Roberts JAF: The risk of recurrence after two children with central nervous system malformations. Lancet i:306–308, 1967.
19. Ingalls TH, Pugh TF, MacMahon B: Incidence of anencephalus, spina bifida, and hydrocephalus related to birth rank and maternal age. Br J Prevent Soc Med 8:17–23, 1954.
20. Goldstein LA, Waugh TR: Classification and terminology of scoliosis. Clin Orthop 93:22, 1973.
21. Lauy NW, Palmer CG, Merritt AD: A syndrome of bizarre vertebral anomalies. J Pediatr 60:1121–1125, 1966.
22. Pochaczeusky R, Ratner H, Perles D, et al.: Spondylothoracic dysplasia. Radiology 98:53–58, 1971.
23. Slabaugh PB, Winter RB, Lonstein JE, Moe JH: Lumbosacral hemivertebrae—a review of twenty-four patients, with excision in eight. Spine 5:234–244, 1980.
24. Uinke TH, White EH: Congenital narrowing of the lumbosacral space. Surg Gynecol Obstet 76:551, 1943.

CHAPTER 2

The Normal and Abnormal Aspects of the Cranio-Vertebral Junction

A. Wackenheim, J.L. Dutreix, and G. Zöllner

It is very important to recall that the cranio–vertebral junction is a key area because it contains the medulla oblongata, the location of life; numerous civilizations chose this structure as the site at which to kill by decapitation. From a clinical point of view, we may be schematic and say that one may distinguish six categories of pathologic patterns.

1. *Pain.* The complexity of movements at the articulations between the occipital condyles and the atlas, and between the atlas and the axis, permit one to understand the many possibilities of articular pain. The frequent minor malformations, except in childhood, are responsible for radicular pain in the C1 and C2 roots. Exceptionally, children may suffer from "flexion pain," due to the flexed position of the head in school. These children may be misunderstood by psychologists when they describe the pain starting after 2 or 3 hours of working at school, interpreted as a device to get out of schoolwork. In fact, it is the position which causes the pain.

2. *Infections.* In the past, especially before the use of antibiotics, an important chapter of pathology was infections. The work of Grisel[1] was devoted to cervico-occipital complications due to infection of the tonsils or abscesses of the pharynx. The main presentation of this pathology is as torticollis due to C1–C2 dislocation (infectious lesions of the ligaments, especially of the transverse ligament). A.W. Sullivan[2] observed that 77% of 56 children suffered this dislocation. The x-ray films demonstrate in all cases a swelling of the soft parts, but it is the forward luxation of head and atlas upon the axis that is the most striking sign seen on a lateral projection. In severe cases, or those detected late, there are destruction of the bones (translucencies, demineralization) so that the epidural space may be infected (epiduritis). In these cases, the sequellae may be serious, necessitating stabilization surgery.

Tuberculous osteoarthritis is not frequent, but it must be suspected in young patients affected with tuberculosis of the lungs, kidney, and so forth.

3. *Rheumatism.* Degenerative arthrosis does not occur in childhood, but we must consider juvenile polyarthritis (Still's disease), illustrated in Fig. 2.17.

4. *Malformations.* In this very important section we consider malformations of the bones and the nervous system. Some of them may coexist in the same patient.

Malformations in childhood, at least those of the bones, are not as complicated as in adults. Many minor malformations do not form because the ossification process is not yet complete. We have, furthermore, to consider that even more severe bone malformations are detected only by chance, i.e., the young patient has no clinical symptoms. We will see examples of basilar invagination and *odontoideum mobile* without clinical symptomatology.

5. *Tumors*. Tumors growing from the bone, meninges, nerve roots, vessels, and medulla cause progressive neurologic signs and require sophisticated imaging investigations for precise anatomic diagnosis.

6. *Trauma*. As in other parts of the human body, the tolerance to trauma is very high in early childhood and adolescence.

Embryology

Osseous development of the cervico-occipital region is more completely understood if it is remembered that, according to different authors, three, four, or five vertebral segments participate in the development of the occipital bone.

The relevant embryologic literature includes Oken (1811), Spix (1815), Goethe (1820), Meckel (1820), Vogt (1842), Remak (1850), Gegenbauer (1872), Froriep (1886), Hayek (1923), Arey (1938), Reiter (1944), and Sensenig (1957). Progressive occipitalization of the upper cervical spine can be said to be the normal evolutionary pattern in humans. This being so, atlanto-occipital assimilation, although considered as a malformation, may be viewed as an early form of progressive evolution. Conversely, the persistence of ossicles between the occipital bone and the atlas may be considered to be a lack of cranialization, i.e., a regressive abnormality (occipital vertebra).

The mechanism of assimilation of protovertebrae 3 to 5 into the occipital bone, first postulated by August von Froriep and termed Froriep's occipitoblast, has found general acceptance (Brocher, 1955). However, Langmann (1965) believed that the most cranial part disappears completely and that only protovertebrae 2 to 4 are assimilated into the occipital bone (Fig. 2.1). In fact the chorda dorsalis extends cranially through the cranio-vertebral junction into the basion, as depicted in Fig. 2.4, and induces normal or abnormal segmentations.

The Occiput

Three types of ossification may be distinguished: (1) the two chordal ossification centers (vertebral origin), forming the basi-occipital and exoccipital parts; (2) the infra-occipital part, corresponding to the secondary ossification centers of the vertebrae; and (3) the supra-occipital part, proceeding from membranous ossification of the skull. Thus the basilar part of the occiput is made up of three embryologic parts, as depicted in Fig. 2.2. The spheno-occipital synchondrosis is usually visible in newborn infants. The persistence of the intrabasilar suture, however, should be considered as a regressive feature. It should be emphasized

Figure 2.1. Diagram of the embryo-logic development of bones of the cervico-occipital area.

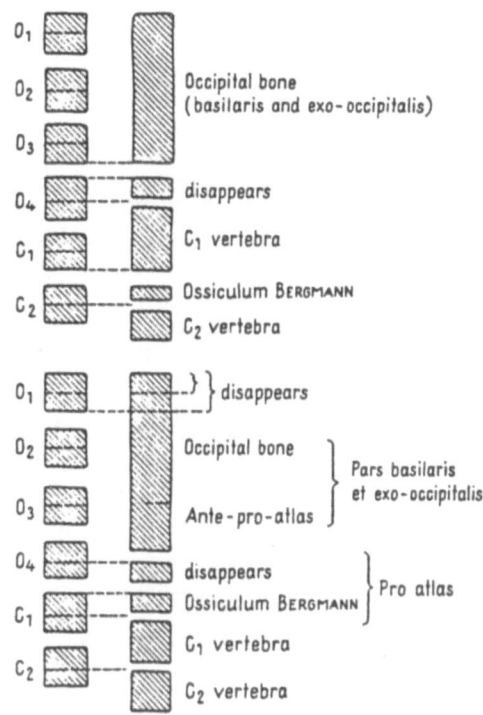

that only the basi-occipital and the lateral masses of the occiput develop from car-tilage, and that changes in cartilaginous ossification will be seen only in these parts. The numerous centers of ossification of the occiput are shown in Fig. 2.2. Certain structures remain visible during childhood: this appearance possesses no pathologic significance.

Several amorphous ossicles may be found between the occiput and the cervical vertebrae, in the cervico-occipital angle proper, which are nonsignificant manifestations of the center of ossification of the occipital vertebra. One of these ossicles, however, forms the ossification center of the odontoid process and is termed Bergmann's ossicle.

The Atlas

The atlas is made up of the caudal sclerotome of the first and the cranial sclero-tome of the second vertebral somite. The body of the atlas, however, fuses with the body of the axis to form the odontoid process. The second unusual feature of ossification of the atlas is that its anterior arch does not arise from the chorda dorsalis, so that no anterior arch can be seen radiologically in newborn infants. In the course of the first year of life, the two secondary centers of ossification of the anterior arch of the atlas appear in the perichordal mesenchyme. The ossifi-

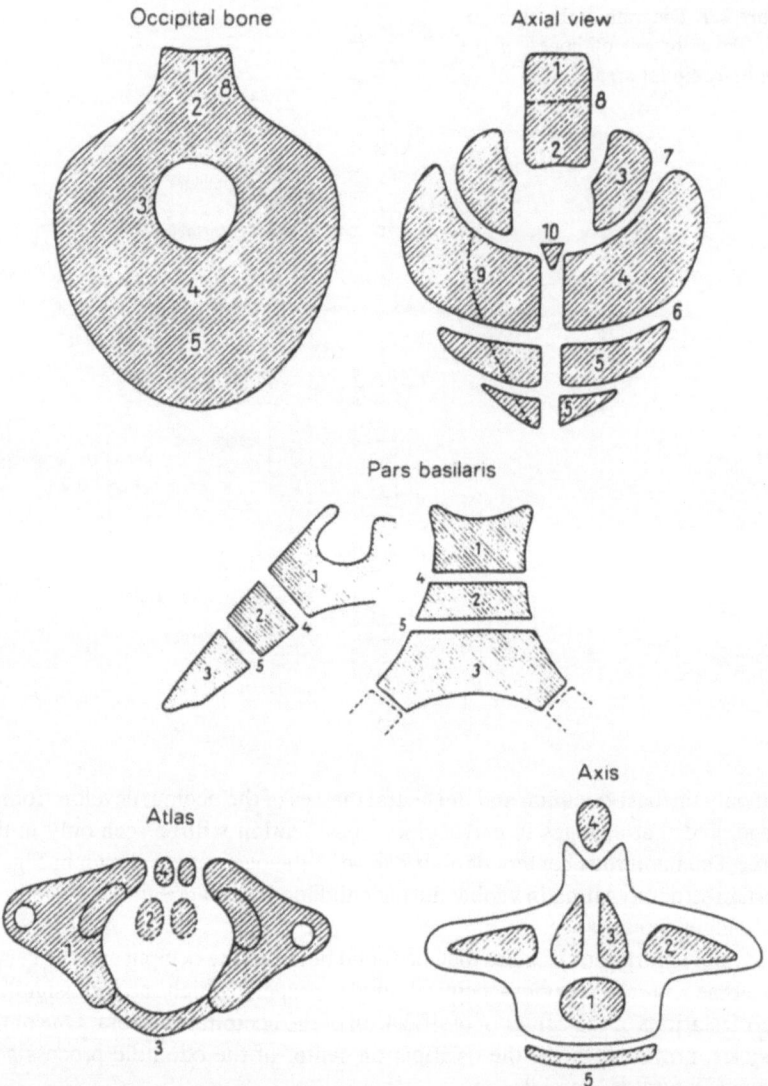

Figure 2.2. Diagram of the ossification centers in the cervico-occipital area. Occipital bone (axial view): 1, basi-oticum; 2, basi-occiput; 3, massa lateralis occipitalis (exo-occipitalis); 4, infra-occipitalis; 5, supra-occipitalis; 6, transverse suture (mendosal); 7, intra-occipital suture (Budin); 8, intrabasal suture; 9, supplementary sutures; 10, Kerkring's ossicle. Pars basilaris: 1, sphenoid part; 2, basi-oticum; 3, basi-occiput; 4, spheno-occipital synchondrosis; 5, intrabasal suture. Atlas (axial view): 1, primary lateral center; 2, primary median centers (primary lateral centers of the odontoid process); 3, primary center of the posterior arch; 4, secondary centers of the anterior arch. Axis (frontal view): 1, primary median center for the body; 2, primary lateral centers for the lateral mass and the posterior arch; 3, primary lateral center (base of the odontoid process); 4, secondary center for the apex; 5, secondary center.

cation centers of the posterior arch fuse later on, sometimes only after the age of 10 years. Thus, the appearance of the atlas during the early years of life are depicted in Fig. 2.2. The transverse process of the lateral masses of the atlas develops early in the embryo; therefore agenesis of either the transverse process or the transverse ligament is evidence of an early congenital malformation.

The Axis

The axis develops from five primary centers of ossification (Fig. 2.2): a *midline center*, appearing between the 4th and 5th months of intra-uterine life; *two symmetrical centers* in the odontoid process, appearing in the 6th month of intra-uterine life, which fuse at birth. However, they may remain nonunited, separated by a less dense area in the midline up to the age of 4 to 6 years; and *two lateral centers*, one for each lateral mass.

Secondary ossification proceeds mainly from two centers: the epiphysis of the body (inferior aspect of the body of the axis) and the apical center of the odontoid process (Bergmann's ossicle) which may be visible radiologically up to the age of 12 years.

Thus, ossification centers in the body of the atlas form not only the odontoid process but also the upper part of the body of the axis.

In Fig. 2.3a–q we schematize the evolution of the radiologic data from birth to the age of 8 years. A normal image at the age of 4 months is demonstrated in Fig. 2.5.

Malformations of the Bones

Basilar Invagination

This malformation is well known in adults, in whom it is often detected in various conditions that may have no correlation with a malformation properly speaking. This is almost a rule during childhood. There are only few cases of neurologic syndromes of the lower brainstem, upper spinal cord, or cranial nerves (IX, X, XI, and XII) leading to radiologic diagnosis of basilar invagination. The roentgenographic features are well known in adults. In childhood, the main signs are revealed in lateral projections of the skull or cervical spine. At first glance, an experienced physician searches for too high a position of the odontoid process and anterior arch of the atlas, with respect to the palato-occipital line (Chamberlain). This criterion is clear enough in the lateral projection. In the frontal projection, one line is sufficient to characterize the disturbed relationship between the skull base and the first vertebra: the bidigastric line (Fischgold). It lies cranial to the bottom of the posterior fossa which is oblique to the midline under the bidigastric line in normal conditions. In cases of basilar invagination, the bottom of the posterior fossa is parallel or even cranially ascending above the bidigastric

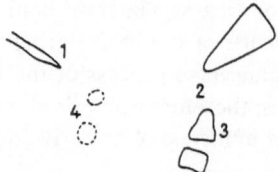

a: Before the age of 6 months. 1, occipital; 2, nonossified odontoid tip; 3, odontoid process; 4, poorly ossified posterior arches of atlas and axis.

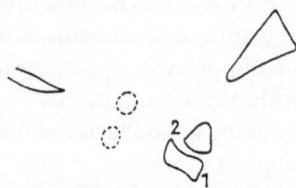

b: Variant of *a*. 1, axis; 2, step formation between the odontoid process and the body of the axis.

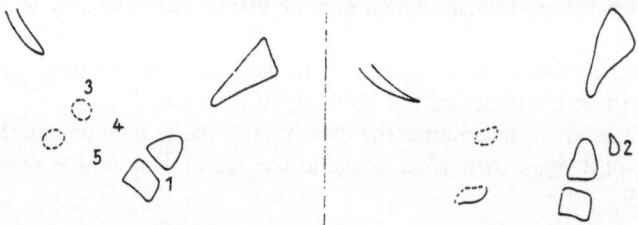

c: At 6 months. 1, persistent disc between the odontoid process and the body of the axis; 2, ossified anterior arch of the atlas; 3, poorly ossified posterior arches of the atlas and axis; 4 and 5, identical antero-posterior diameters of atlas and axis.

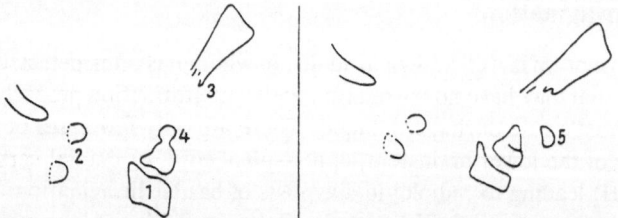

d: From 6 months to 1 year. 1, body of the axis; 2, ossified posterior arches of atlas and axis; 3, nonossified basion; 4, progressive ossification of the tip of the odontoid process; 5, anterior arch of the atlas.

Figure 2.3. Diagram of midline sagittal tomograms in children.

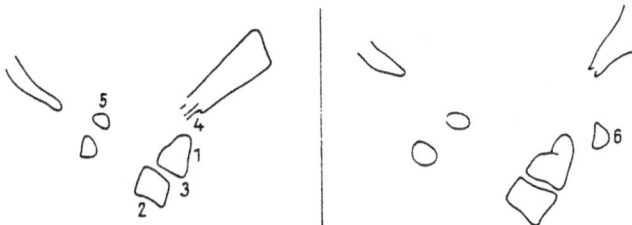

e: At 1 year. 1, odontoid process; 2, body of the axis; 3, persistent C1–2 disc between the odontoid process and the body of the axis; 4, nonossified basion; 5, posterior arch of the atlas; 6, anterior arch of the atlas.

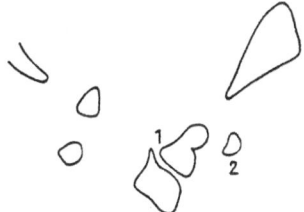

f: At 18 months. 1, persistent step formation between the odontoid process and the body of the axis; 2, anterior arch of the atlas.

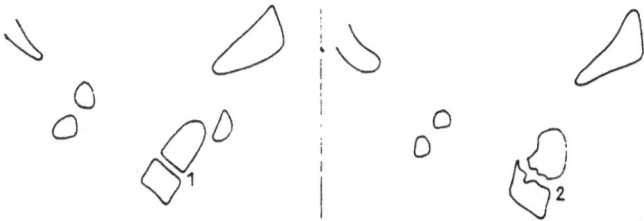

g: Variant of *f*. Regular (1) or irregular (2) margins of the persistent space between the odontoid process and the body of the axis.

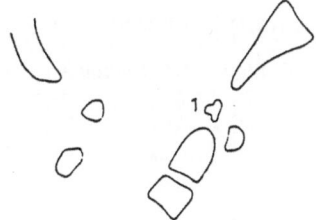

h: At 2 years. 1, free ossification center of the tip of the odontoid process.

Figure 2.3. *Continued.*

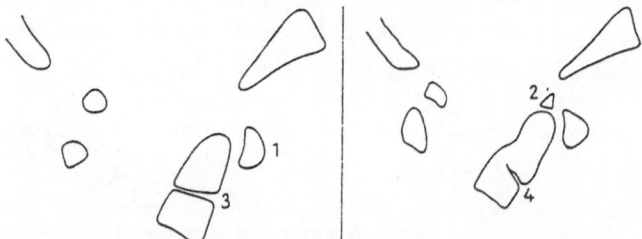

i: At 2 years and 6 months. 1, anterior arch of the atlas; 2, apical ossification center of the odontoid process; 3 and 4, progressive narrowing of the space between the odontoid process and the body of the axis.

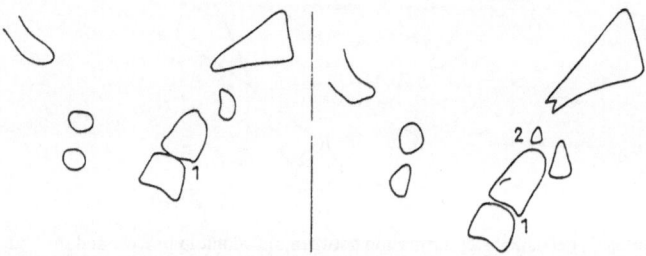

j: At 3 years. 1, persistent but narrowed space between the odontoid process and the body of the axis; 2, apical ossification center of the odontoid process.

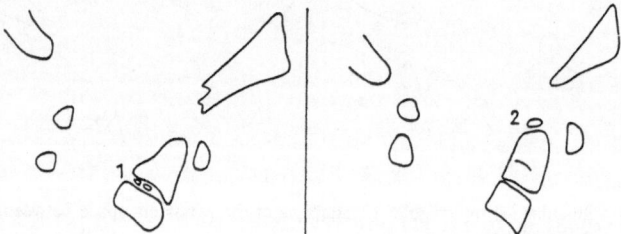

k: At 3 years and 6 months. 1, irregularly distributed ossicles in the space between the odontoid process and the body of the axis; 2, apical ossification center of the odontoid process.

Figure 2.3. *Continued.*

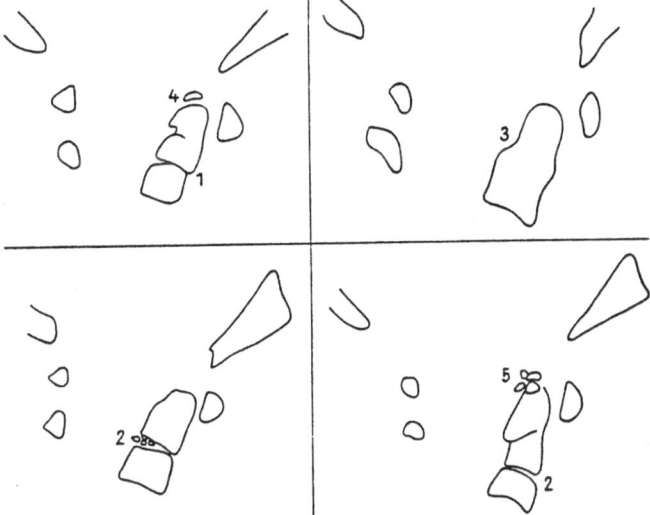

l: At 4 years. 1, very narrow space between the odontoid process and the body of the axis with step formation; 2, progressive ossification of the space between the odontoid process and the body of the axis; 3, completely ossified space, with step formation on the posterior aspect; 4, apical ossification center of the odontoid process; 5, multiple apical ossification centers of the odontoid process.

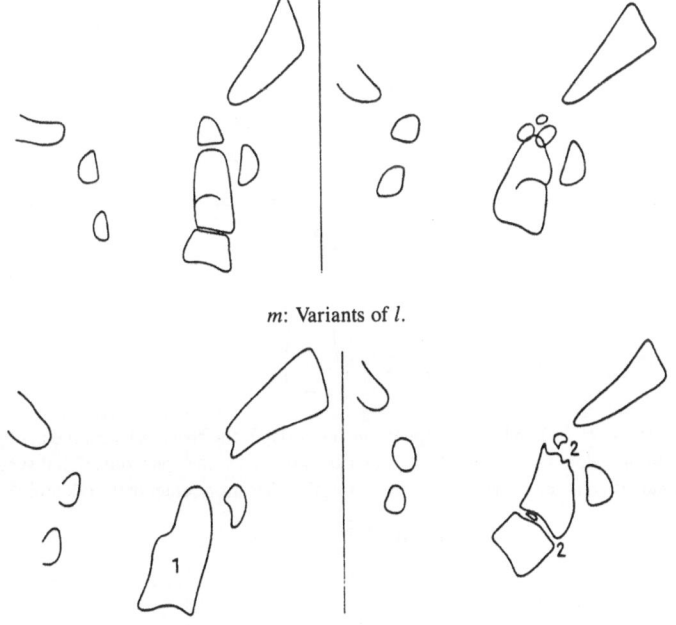

m: Variants of *l*.

n: From 4 to 5 years. 1, completely ossified axis; 2, uncompletely ossified axis.

Figure 2.3. *Continued.*

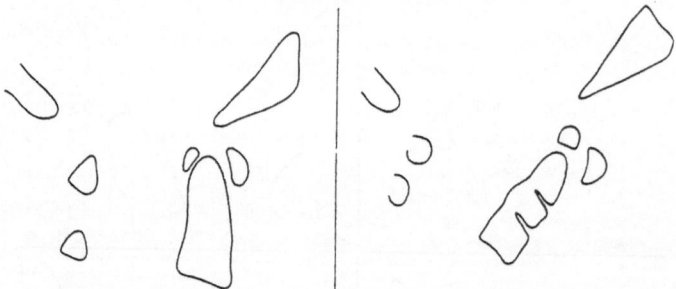

o: ·From 5 to 6 years. 1, persistent apical ossification center of the odontoid process and persistent clefts at the level of the C1–2 disc.

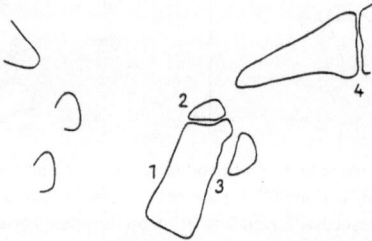

p: From 6 to 7 years. 1, complete fusion between the odontoid process and the body of the axis; 2, unfused apical ossification center of the odontoid process; 3, persistence of a large space between the anterior arch of the atlas and the odontoid process, the spheno-occipital synchondrosis remaining nonossified (4).

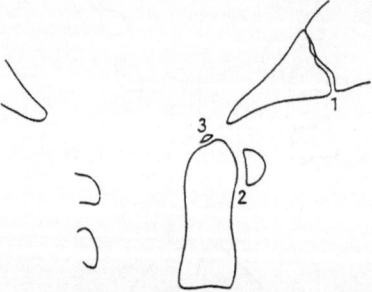

q: Eight years and over. 1, spheno-occipital synchodrosis; 2, the space between the anterior arch of the atlas and the odontoid process is still larger than in adults, the spheno-occipital synchondrosis remains nonossified (1) and persists an unfused apical ossification center of the odontoid process (3).

Figure 2.3. *Continued.*

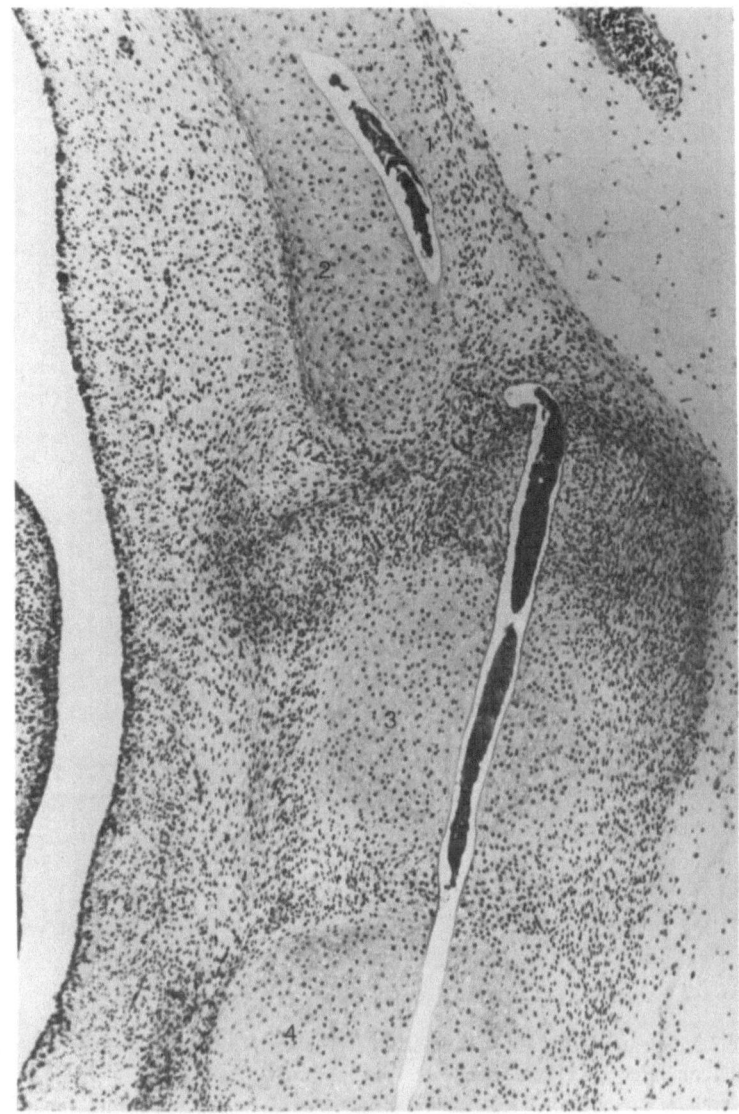

Figure 2.4. Sagittal section of a human embryo (24 mm crown–rump length; stage 21). 1, notochord; 2, basi-occiput; 3, dens axis; 4, corpus axis. (Courtesy of Prof. Dr. B. Christ, Institute of Anatomy, Ruhr-University Bochum.)

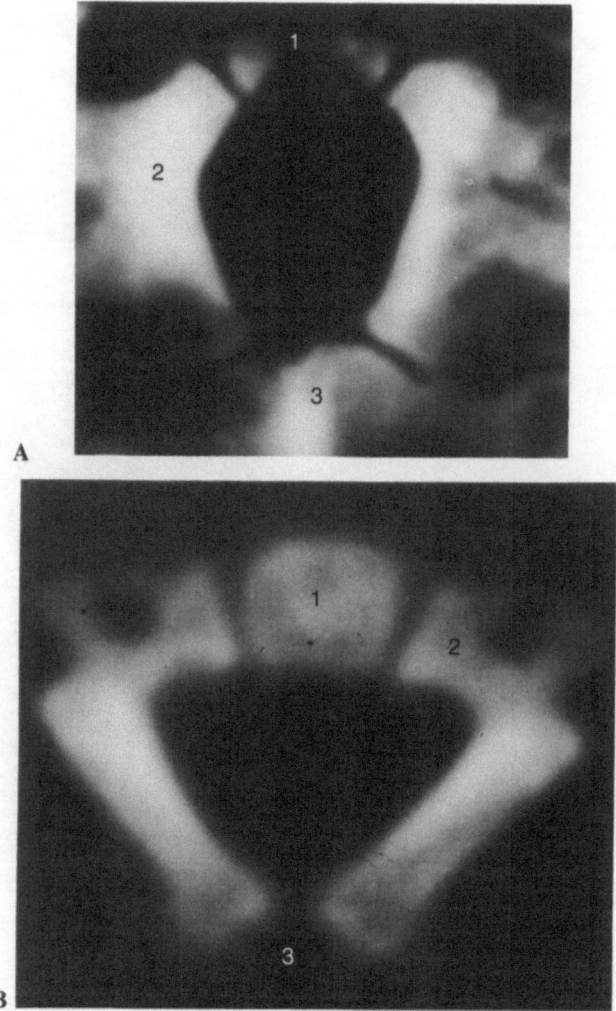

Figure 2.5. Normal ossification of the cranio-vertebral junction in a 4-month-old girl. **A**: occiput (compare with Fig. 2.2 above). 1, basi-occiput; 2, exo-occiput; 3, infra-occiput. **B**: Axis vertebra. 1, vertebral body; 2, lateral masses with foramen transversarium; 3, nonfused posterior arch.

line. Other lines may be useful but not indispensable for the practical work. In a frontal view, the bimastoid line (Fischgold) gives the same information as the bidigastric line; the intervestibular line (Wackenheim) allows one to demonstrate the lateral predominance of the basilar invagination. The Schmidt–Fischer angle gives a criterion for the degree of platycondylia. In the lateral view, the suboccipito-palatine line (McGregor) gives the same information as Chamberlain's line. The basilar line (Wackenheim) demonstrates the posterior displace-

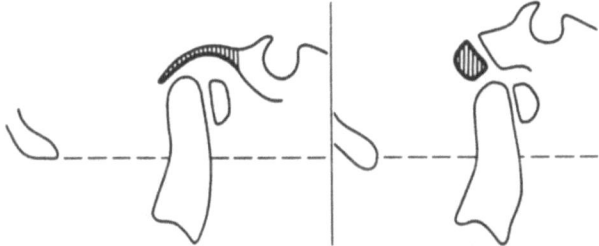

Figure 2.6. Two types of basilar invagination. *Left*: Hypoplasia of the basi-occiput. *Right*: Free ossicle (basi-oticum).

ment of the odontoid, whereas the line of the foramen magnum gives the limit that is passed when the dens is luxated upward.

For the understanding of basilar invagination, one must remember that the entity consists of an underdeveloped (hypoplastic) basi-occiput and that this hypoplasia may have various forms. Classically, we have to distinguish an anterior (basi-occipital), a posterior (squamous), a lateral (condylar), a unilateral, and a diffuse form. The most important form is the anterior one. This form may be divided into two different morphologic variances (Fig. 2.6). Let us first review some developmental and historical data.

The basilar part of the occipital bone is generally called basi-occipital. Another denomination is *pars basilaris ossis occipitalis*. In 1903 Le Double[3] devoted a large chapter to the basi-occiput and recalled the works of P. Albrecht,[4] Henle,[5] and Legge.[6] The authors described one of the three anomalies of our patient, i.e., hypoplasia or even the absence of the basilar part of the occipital bone. Another anomaly is the presence of a supplementary fissure illustrated in the drawing taken from Le Double[3] in Fig. 2.7. P. Albrecht[4] first described this transverse segmentation in a case in 1878 and again in 1883. Later, Morselli (1888), Rossi (1891), and Staurenghi (1894) reported other cases and Le Double reviewed the total number of cases described up to 1903 at 10.[3] The occurrence is approximately one per thousand and concerns exclusively the transverse segmentation with the presence of an independent ossicle named *basioticum*, anterior basi-occipit, pre-basi-occiput, anterior centrum of the basi-occiput or even *pars basilaris occipitalis duplex*. Henle[5] reported a case of *basi-occipitalis* measuring only 6 mm in length and recalled that Schwegel published two cases of adult skull with transverse fissure located midway between the spheno-occipital synchrondrosis and the basion.

Legge[6] found two skulls out of 760 in which the basilar part of the occipital bone was absent. This anomaly seems to be the same as in our case but we have no information about the spheno-occipital synchondrosis in Legge's case. Le Double also recalls several works about longitudinal segmentation of the basi-occiput and the possibility of association of transverse and longitudinal segmentation, responsible for cross-like segmentation in animals. He was particularly

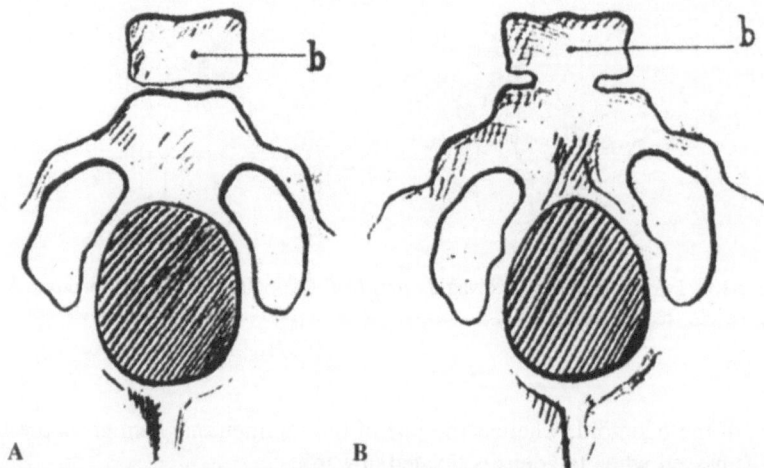

A   B

Figure 2.7. Drawing from Le Double. **A**: Segmentation of the basi-occiput into two parts. **B**: Lateral fissures corresponding to an incomplete segmentation of the basi-occiput. The free segment or distal part is called basi-oticum.

interested in the transverse segmentation of the basi-occiput. He recalls the opinion of Calori,[7] that the sphenoidal part of the clivus may also be transversally segmentated by a fissure at the level of the bottom of the sella turcica. Thus, Calori[7] believes that the sphenoidal clivus, as well as the basi-occiput, each develop from two ossification centers considered as a complex of "spondylo-centers," i.e., arising from the *chorda dorsalis*. In fact, two general theories may be discussed: (1) Calori's, which tends to localize the segmentation process up to the dorsum sellae and (2) Staderini and others who limit the segmentation process to the basi-occiput. In our patient, we demonstrate the transitory supplementary fissure of this kind of segmentation of the basi-occiput.

In 1926, Madame J. Déjérine[8] described a case of aplasia of the basi-occiput without mentioning Legge's case.[13] She emphasized the atrophy of the spongiosa. Indeed, the autopsy demonstrated that the cancellous bone was absent from the basi-occiput which was formed by two layers of compact bone. Madame Déjérine notes, furthermore, the angulation of the spheno-occiput, the sphenoidal part being vertical and the occipital part horizontal. The author described no anomaly of the spheno-occipital synchondrosis. There are various associated anomalies of the nervous system in this case of Madame Déjérine. She concluded that the primary feature was aplasia of the cancellous bone of the basilar part of the occipital bone.

In 1932, Adam-Falkiewiczova and Nowiki[9] published a case similar to Madame Déjérine's. G. Bodechtel and H.U. Guizetti[10] published another case in 1933, and recalled the similarity of their findings with those of Adam-Falkiewiczova and Nowiki and Déjérine. In the case described by Bodechtel, there was marked hypoplasia of the clivus Blumenbrachii. The missing part of the clivus was replaced by very hard tissue. In 1936, G. De Morsier and R. Junet[11] published a case of complete aplasia of the basilar part of the occiput. This case is very similar to the description of Madame Déjérine, but the authors mention nothing about the spheno-occipital synchondrosis. There have been numerous subsequent publications of identical cases of marked hypoplasia of the basi-occiput which is thin, short, and elevated but attached to the sphenoidal clivus. In our opinion, the best description of the anomaly is that of Madame Déjérine. It represents a clinico-radiologic entity. The majority of neuroradiologists examine approximately one such case once a year.

In 1857, R. Virchow[12] created the term "basilar impression," and it was adopted by Schuller in 1911.[13] Since that time, radiologists use this very imprecise terminology without description of the real radio-anatomic conditions, so that the term covers various anomalies of the posterior part of the base of the skull. Schmidt and Fischer[14] and Klaus[15] already criticized the general concept of basilar impression. It is at present obvious that we have to go back to a more precise radiologic study in each case. As we said, our patient had also a third anomaly, the persistence of the spheno-occipital synchondrosis. J. Lang[16] recalls that the spheno-occipital synchondrosis ossifies from the intracranial margin to the extracranial, and that it is closed in men between 13½ and 18½ years and earlier in women, between 12¼ and 16 years. The sphenoidal bone in median sagittal section may demonstrate another synchondrosis, in front of the sella turcica, the intrasphenoidal synchondrosis. The course of this synchondrosis is parallel to the synchondrosis spheno-occiputalis. The intrasphenoidal synchondrosis disappears in the perinatal period. In our patient, as we will see, the synchondrosis spheno-occipitalis persists definitively. It also persisted without other anomalies in the father of the patient. J. Lang considers that this persistence is "außerordentlich selten," i.e., "extraordinarily seldom." He recalls also that this synchondrosis is considered as the anterior limit of the "Wirbelschädel," i.e., the cranial bones of vertebral origin.

We have had the opportunity to observe the radiologic evolution of a case over 18 years (from the ages of 2 to 20 years).[17] This patient associates three radio-anatomic anomalies: (1) a transitory supplementary fissure of the basi-occiput, corresponding to the description of Le Double, (2) persistence of the spheno-occipital synchondrosis, and (3) hypoplasia of the basi-occiput responsible for marked basilar impression.

Transitory Supplementary Fissure of the Basi-Occiput

The detailed evolution in one case is shown in Figs. 2.8 and 2.9. It appears that the supplementary fissure of the basi-occiput ossifies between 2 and 4 years. As we have seen, these fissures are quite frequent (Albrecht, Morselli, Rossi, Staurenghi, Legge, Henle, Le Double ...). The originality of our images consists in the demonstration of the fissure and of its ossification, whereas the spheno-occipital synchondrosis does not ossify.

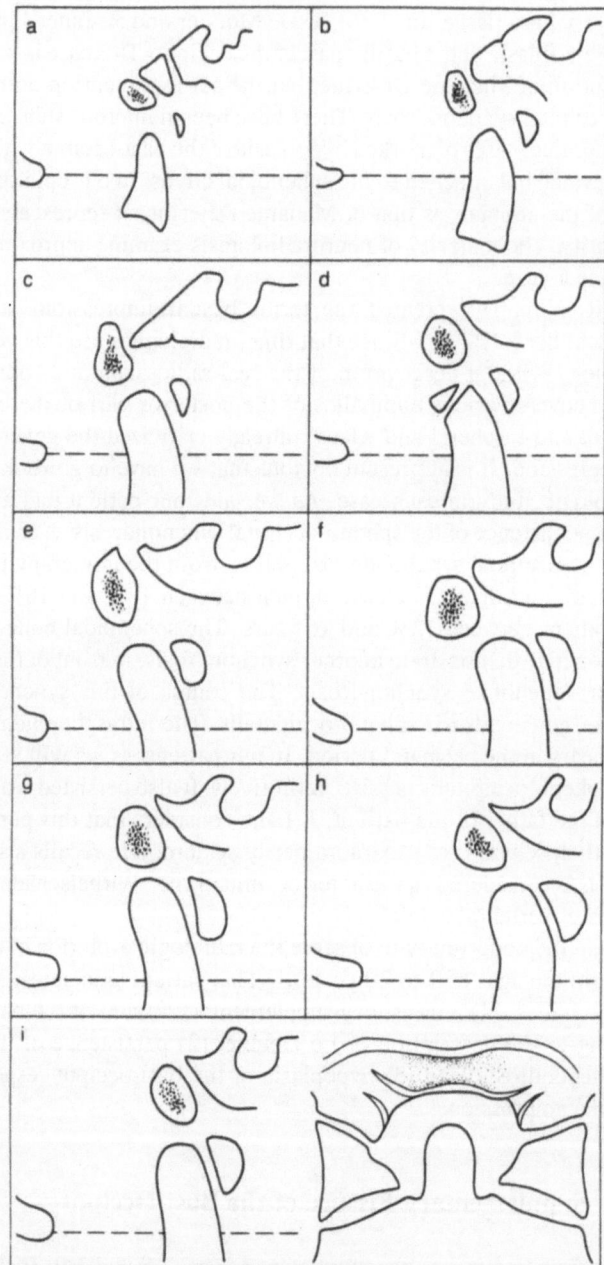

Figure 2.8. Basilar invagination. Schematic evolution in the lateral view from the age of 2 to 20 years. a: 2 years; b: 4 years; c: 9 years; d 10 years; e: 12 years; f: 13 years; g: 14 years; h: 15 years; i: 20 years.

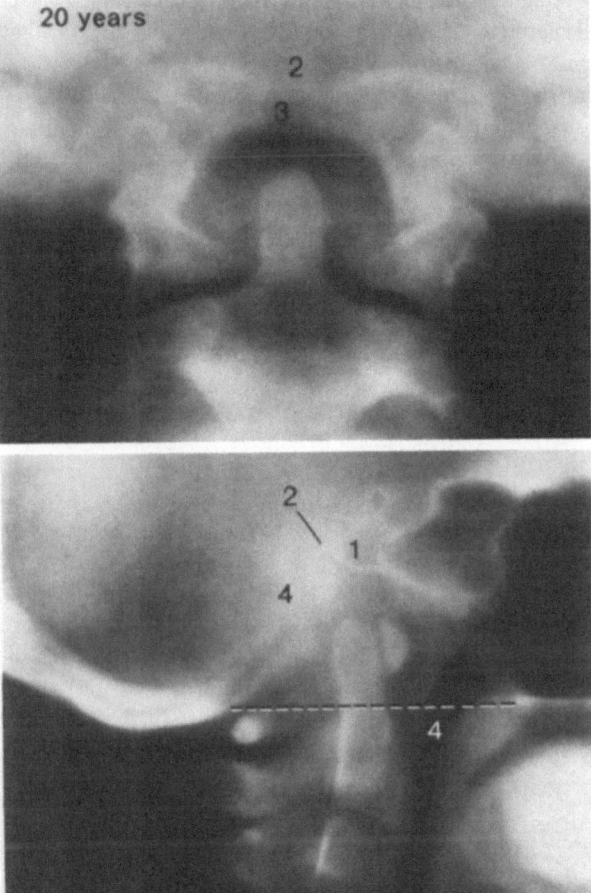

Figure 2.9. Basilar invagination. Tomograms corresponding to the terminal stage depicted in Fig. 2.8. 1, sphenoidal body; 2, spheno-occipital synchondrosis; 3, lower part of the basi-occiput; 4, palato-occipital line (Chamberlain).

Persistence of the Spheno-Occipital Synchondrosis

This, the second main sign of the malformation we describe, is very clearly demonstrated in all the films. The same anomaly exists in the father of our patient, in association with a short, rounded basion, similar to a minor form of *condylus tertius*. The mother has a normal cervico-occipital region.

Hypoplasia of the Basi-Occiput Responsible for Marked Basilar Impression

To characterize the degree of basilar impression, the whole odontoid peg and the anterior arch of the atlas lie above the palato-occipital line of Chamberlain, a topographic anomaly of approximately 2 cm. The basi-occiput is very short and very dense. In a sagittal median tomogram, it is seen as a rounded section that has lost its normal shape (Fig. 2.9). In a frontal tomogram passing through the occipital condyles and the basi-occiput, it appears that the cortex of the basi-occiput is very thick, both at the cranial and the caudal aspects (Fig. 2.9).

Clincally, our patient is of normal intelligence, but complains of epileptic seizures without a particular aura and without specific EEG pattern. There are neither objective neurologic disturbances nor functional deficiency of any neurophysiologic system.

Transitional Anomalies of the Cranio-Vertebral Junction

These anomalies may be divided into two main categories: those that are due to the assimilation of the first vertebra and those with persistence of primitive vertebrae (occipitalization and vertebralization).

Occipitalization (Fig. 2.10)

This is the most pathogenic malformation in adults and is generally well tolerated during childhood, although it is very often associated with syringomyelia. The radiologic examination has to determine the type of occipitalization: total, partial, of the anterior or posterior arch or of both, with symmetric or asymmetric involvement of the lateral parts. The main investigation concerns the size of the foramen magnum and of the vertebral canal. Indeed, the former may be stenotic because of fusion with the atlas. The latter may also be narrowed because of the

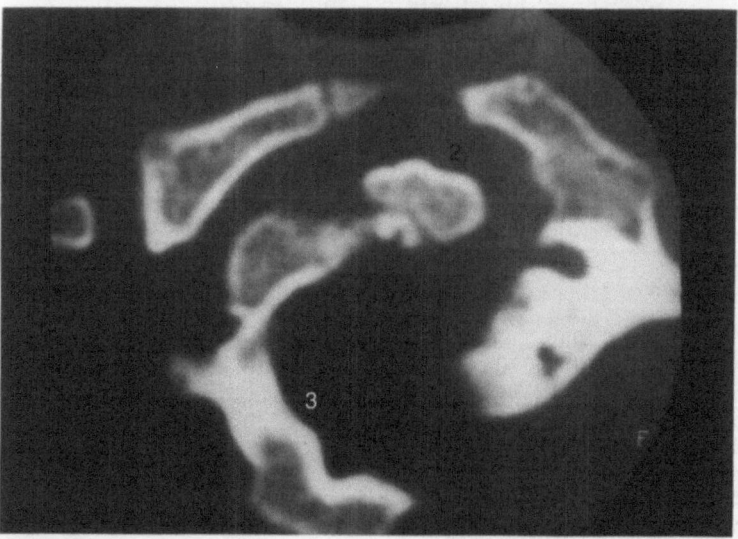

Figure 2.10. Occipitalization of the atlas with aplasia of the transverse ligament. 1, fused atlas with the occiput; 2, odontoid process; 3, posterior arch of the axis.

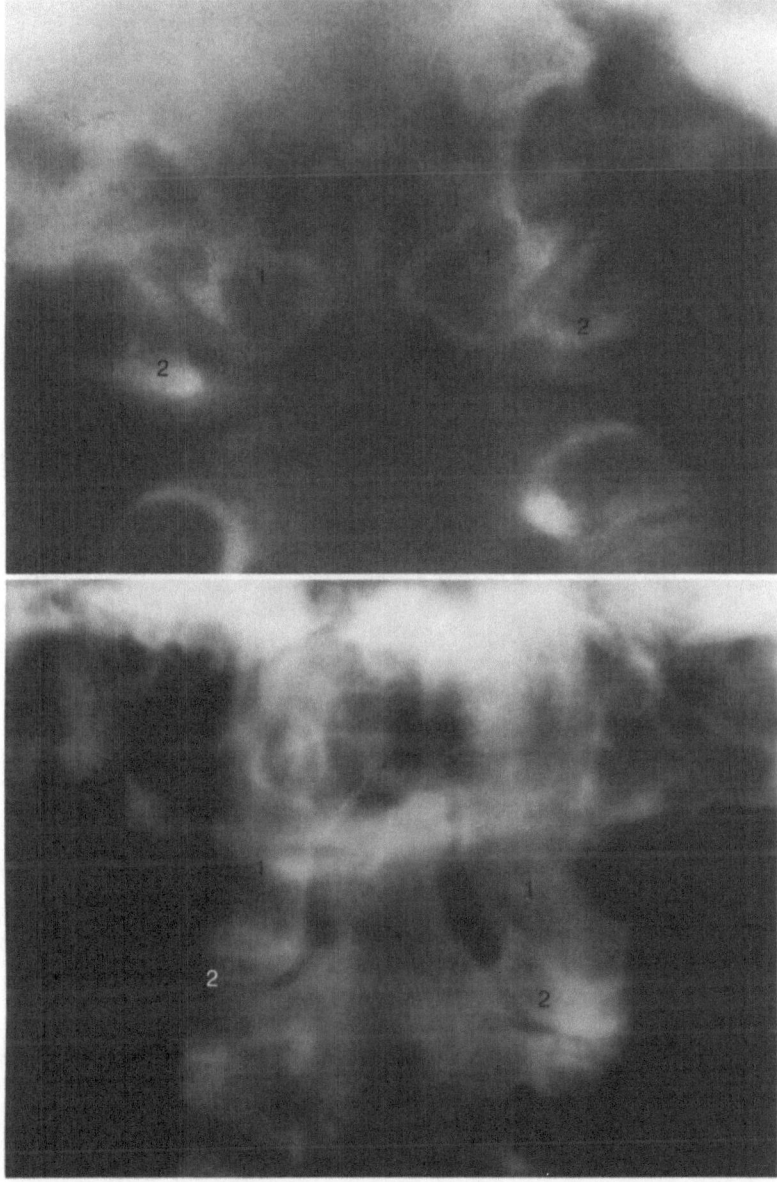

Figure 2.11. Two cases of vertebralization of the occipital condyles. 1, peninsula-shaped occipital condyles; 2, lateral masses of the atlas.

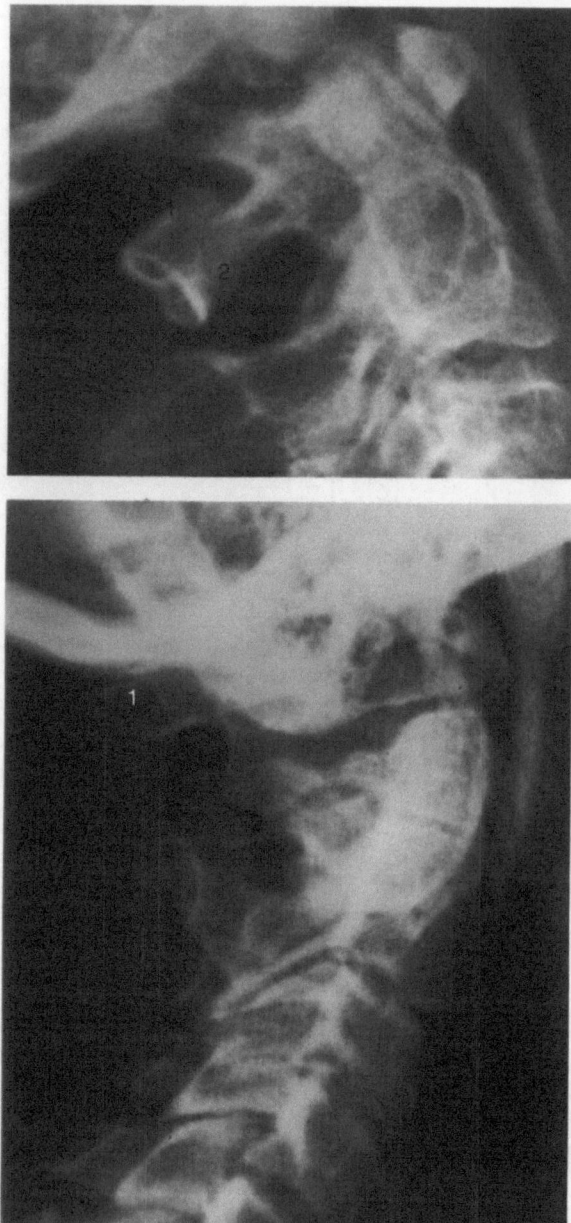

Figure 2.12. Two cases of vertebralization of the occipital with double posterior arch of the atlas. 1, cranial posterior arch of the atlas; 2, caudal posterior arch of the atlas.

posterior location of the odontoid process. In cases of occipitalization of the atlas, there is a variable incidence in the development of the transverse ligament. When completely absent, the axis is luxated posteriorly and eventually cranially. In minor cases, the ligament is weakened and elongated so that the dislocation of the axis is less marked. The transverse ligament can be demonstrated by CT or NMR. These procedures may also detect an associated syringomyelia or a cord compression.

Vertebralization (Figs. 2.11 and 2.12)

When the normal process of integration of the provertebrae into the occipital bone is not perfect, we may find images of supplementary ossicles between the occiput and the atlas. These supplementary ossicles were called "manifestation of the occipital vertebra." We described another variety called vertebralization.

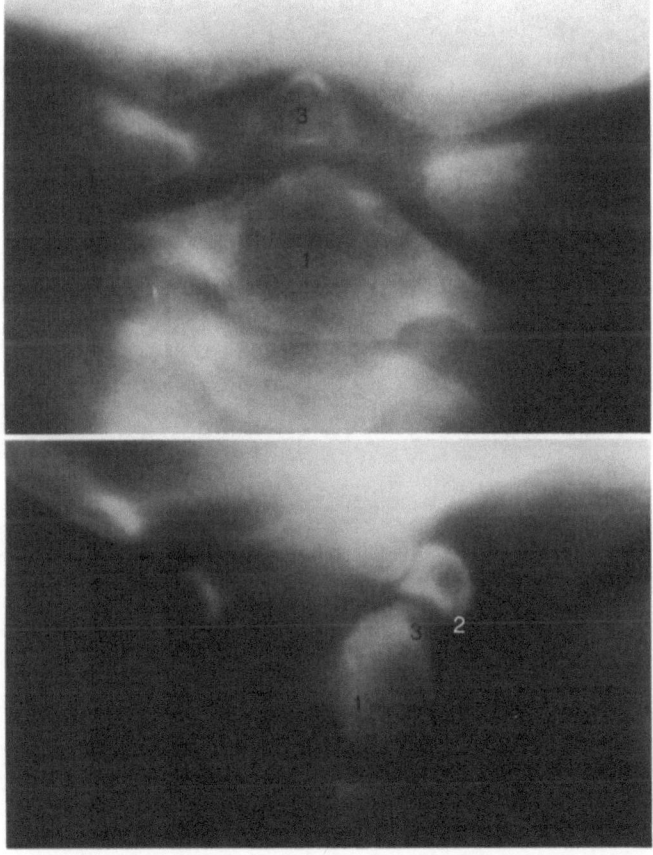

Figure 2.13. Odontoideum mobile. 1, massive and rounded upper aspect of the body of C2; 2, hypertrophic anterior arch of the atlas; 3, spheric free odontoid ossicle.

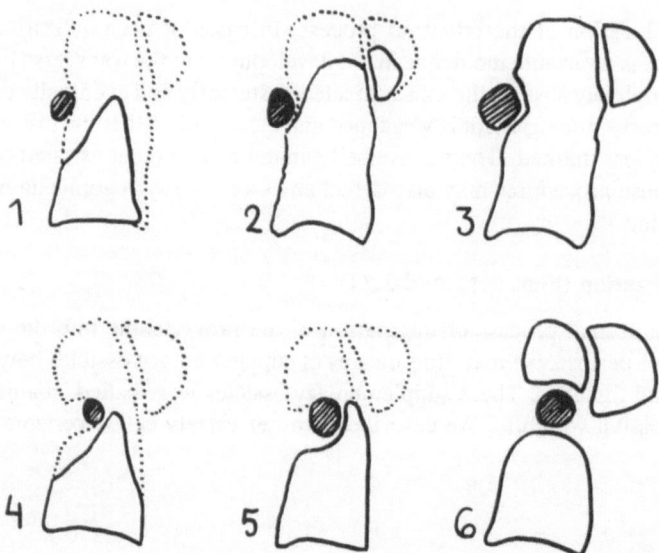

Figure 2.14. The normal transverse ligament is located behind the posterior aspect of the odontoid process (1 and 2) and provokes a small concavity (3). The too short transverse ligament is located too anteriorly and may be responsible for the ossification disturbance which separates the odontoid tip from the axis body (4, 5, and 6).

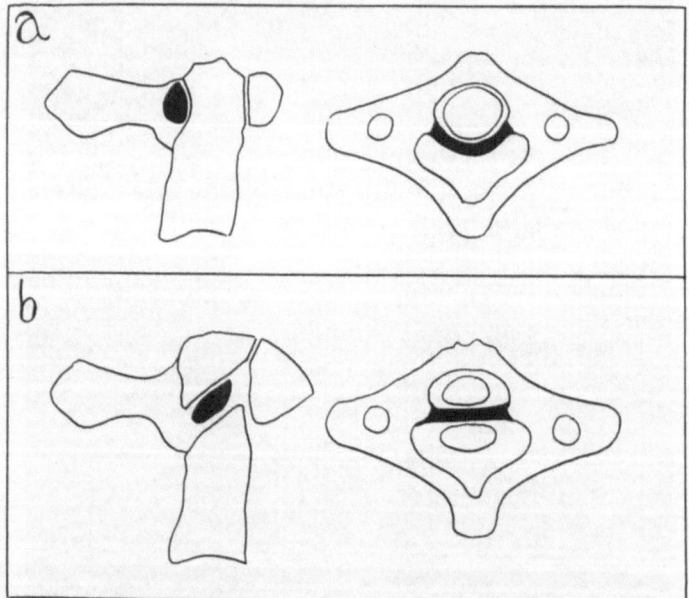

Figure 2.15. *a*: Normal transverse ligament. *b*: Too short transverse ligament.

In these cases, the occipital condyles mimic a supplementary lateral mass of the atlas. They may also go along with a double posterior arch of the atlas.

Mobile Odontoid

This malformation consists in nonfusion of the cranial part of the odontoid process with the caudal part (Fig. 2.13). The causes of this lack of fusion are unknown. In 1986,[18] we observed an adult with too short a transverse ligament and proposed the possibility of a section of the odontoid process during ossification by the shortened ligament (Figs. 2.14 and 2.15). During childhood, the *odontoideum mobile* is generally clinically silent. Neurologic changes occur in adults (cervical myelopathy) and necessitate surgical procedures for stabilization).

Block Vertebrae (Fig. 2.16)

In the field of the cranio-vertebral junction there exist equivalences of the block-vertebrae of the middle and lower cervical spine. We may distinguish the following varieties: the occipitalization of the atlas is a block vertebra between the primitive vertebrae (basi-occiput) and the atlas; the block between the anterior arch of the atlas and the odontoid process[19]; block of the posterior arches of C1 and C2; block vertebrae C2–C3. Combined malformations may be observed.

Dehiscence and Split Atlas

The dehiscence of the posterior arch of C1 is frequent (spina bifida). When associated with a dehiscence of the anterior arch, the condition is called split atlas. Both anomalies (anterior and posterior dehiscence) may also be observed in association with other malformations (Fig. 2.16b).

C1–C2 Dislocation (Figs. 2.17 and 2.18)

This condition is due to aplasia or malformation of the ligaments, especially of the transverse ligament, or to malformations of the bone associated with these ligamentous malformations. In the past it was difficult to have a precise view of the anatomic conditions, but the recent imaging of CT and MRI allow one to demonstrate the image of the transverse ligament. As depicted in Fig. 2.18, the dislocation is a ventro-dorsal displacement between C1 and C2, the atlas being fused to the skull. It is very easy to recognize the anterior displacement of the skull and atlas with respect to the axis because of the basilar line.[20] During childhood, as long as the ossification process is not finished, there is an increased space between the anterior arch of the atlas and the odontoid process but the tip of the odontoid is located in front of the basilar line, contrary to cases of dislocation.

Clinically, the C1–C2 dislocation may determine a more or less severe cord compression syndrome and necessitate surgical stabilization, generally of the

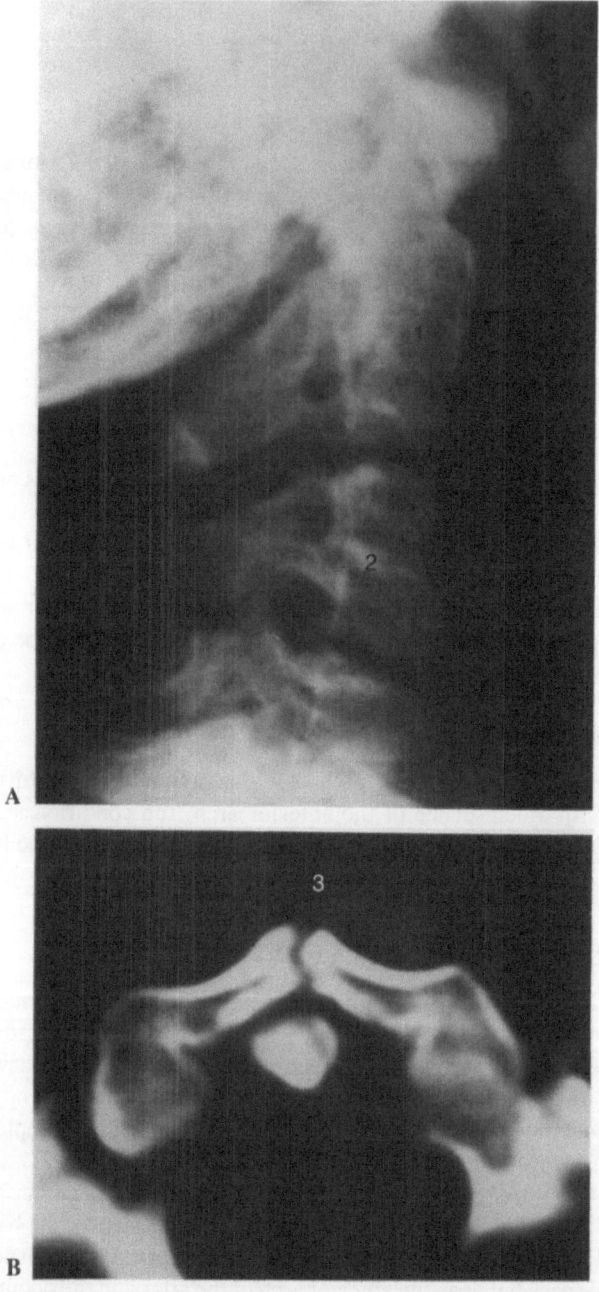

Figure 2.16. Association of malformations in a 9-year-old girl. **A**: 1, C1–C2 block vertebra; 2, C3–C4 block vertebra; 3, plump atlas (see *b*). **B**: Nonfused anterior arch of the atlas responsible for the blurred image of the anterior arch of the atlas (3).

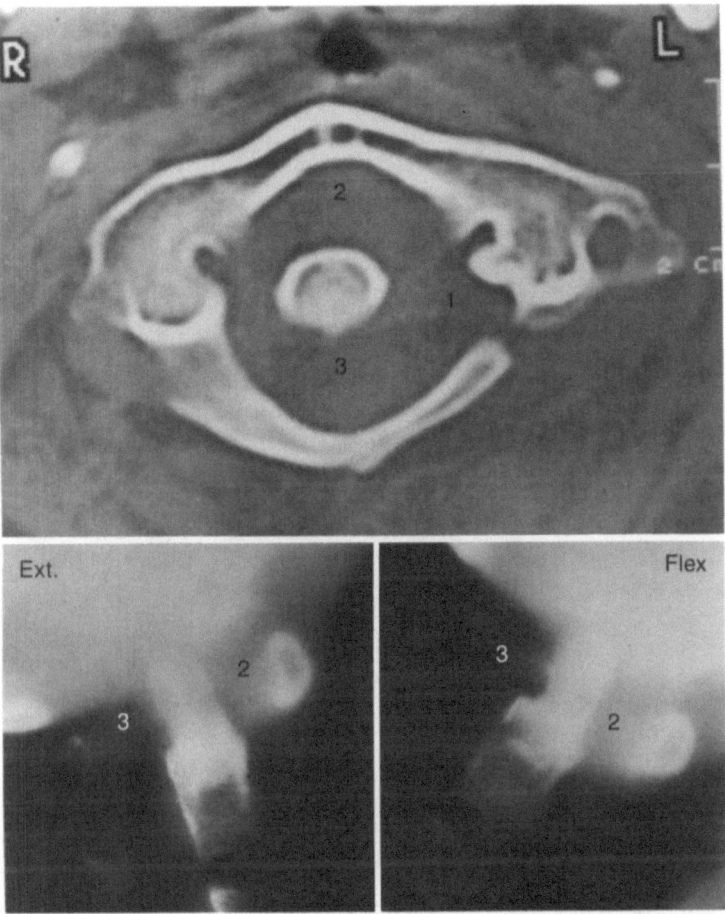

Figure 2.17. Still's disease. Destroyed ligamentum transversum responsible for large dislocation between the atlas and the odontoid process. 1, destroyed ligamentum transversum; 2, C1–C2 dislocation; 3, reduced anterio-posterior diameter of the vertebral canal responsible for the spinal compression.

three levels (occipital–atlas–axis). Out of the malformation, the dislocation is a complication of infection, rheumatism, trauma, or any other destructive process of the ligamentary system in the cervico-occipital region. Let us recall that aplasia of the transverse ligament may be observed in cases of Down's syndrome and Recklinghausen's disease.

Miscellaneous

In this short chapter it is impossible to report all varieties of malformations that are reported in the literature.[20] Let us nevertheless recall that one of the impor-

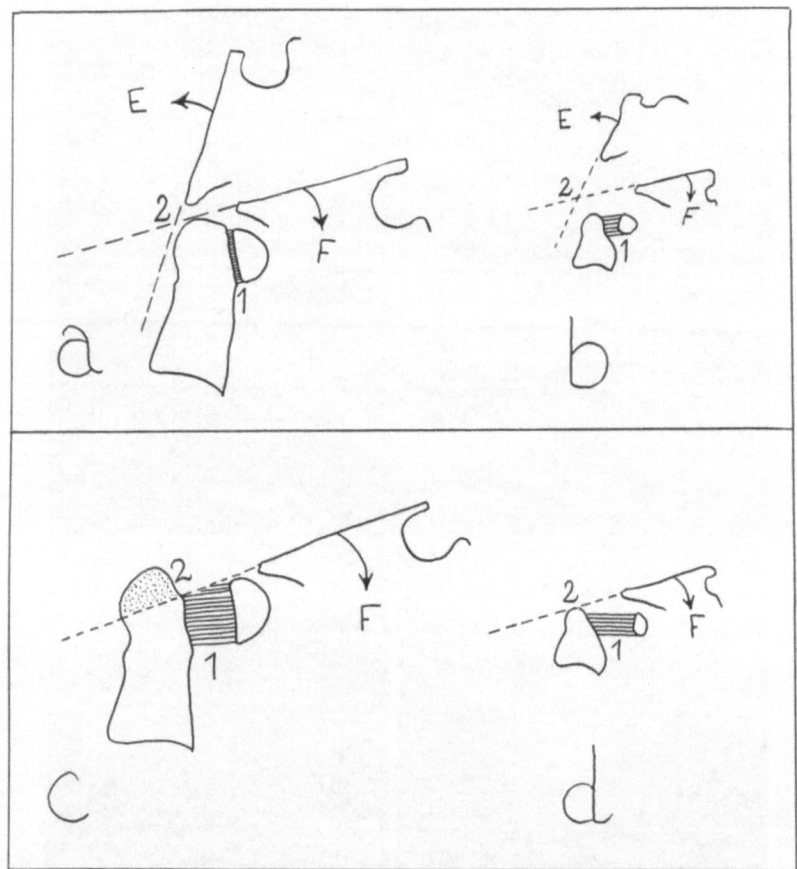

Figure 2.18. C1–C2 dislocation. Normally in an adult (a) or during childhood (b) the flexion (F) and extension (E) movement do not modify the distance between the anterior arch of the atlas and the odontoid process (1) or the relationship between the odontoid tip and the basilar line (2). In case of C1–C2 dislocation in an adult (c) or during childhood (d), the flexion movement (F) modifies both parameters (1 and 2).

tant pathogenic situations is stenosis of the cervico-occipital canal, and that this condition may be the result of many very different anomalies associated with malformations, bone diseases, sequellae of injuries, and so on.[21-28]

Malformations of the Soft Parts

More and more anatomic details in this field are recognized as the result of imaging by magnetic resonance of the soft parts (Fig. 2.19).

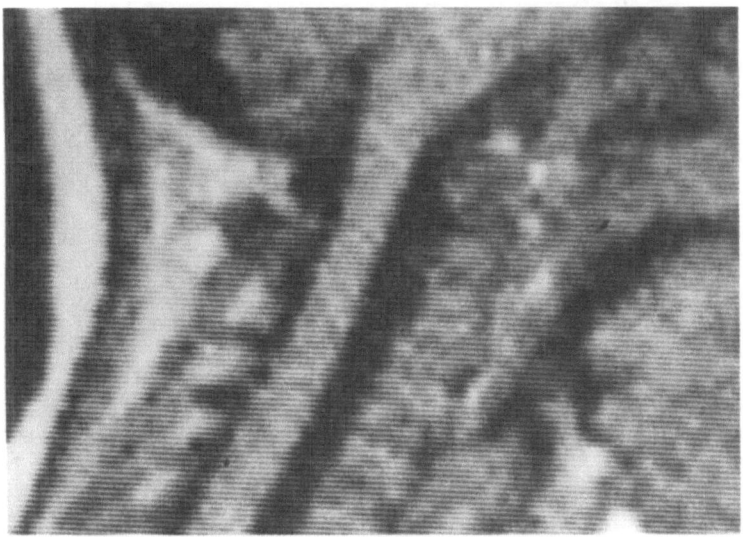

Figure 2.19. Normal MRI of the cranio-vertebral junction. The tonsils, medulla oblongata, and cervical spine are perfectly demonstrated whereas the bones are more or less blurred.

Chiari Malformations (Fig. 2.20)

In the medical literature one distinguishes three types that represent three degrees of the malformation:

Type I: There is just a lower position of the cerebellar tonsils. This type has no practical incidence during childhood.

Type II: This is a more severe malformation: the tonsils, medulla oblongata, and the IVth ventricle are located below the foramen magnum so that the upper brainstem is elongated. This malformation may be associated with a lumbar spina bifida and meningomyelocele, hydrocephalus, and various cerebral and spinal malformations. The lumbo-sacral meningomyelocele and the hydrocephalic or hydromyelic complications necessitate surgical treatment.

Type III: This is the most severe degree, and generally not compatible with life. These patients have a large encephalomeningomyelocele in the cervico-occipital region with syringomyelia and vascular malformations.

Syringomyelia and Hydromyelia

This condition may exist without other malformations. In both cases we have to localize the cysts (syringomyelic cysts or hydromyelic dilation of the ependymal canal), with magnetic resonance imaging (MRI), the ideal method of demon-

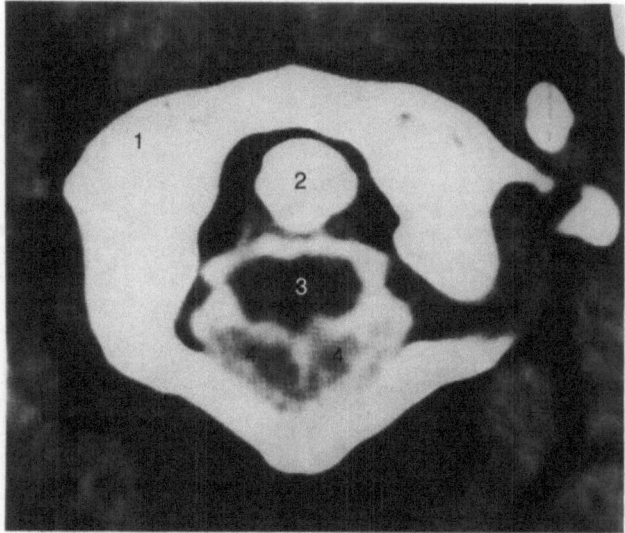

Figure 2.20. Arnold–Chiari malformation. 1, atlas; 2, odontoid process; 3, medulla oblongata; 4, tonsils.

strating them in childhood. The radiologic examination must demonstrate the cranial and caudal pole of the cysts.[23,24,29-34]

Dandy–Walker Syndrome

In this case, the IVth ventricle is dilated as a consequence of narrowed foramina of Magendie and Luschka. The dilation may become very large and occupy a great part of the posterior fossa (Figs. 2.21 and 2.22).[35,36]

Meningomyeloceles

Apart from the Chiari malformation, encephaloceles, myeloceles, and meningoceles may occur as autonomous malformations and adopt various degrees.[37-41] In all these cases, the contribution of CT and MRI is at present predominant to recognize the content of these herniae. Indeed, they may be associated with tumors (teratomas, lipomas). Angioscanning is very helpful to detect hypervascularization and associated angiomas.

Polyarthritis (Still's Disease) (Fig. 2.17)

The main complication of this pathologic condition is the destructive lesion of the transverse ligament which has the same roentgenographic features as in adults, i.e., the erosion of the posterior aspect of the odontoid process and the

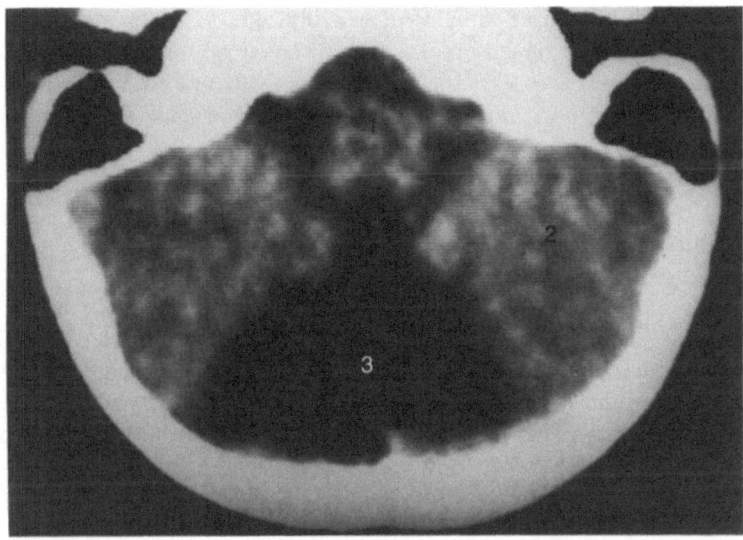

Figure 2.21. Enlarged cisterna magna (megacistern) in a 3-year-old girl. 1, brainstem; 2, cerebellum; 3, cisterna magna.

forward luxation of the skull and atlas. In severe cases, one may also observe a cranial luxation of the axis which penetrates into the foramen magnum. Generally, the dislocation is stable during the evolution of the disease.

Computed tomography (CT) is usually informative enough so that nuclear magnetic resonance (NMR) becomes not compulsory. If a dislocation is

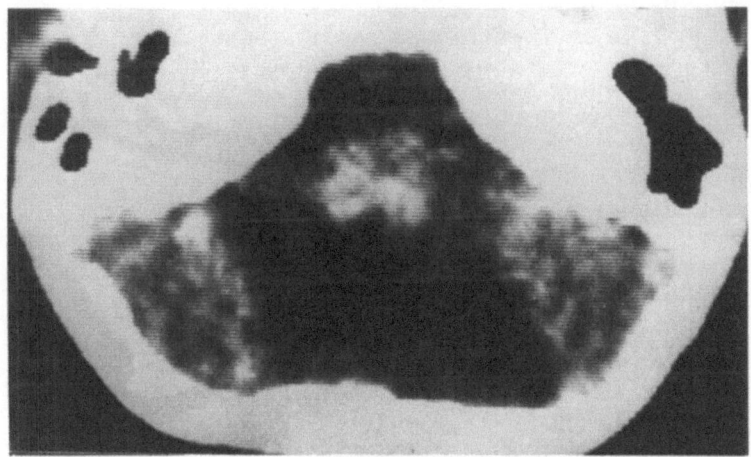

Figure 2.22. Dandy–Walker syndrome in a 3-year-old girl.

detected, the immobilization by a collar is indicated. In cases with neurologic complications, motor or sensory, the therapy has to be surgical, to stabilize the lesion. In these special cases of rheumatic disease with more or less bone destruction and articular alterations, the surgery has to be oriented according to each particular case.[42-44]

Infections

Infections of the cranio-vertebral area have become more and more rare. Indeed, tuberculosis[45] is in general regression and the infections of the pharyngeal area are usually cured before the stage of complications at the level of the bones and joints. One may, however, still see cases of infection, of the so-called Grisel syndrome described in 1930.[1,46] The radiologic image is characterized by osteolysis,

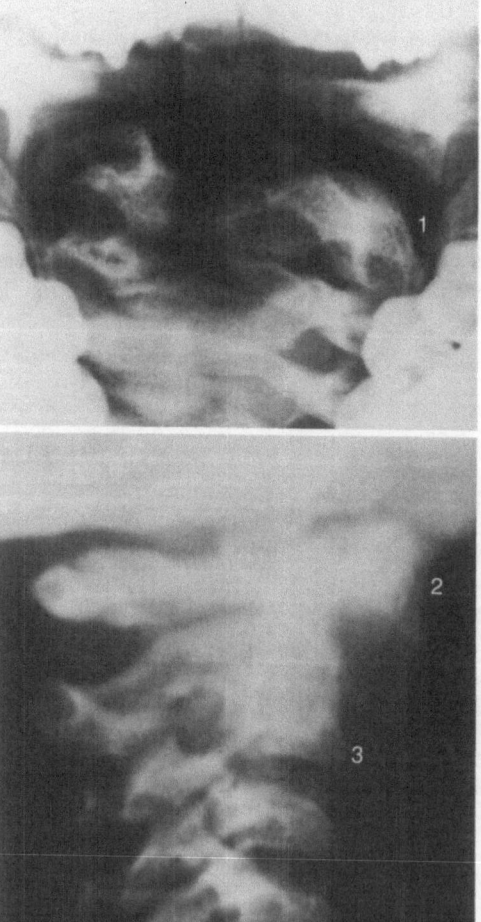

Figure 2.23. Grisel's syndrome. 1, rotation of the axis; 2, blurred limits of the atlas; 3, thickened soft parts in front of the axis.

alterations of the articular interspaces, and various kinds of dislocations (lateral, ventrodorsal, and cranio-caudal). In Fig. 2.23, we report such a case.

Metabolic and Developmental Changes

Here, we emphasize the mucopolysaccharidoses that are characterized by under-development of the odontoid process (Fig. 2.24). These children have to be treated by surgery when they suffer from neurologic signs of cord compression. This condition is usually due to instability, but may also be determined by nar-rowness of the cranio-vertebral canal, or even by both. Developmental anomalies concerning diseases of the bones such as osteogenesis imperfecta, avitaminoses, and osteomalacias are not very frequent and generally do not involve particularly the cranio-vertebral junction.[47-50]

Injuries

Injuries of the cranio-vertebral junction are particularly well tolerated during childhood[20,51-59] Later on, when the bones are developed, the traumatic condi-tions are the same as those of the adult. A highly recommended monograph of traumatic lesions has been published by J.C. Dosch.[61]

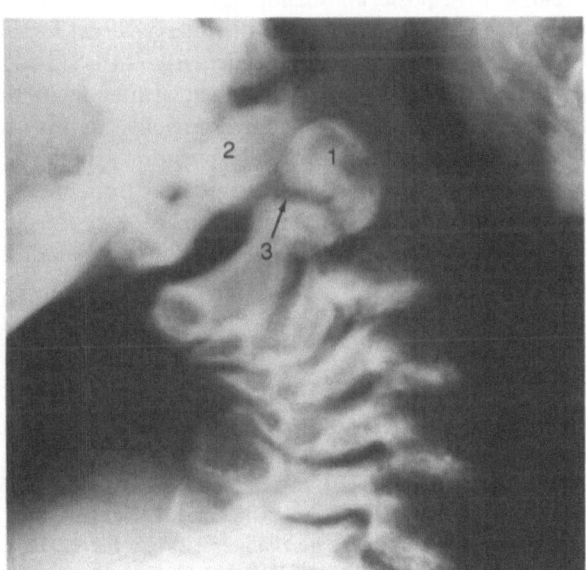

Figure 2.24. Morquio's disease with agenesis of the odontoid process. 1, body of the axis; 2, lateral mass of the atlas; 3, synchondrosis between the body and the posterior arch of the axis.

Tumors

In the cranio-vertebral region we have to consider a specific tumor that develops on vestiges of the chorda dorsalis: the chordoma.[62,63] In Fig. 2.4, we recall the course of the chorda dorsalia in the ventral part of the transitional area. Chordomas develop at this level and induce heterogeneous images of osteolysis and calcifications. They behave as tumors of the base of the skull in the posterior fossa. Among chordomas, the location at the level of the cranio-vertebral junction is more frequent in children than at the level of the lumbo-sacral region which is more frequent in adults.

Eosinophilic granulomas, benign osteoblastomas, aneurysmal cysts, and osteoid osteomas are not frequent at the level of the cranio-vertebral junction. Malignant tumors, as metastases, have no particular semiology. Both are not frequent in the cranio-vertebral junction.

Apart from the bone tumors,[64] the cranio-vertebral junction may be involved by congenital tumors such as dermoid and epidermoid cysts, lipomas, and teratomas, as well as tumors of the nervous structures (ependymoma, glioma, neuroblastoma, ganglioneuroma, medulloblastoma, neurinoma) and of the meninges (meningioma).[40,65,66] All these tumors are easily demonstrated by CT and MRI and necessitate surgical cure.

Let us say some words about the neurofibromatosis of von Recklinghausen, who was a professor of pathology in Strasbourg. This disease determines anomalies of the bones (enlargement of the foramen magnum and of the cervical canal with or without scalloping of the vertebral bodies), as well as anomalies of the dura mater (ectasia with posterior scalloping) and of the meninges (radicular cysts and diverticulae with enlargement of the intervertebral formina). The disease is also responsible for neurinomas, particularly of the C3 root.

In the cranio-vertebral area, we have to pay special attention to the ependymal canal. Two conditions, syringomyelia and hydromyelia, are very easily demonstrated by MRI, but one has to be careful in the positioning of the patient because these cavities may collapse when the CSF drops away from the cranio-vertebral region. In childhood, the dilation of the ependymal canal or the presence of cystic cavities generally accompany other malformations (occipitalization, Chiari, large cervical canal).[23,29-31,33,34]

References

1. Grisel P: Enucléation de l'atlas et torticolis nasopharyngien. Presse Med 38:50-52, 1930.
2. Sullivan AW: Subluxation of the atlanto-axial joint. J Pediatrics 35:451, 1949.
3. Le Double AF: Traité des variations des os du crâne de l'homme et de leur signification au point de vue de l'Anthropologie zooligique. Vigot Frères, Paris, 1903/1919.
4. Albrecht P: Anat Anz Leipzig, 1879 and Bult de la Soc d'Anthrop de Bruxelles, 1885.
5. Henle FGJ: Anatom TIS 103 (given by Le Double).

6. Legge F: Varieta della osse del cranio e della faccia in alcuni crani Camerinesi, 1883, (nach Le Double).
7. Calori L: Sulle varie particolarità osteol. Mem d'Acad d Sci Bologna, 301, 1892.
8. Déjérine J: Dystrophie osseuse par aplasie de la substance spongieuse du corps basilaire de l'occipital. Rev Neurol 2:181-300, 1926.
9. Adam-Falkiewiczova St, Nowicki W: Internationaler Neurologen Kongress, Bern 1931. Zentralb Neuchir 61:472, 1934.
10. Bodechtel G, Guizetti UH: Pseudotumeur cerebri, bedingt durch eine röntgenologisch Faßbare Anomalie des Hinterhauptloches mit Verlagerung der beiden oberen Halswirbel. Z Gesamt Neurol Psychiatr 143:470, 1933.
11. Morsier DeG, Junet R: L'aplasie de la lame basilaire de l'os occipital avec syndrome clinique de tumeur de la fosse postérieure. Rev Neurol 2:1483-1492, 1936.
12. Virchow R: Untersuchungen über die Entwicklung des Schädel-grundes. Reimer, Berlin, 1857.
13. Schuller A: Zur Roentgendiagnose der basilaren Impression des Schädels. Wien Med Wochenschr 61:2594, 1911.
14. Schmidt H, Fischer E: Die okzipitale Dysplasie. Thieme, Stuttgart, 1960.
15. Klaus E: Die basiläre Impression. S Hirtzel, Leipzig, 1969.
16. Lang J: Klinische Anatomie des Kopfes. Springer-Verlag, Berlin, 1981.
17. Wackenheim A: Hypoplasia of the basi-occipital bone and persistence of the spheno-occipital synchondrosis in a patient with transitory supplementary fissure of the basi-occipital. Neuroradiology 27:226-231, 1985.
18. Wackenheim A, Burguet JL, Sick H: Section of the odontoid process by a shortened transverse ligament (a possible etiology for the mobile odontoid). Neuroradiology 28:281-282, 1986.
19. Wackenheim A: C1/2 block vertebra, fusion of the anterior arch of the atlas with the axis, follow-up of the fusion in a child. Neuroradiology 16:416-417, 1978.
20. Wackenheim A: Roentgen Diagnosis of the Cranio-Vertebral Region. Springer-Verlag, Berlin, 1974.
21. Aboulezz AO, Sartor K, Geyer CA, Gado MH: Position of cerebellar tonsils in the normal population and in patients with Chiari malformation: a quantitative approach with MR Imaging. J Comput Assist Tomogr 9:1033-1036, 1985.
22. Bamberger-Bozo C: Malformation de Chiari II. Arnold–Chiari de la littérature. J Neuroradiology 9:47-70, 1982.
23. De la Paz RL, Brady TJ, Buonanno FS: Nuclear Magnetic Resonance imaging of Arnold-Chiari type I malformation with hydromyelia. J Comput Assist Tomogr 7:126-129, 1983.
24. Forbes WStC, Isherwood I: Computed tomography in a syringomyelia and the associated Arnold–Chiari type I malformation. Neuroradiology 15:73-78, 1978.
25. Naidich TP, Pudlowski RM, Naidich JB: Computed tomography signs of Chiari II malformation: skull and dural partitions (part I). Radiology 134:65-71, 1980. Midbrain and cerebellum (part II). Radiology 134:391-398, 1980. Ventricles and cisterns (part III). Radiology 134:657-663, 1980.
26. Naidich TP: Aspects tomodensitométriques des lésions crânio-cervicales de la malformation de Chiari II. Corrélations anatomo-tomodensitométriques. J Neuroradiol 8:207-227, 1981.
27. Naidich TP, McLone DG, Fullin KH: The Chiari II malformation: part IV. The hindbrain deformity. Neuroradiology 25:179-197, 1983.

28. Park TS, Hoffman HJ, Hendrick EB, Humphreys RP: Experience with surgical decompression of the Arnold-Chiari malformation in young infants with myelomeningocele. Neurosurgery 13:147–152, 1983.

29. Aboulker J: La syringomyélie et les liquides intra-rachidiens. Neurochirurgie 25 (Suppl 1): , 1979.

30. Aubin ML, Vignaud J, Jardin C: Computed tomography in 75 clinical cases of syringomyelia. AJNR 2:199–204, 1981.

31. Bonafe A, Manelfe C, Espagno J, Guiraud B, Rascol A: Evaluation of syringomyelia with metrizamide computed tomography myelography. J Comput Assist Tomogr 4:797–802, 1980.

32. Cahan LD, Benison JR: Considerations in the diagnosis and treatment of syringomyelia and the Chiari malformation. J Neurosurg 57:24–31, 1982.

33. Kokmen E, Marsh WR, Baker HL: Magnetic resonance imaging in syringomyelia. Neurosurgery 17:267–270, 1985.

34. Yeates A, Brant-Zawadzki M, Norman D: Nuclear magnetic resonance imaging of syringomyelia. AJNR 4:234–237, 1983.

35. Kojima T, Waga S, Shimizu T: Dandy–Walker cyst associated with occipital meningocele. Surg Neurol 17:52–56, 1982.

36. Lehman RM: Dandy–Walker syndrome in consecutive siblings: familial hindbrain malformation. Neurosurgery 8:717–719, 1981.

37. Babcock DS, Han BK: Cranial sonographic findings in meningomyelocele. AJR 136:563–569, 1981; AJNR 1:493–499, 1980.

38. Fenstermaker RA, Roessmann U, Rekate HL: Fourth ventriculoceles with extracranial extension. J Neurosurg 61:348–350, 1984.

39. Marar BC, Orth MC, Balachandran N: Nontraumatic atlanto-axial dislocation in children. Clin Orthop 92:220–226, 1973.

40. Parker Mickle J, McLennan JE: Malignant teratoma arising within a lipomeningocele. J Neurosurg 43:761–763, 1975.

41. Zimmerman RD, Breckbill D, Dennis MW, Davil DO: Cranial CT finding in patients with meningomyelocele. AJR 132:623–629, 1979.

42. Bonneville JF: En savoir plus sur le rachis cervical. Masson, Paris, 1980.

43. Debre R, Broca R, Cremieux M: Maladie de Still à début cervical. Bulletin de la Société de Pédiatrie de Paris. 234, 1932.

44. DiMeglio A, Ferran JL, Lutter L: Rachis cervical et arthrite chronique juvénile, in l'arthrite chronique juvénile. Masson, Paris, 1984, pp 74–85.

45. Bailey H, Sister Mary Gabriel, Hodgson AR, Shin JS: Tuberculosis of the spine in children. J Bone Joint Surg 54:1633–1657, 1972.

46. Mozziconacci P, Abramovici M, Hassan M, Hayem F: Luxations atloido-axoidienne rhumatoide et syndrome de Grisel. Ann Pédiatr 20:405–418, 1973.

47. Friedman WA, Mickle JP: Hydrocephalus in achondroplasia: a possible mechanism. Neurosurgery 7:150–153, 1980.

48. Maroteaux P: Maladies osseuses de l'enfant. Flammarion, Paris, 1974.

49. Pueschel SM, Scola FH, Perry CD, Pezzullo JC: Atlantoaxial instability in children with Down's syndrome. Pediatr Radiol 10:129–132, 1981.

50. Watts RWE, Spellacy E, Kendall BE, Du Boulay G, Gibbs DA: Computed tomography studies on patients with mucopolysaccharidoses. Neuroradiology 21:9–23, 1981.

51. Barcat E, Rigault P, Padovant JP, Martin P: Fractures et luxations du rachis cervical chez l'enfant. Ann Chir Infant 17:197–212, 1975.

52. Chagnon S, Blery M: Entorses et luxations du rachis cervical chez l'enfant. J Radiol 63:465–470, 1982.
53. Chagnon S, Blery M: Les lésions traumatiques du rachis chez l'enfant. Cours de perfectionnement post-universitaire. Paris, 1984.
54. Duncan AW, Stanley P, Isaacson J: Fracture– dislocation of the cervical spine in the newborn. AJR 135:868, 1980.
55. Kaiser MC, Pettersson H, Harwood-Nash DC, Fitz CR, Chuang S: CT for trauma of the base of the skull and spine in children. Neuroradiology 22:27–31, 1981.
56. McPhee IB: Spinal fractures and dislocations in children and adolescents. Spine 6:533–537, 1981.
57. Pennecot GF, Leonard P, Peyrot des Gachons S, Hardy JR, Pouliquen JC: Traumatic ligamentar instability of the cervical spine in children. J Pediatr Orthop 4:339–345, 1984.
58. Savader SJ, Martinez C, Reed Murtagh F: Odontoid fracture in a nine-month-old infant. Surg Neurol 24:529–532, 1985.
59. Sherk HH, Nicholson JT, Chunk SMK: Fractures of the odontoid process in young children. J Bone Joint Surg 60:921–924, 1978.
60. Wackenheim A: La dynamique de l'odontoide mobile. J Radiol Electrol 592:107–108, 1978.
61. Dosch JC: Trauma. Springer-Verlag, Berlin, 1985.
62. Meyer JE, Oot RF, Lindfors KK: CT appearance of clival chordomas. J Comput Assist Tomogr 1:34–38, 1986.
63. Wold LE, Laws ER: Cranial chordomas in children and young adults. J Neurosurg 59:1043–1047, 1983.
64. Lichtenstein L: Bone tumors. Mosby, St. Louis, 1972.
65. Holliday PO III, Davis C, Angelo J: Multiple meningiomas of the cervical spinal cord associated with Klippel-Feil malformation and atlanto-occipital assimilation. Neurosurgery 14:353–357, 1984.
66. Jeanmart L: Tumors. Springer-Verlag, Berlin, 1986.

Bibliography

Adam R, Greenberg JO: The mega cisterna magna. J Neurosurg 48:190–192, 1978.
Arredondo F, Haughton VM, Hemmy DC, Zelaya B, Williams AL: The computed tomographic appearance of the spinal cord in diastematomyelia. Radiology 136:685–688, 1980.
Anderson FM: Occult spinal dysraphism: a series of 73 cases. Pediatrics 55:826–835, 1975.
Bewermeyer H, Dreesbach HA, Hunermann B, Heiss WD: MR imaging of familial basilar impression. J Comput Assist Tomogr 8:953–956, 1984.
Byrd SE, Harwood-Nash DC, Fitz CR, Rogovitz DM: Computed tomography in the evaluation of encephaloceles in infants and children. J Comput Assist Tomogr 2:81–87, 1978.
Caffey J: Pediatric X Ray Diagnosis. Year Book Medical Publishers, Chicago and London, 1978.
Chagnon S, Labrune M: Le rachis de l'enfant. Feuillets Radiol 21:7–46, 1981.
Dorne HL, Just N, Lander PH: CT recognition of anomalies of the posterior arch of the atlas vertebra: differentiation from fracture. AJNR 7:176–177, 1986.

Dublin AB, McGahan JP, Reid MH: Value of computed tomographic metrizamide myelography in the neuroradiological evaluation of the spine. Radiology 146:79–86, 1983.

Fischgold H, Metzger J, Legré J, Djindjian R, Engel P: Neuroradiologie, canal rachidien, moelle et racines, in traité de radiodiagnostic. Tome 15, Masson, Paris, 1971.

Frank E, Berger T, Tew JM: Basilar impression and platybasia in osteogenesis imperfecta tarda. Surg Neurol 17:116–119, 1982.

Gardeur D: Pathologies Malformatives et Néonatales, in Tomodensitométrie Intra-Crânienne. Livre VI, Marketing, Paris, 1983.

Gehweiler JA, Daffner RH, Roberts L: Malformations of the atlas vertebra simulating the Jefferson Fracture. AJR 140:1083–1086, 1983.

Gras M, Bourbotte G, Boluix B, Castan P, Pous JG, Dimeglio A, Frerebeau P: Scolioses malformatives avec ou sans dysraphie spinale occulte. A propos de 82 observations de l'enfant. J. Radiol 63:383–395, 1982.

Hamilton, Boyd, Mossmans: Human Embryology, Williams & Wilkins, Baltimore, 1978.

Hammock MK, Milhorat TH: Cranial Computed Tomography Infancy and Childhood. Williams & Wilkins, Baltimore, 1981.

Han JS, Huss RG, Benson JE, Kaufman B, Yoon YS, Morrison SC, Alfidi RJ, Rekate HL, Ratcheson RA: ME Imaging of the skull base. J Comput Assist Tomogr 8:944–952, 1984.

Han JS, Kaufman K, El Yousef SJ: NMR imaging of the spine. AJNR 4:1151–1159, 1983; AJR 141:1137–1145, 1983.

Han JS, Benson JE, Yoon YS: Magnetic resonance imaging in the spinal column and cranio-vertebral junction. Radiol Clin North Am 22:805–827, 1984.

Han JS, Bonstelle CT, Kaufman B: Magnetic resonance imaging in the evaluation of the brainstem. Radiology 150:705–712, 1984.

Harwood-Nash CC, Fitz CR: Neuroradiology in Infants and Children. Mosby, St. Louis, 1976.

Harwood-Nash DCF, Fitz CR, Margareta Resjo I, Chuang S: Congenital spinal and cord lesions in children and computed tomographic metrizamide myelography. Neuroradiology 16:69–70, 1978.

Harwood-Nash DC: Tomodensitométrie des anomalies cérébrales chez le nouveau-né. J Neuroradiol 8:125–142, 1981.

Harwood-Nash DC: Techniques neuroadiologiques pédiatriques. J Neuroradiol 8:73–91, 1981.

Harwood-Nash DC, Fitz CR: Neuroradiology in infants and children. Mosby, St. Louis, 1976.

Haughton VM, Williams AL: Computed Tomography of the Spine. Mosby, St. Louis, 1982.

Hawkes RC, Holland GN, Moore WS: Craniovertebral junction pathology: assessment by NMR. AJNR 4:232–233, 1983.

Henrys P, Lyne ED, Lifton C, Salciccioli G: Clinical review of cervical spine injuries in children. Clin Orthop Relat Res 129:172–176, 1977.

Holt JF: Neurofibromatosis in children. AJR 130:615–639, 1978.

Hunter GA: Non-traumatic displacement of the atlanto-axial joint. J Bone Joint Surg 50B:44–51, 1968.

Just NWM, Goldenburg M: Computed tomography of the enlarged cisterna magna. Radiology 131:385–391, 1979.

Kaiser MC, Pettersson H, Harwood-Nash DC, Fitz CR, Armstrong E: Direct coronal CT of the spine in infants and children. AJNR 2:465–466, 1981.

Kaufman RA, Dunbar JS, Botsford JA, McLaurin RL: Traumatic longitudinal atlanto-occipital distraction injuries in children. AJNR 3:415–419, 1982.

Labrune M, Chagnon S: Le rachis de l'enfant. Feuillets Radiol 21:47–54, 1981.

Levine RS, Geremia GK, McNeill TW: CT demonstration of cervical diastematomyelia. J Comput Assist Tomogr 9:592–594, 1985.

McGinnis BD, Brady TJ, New PFJ: Nuclear magnetic resonance imaging of tumors in the posterior fossa. J Comput Assist Tomogr 7:575–584, 1983.

McRae DL: Bony abnormalities in the region of the foramen magnum: correlation of anatomic and neurologic findings. Acta Radiol (Stockh) 40:335, 1953.

Martin K, Krastel A, Hamer J, Banniza UK: Symptomatology and diagnosis of diastematomyelia of children. Neuroradiology 16:89–90, 1978.

Martin N, Gaston A, Brugieres P, Guilbeau JC, Marsault C, Nahum H: Bilan radiologique actuel des dysraphismes. Feuillets Radiol 25:331–344, 1985.

Matsumara M, Nojiri K, Yumoto Y: Persistent primitive hypoglossal artery associated with Arnold-Chiari type I malformation. Surg Neurol 24:241–244, 1985.

Miller JH, Reid BS, Kemberling CR: Utilization of ultrasound in the evaluation of spinal dysraphism in children. Radiology 143:737–740, 1982.

Modic MT, Weinstein MA, Pavlicek W: Magnetic resonance imaging of the cervical spine. Technical and clinical observations. AJR 141:1129–1136, 1983.

Nagib MG, Maxwell RE, Chou SN: Identification and management of High-risk patients with Klippel-Feil syndrome. J Neurosurg 61:523–550, 1984.

Naidich TP, Epstein F, Lin JP, Kricheff II, Hochwald GM: Evaluation of pediatric hydrocephalus by computed tomography. Radiology 119:337–345, 1976.

Newton TH, Potts DG: Computed Tomography of the Spine and Spinal Cord. Clavadel Press, San Anselmo, 1983.

Osborne D, Triolo P, Dubois P: Assessment of cranio-cervical junction and atlanto-axial relation using metrizamide-enhanced CT in flexion and extension. AJNR 4:843–845, 1983.

Park TS, Cail WS, Maggio WM, Mitchell DC: Progressive spasticity and scoliosis in children with myelomeningocele. J Neurosurg 62:367–375, 1985.

Pennecot GF, Gouraud D, Hardy JR, Pouliquen JC: Roentgenologic study of the stability of the cervical spine in children. J Pediatr Orthop 4:346–352, 1984.

Petterson H, Harwood-Nash DC: CT and Myelography of the Spine and Cord. Springer-Verlag, Berlin, 1982.

Probst FP, Brun A: Recurrent meningoencephalitis and ascending myelitis caused by dermal sinus tract of extraordinary length. Neuroradiology 19:161–165, 1980.

Raybaud C, Jiddane M, Garnier JM, Gondim-Oliveira J: Neuroradiologie pédiatrique (aspects spécifiques). Encyclopédie Médico Chirurgicale Paris, Radiodiagnostic II, 31621 A10 et A20, 12-1983.

Resjo IM, Harwood-Nash DCF, Fitz CR, Chuang S: Normal cord in infants and children examined with computed tomographic metrizamide myelography. Radiology 130:691–696, 1979.

Resjo IM, Harwood-Nash DC, Fitz CR, Chuang S: Computed tomographic metrizamide myelography in spinal dysraphism in infants and children. J Comput Assist Tomogr 2:549–558, 1978.

Rougerie J: Les Compressions Médullaires non Traumatiques de l'Enfant. Masson, Paris, 1973.

Sauser G: Intrakraniale Manifestation des letzten Occipital-Wirbels. Z Anat Entwickl Gesch 104:159–168, 1935.

Sauvegrain J: Radiologie des affections ostéoarticulaires de l'enfant. Journées de radiologie pédiatrique. Hôpital Trousseau, Paris, 1979.

Sauvegrain J, Mareschal JL: Malformations de la charnière crânio-cervicale chez l'enfant. A propos de 35 observations. Ann Radiol 15:263–277, 1972.

Schuller A: The diagnosis of "basilar impression." Radiology 34:214, 1940.

Scotti G, Musgrave MA, Harwood-Nash DC, Fitz CR, Chuang SH: Diastematomyelia in children: metrizamide and CT metrizamide myelography. AJR 135:1225–1232, 1980.

Smith MT, Huntington HW: Inverse cerebellum and occipital encephalocele. A dorsal fusion defect uniting the Arnold–Chiari and Dandy–Walker spectrum. Neurology 27:246–251, 1977.

Stark GD: Spina bifida. Blackwell, Oxford, 1977.

Suss RA, Zimmerman RD, Leeds NE: Pseudospread of the atlas: false sign of Jefferson fracture in young children. AJR 140:1079–1082, 1983.

Swischuk LE: Anterior displacement of C2 in children: physiologic or pathologic? A helpful differentiating line. Radiology 122:759–763, 1977.

Taveras JM, Wood EH: Diagnostic neuroradiology. Williams & Wilkins, Baltimore, 1976.

Trial R, Bacques O, Plainfossé MC, Blery M, Chevrot A: Traité de Radiodiagnostic n° 12, os et Articulations. Pathologie Régionale. Masson, Paris, 1983.

Wackenheim A: Occipitalization of the ventral part and vertebralization of the dorsal part of the atlas with insufficiency of the transverse ligament. Neuroradiology 24:45–47, 1982.

Woodring JH, Selke AC, Duff DE: Traumatic atlantooccipital dislocation with survival. AJR 137:21–24, 1981.

Yanai Y, Tsuji R, Ohmori S, Kubota S, Nagashima C: Foramen magnum syndrome caused by a dolichoodontoid process. Surg Nerol 24:95–100, 1985.

Young IR, Burl M, Clarke GJ: Magnetic resonance properties of hydrogen: imaging the posterior fossa. AJR 137:895–901, 1981.

CHAPTER 3

Chiari Malformations

Concezio Di Rocco and Mario Rende

Under the eponymous definition of *Chiari's malformations* are grouped a variety of hindbrain anomalies, which actually differ considerably in terms of embryogenic defect, pathogenesis, clinical manifestations, treatment, and outcome.

Since the earliest description of these anomalies about a century ago, they have been the subject of continuous controversy; even today the discussion is open, especially concerning their physiopathogenetic interpretation, and to a lesser extent, their correct management.

In clinical practice, however, only one type, namely that described by Chiari as type II malformation, has assumed a particular importance because of its relative frequency and its almost constant association with a defect of neural tube closure and hydrocephalus.

Historical Background and Definition

In 1891,[1] and more extensively in 1896,[2] Chiari reported on different types of caudal herniation of cerebellum and brainstem structures, which he considered to be the result of a congenital hydrocephalus. The author[1] first defined three and subsequently[2] four types of conditions (Fig. 3.1). Apparently Chiari's main concern was to organize the malformations of the structures of the posterior cranial fossa systematically, by taking into account the position of the cerebellum and lower brainstem in relation to the foramen magnum and upper cervical canal, as the principal criterion of severity.

The *type I malformation* was found by Chiari in 14 subjects with hydrocephalus, in most cases due to tuberculous meningitis, and in carcinomatous meningitis. The most evident characteristic was the dislocation of the cone-shaped tonsils and the medial aspect of the posterior lobe of the cerebellum into the upper cervical vertebral canal. The medulla appeared elongated in several patients, though still confined within the posterior cranial fossa. The *normal* position of the medulla oblongata in this type of malformation can actually be appreciated indirectly by evaluating Chiari's original drawing[2] in which the upper cervical nerves do not run upward to their exit foramina, and the hypoglossal nerve actually runs downward.

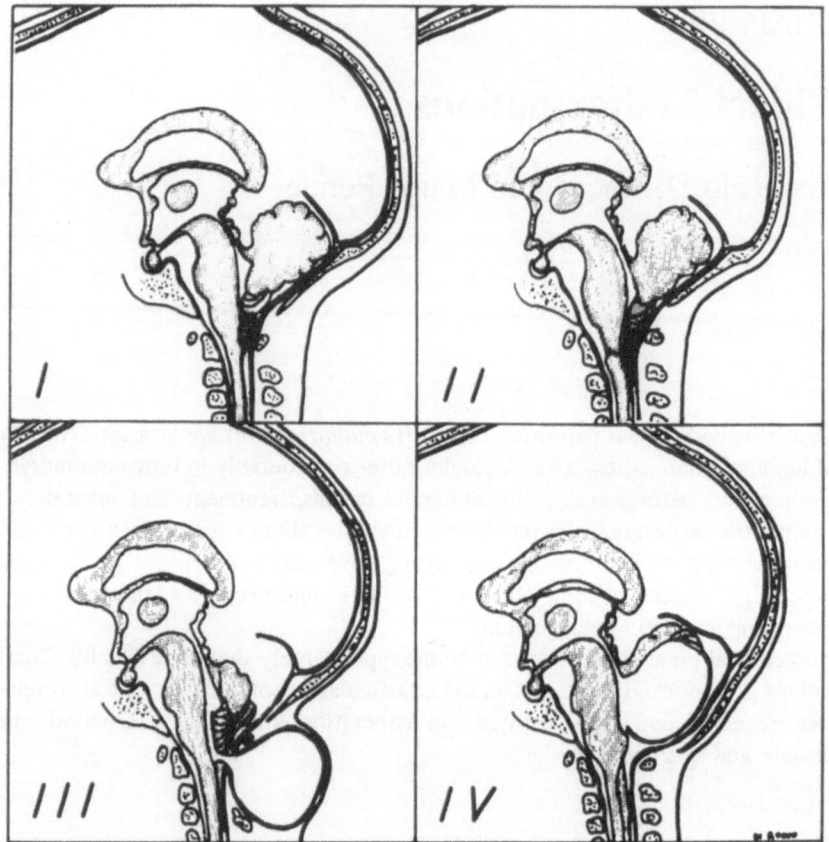

Figure 3.1. Schematic representation of the four types of Chiari malformations.

The *type II malformation* was described by Chiari in seven hydrocephalic infants, all of them with spina bifida. This type of malformation includes the dislocation of the inferior vermis into the upper part of the cervical spinal canal, and the caudal displacement of the lower pons and medulla as well as the IVth ventricle. The last structure is peculiarly elongated, so that its opening may be located within the cervical canal. Again, the caudal dislocation of the brainstem structures may be noted in Chiari's original depiction of the condition,[2] as the first six cervical nerves run upward and the lower extremity of the IVth ventricle lies at the level of the origin of the first cervical nerve.

The most severe degree of caudal displacement of the brainstem and cerebellum was reported by Chiari as combined with the herniation of the cerebellar structures through the foramen magnum into a bifid upper cervical vertebral canal. This *type III malformation* allowed the *distended cerebellum and IVth ventricle to form a sac-like encephalocele at the base of the skull.*

The *type IV malformation* was added by the author to the first three types in the article published in 1896,[2] in which two cases characterized by an extreme hypoplasia of the cerebellum were described. In one of these cases there was an associated dilation of the IVth ventricle.

With the exception of the last type of malformation in which the cerebellum and the brainstem lie completely within the posterior cranial fossa, Chiari's classification of the first three types of malformations obviously is expressive of his opinion that the caudal displacement of cerebellar and brainstem structures, as well as their abnormal development, reflect directly the hydrostatic forces of the concomitant hydrocephalus. In other words, Chiari rejected the alternative explanation of a complex cerebral maldevelopment, which had been advocated 13 years before by Cleland.[3] Cleland's description of his first specimen in *Hydrocephalus and Spina Bifida in an Infant Born at Full Time*, representing an accurate report on the malformations of neuroectodermal and mesodermal origin which can be found in association with a meningomyelocele, was actually consistent with the Chiari type II malformation. The author, in fact, had noted (and clearly depicted in Fig. 6 of his article[3]) that "the laminated tubercle (nodule) hangs down from an exaggerated *velum posticum*, as an appendix ¾ inch in length lying in the prolonged 4th ventricle." Cleland also mentioned the coexisting hydrocephalus ("the corpus callosum and fornix had been destroyed by the distending effusion") as well as some of the cerebral anomalies which today are known to be typical in subjects with myelodysplasia ("the corpora quadrigemina were curiously altered in shape, the testes being projected above the nates, and the nates being flattened, probably by pressure of distended hemispheres"; "the inferior (cerebellar) vermiform process extends up so far, that what appears to be pyramid touches the corpora quadrigemina, while the uvula looks backward"). In interpreting the cause of the failure of the neural tube closure, Cleland appears deeply influenced by the memoir published by Lebedeff in 1881,[4] dealing with various specimens of anomalous brain and spinal cord in the embryo chick. Commenting on the bearing of these anomalies on anencephaly in human subjects, Lebedeff concluded that an open condition of the cerebrospinal canal was related to an overgrowth of the cerebrospinal axis.

Cleland, however, did not deny the possibility of a rupture of an already fused neural tube secondary to an embryonic cerebral or spinal fluid accumulation as proposed by Forster[5] and Ahlfeld,[6] when he postulated that "it is perhaps more likely that distention of the (spinal) canal, after closure, caused its dilation above, and led to its rupture below in very early development"). The author, however, excluded that the caudal displacement and abnormal shape of the cerebellar vermis he had observed in his specimen could depend on the pressure exerted from above because of the ventricular dilation, as "the hydrocephalus was obviously of much later origin, when the different parts of the brain were already formed." Actually, Cleland's explanation of the anomalies of the structures of the posterior cranial fossa may be considered just opposite to that of Chiari, i.e., the result of the absence of a pressure limiting the normal development of the cerebellum ("The most extraordinary instance of enlarged structure is, however, the enormous laminated tubercle. . . . Here is a structure in ordinary circumstance closely pressed on by other parts, which in this instance (specimen I) has obviously hung in a larger space caused by effusion of fluid. . . . The laminated tubercle hanging free in this fluid has been very differently situated from what is when its growth is resisted by solid structures.").

In 1894, Arnold[7] reported on the pathologic findings detected at autopsy in an infant with a sacro-coccygeal tumor and spina bifida. Though he gave more attention to the description of the spinal tumor, the author also mentioned the displacement of the cerebellum downwards into the upper cervical spinal canal. Neither hydrocephalus nor abnormalities of the brainstem were noted. Working in Arnold's laboratory, in 1907 Schwalbe and Gredig[8] gave a detailed account on the brainstem and cerebellar changes, evaluated through serial sections in four of their own cases, with hindbrain anomalies consistent with the Chiari type II malformation; they also summarized the characteristics of all previous cases recorded in the literature. In spite of the fact that they were aware of the first three cases described by Chiari in 1891, Schwalbe and Gredig gave credit to Arnold as having made the first description of the condition and coined the definition "Arnold'sche und Chiari'sche Missbildung," i.e., Arnold–Chiari malformation.

Though incorrect, as Arnold had not added any significant observation to those made by Chiari, the eponym became popular, and several cases of Chiari type II malformation were subsequently reported under the double name definition until the late 1960s.[9-21] Since the early 1970s, however, Arnold's name was progressively abandoned by several authors.[22-30]

Physiopathogenic Interpretations

After Chiari's original suggestion, the variety of anomalies of the structures of the posterior cranial fossa he subsequently described was long considered merely to represent a different degree of the same pathologic process. However, the lack of an indisputable unitary physiopathogenic interpretation of the entire spectrum of malformations accounted for the opinions of those who regarded each type of Chiari malformation as a specific pathologic process, characterized by different clinical expressions and a variable association with the other types of malformations.

Although several studies were carried out to improve the understanding of Chiari type I and type II malformations, Chiari type III and IV malformations received very little attention, either because of their limited clinical significance or because they were more correctly identified with other nosographic entities. Indeed, Chiari type III malformation is only rarely compatible with postnatal life; recently, it has been proposed that it represents a severe form of Klippel–Feil syndrome.[31,32] Besides constituting the smallest group in Chiari's series, Chiari type IV malformation appeared early on to be also the less homogeneous and the most difficult to be related to the other types of anomalies.

At least one of the two cases of Chiari's original series would today be classified as a Dandy–Walker cyst.[33]

Also, Chiari type I and type II malformations hardly fit into a unitary frame. Chiari type I malformation is, in fact, usually found in adolescence and adulthood in association with an acute or chronic state of intracranial pressure; the spinal cord, except in the possible presence of a spinal cavitation,[34] and the supratentorial cerebral structures are normal; the dentate ligaments and cervical nerve roots maintain a normal position. On the other hand, the caudal descent of the inferior cerebellar vermis, the IVth ventricle, the medulla oblongata, and the last cranial and first spinal nerves, which is typical of Chiari type II malformation, occur more frequently in infancy and childhood, and are almost always associated with a defect of spinal tube closure. Increased intracranial pressure is not necessarily present, as the condition can be detected even in subjects who have undergone a cerebrospinal fluid (CSF) shunting procedure at a very early age. Associated cerebral anomalies are nearly always present as are mesodermal defects of the skull. Finally, anomalies of the cardiovascular, gastrointestinal, and genitourinary systems may be noticed in about a tenth of the cases.[34]

A considerable number of hypotheses have been proposed to explain the entire spectrum of Chiari's malformations in a unitary manner. They can be schematically divided into three main groups: (1) the "hydrodynamic" theories, based on the existence of a pressure gradient between the cranial and the spinal spaces; (2) the "mechanical" theories, which indicate as a principal causative factor a block in the circulating CSF at the foramen magnum, and (3) the "maldevelopmental" theories, which consider the deformities of the structures of the posterior cranial fossa as being only the localized expression of generalized dysembryogenetic pathologic processes, which interests the whole organism.

"Hydrodynamic" Theories

Primary Hydrocephalus

This hypothesis postulates that a primitive embryonal hydrocephalus causes the caudal dislocation and the progressive extrusion of the posterior cranial fossa structures out of the skull. First advanced by Chiari, the hypothesis was again propounded by Gardner[32,35] in an attempt to identify in only one factor—the failure of the primitive rhombic roof to become permeable during fetal development—the cause of the dilation of the cerebral ventricles, the caudal migration of the hindbrain, and eventually the dilation or rupture of the central spinal canal. According to Gardner the combined effects of the progressive accumulation of the fluid within the supratentorial ventricular system, and the mechanical stresses due to pulsations of the choroid plexus within the lateral and IVth ventricles, determine the characteristics of the resulting formative and positional anomalies of the brainstem and cerebellum, which are typical of Chiari's malformations. In Chiari type I malformation, the caudal migration of the cerebellum would be opposed by the CSF pulsations within the IVth ventricle;

conversely, in the Chiari type II malformation, the opposing effect of such pulsatile forces would be lost, as the changes in CSF volume they induce are compensated for by the spreading of CSF throughout the opening of the associated meningomyelocele.

Although this theory would provide a sound explanation for the occurrence of phenomena such as the frequent association with hydromyelia and syringomyelia, present in Chiari type I malformation,[23,36] and the caudal displacement of the tentorium and the reduced size of the posterior cranial fossa observed in Chiari type II malformation, it cannot be applied to those cases of Chiari malformations without hydrocephalus.[37]

The value of the theory is also limited by evidence of the obvious descent of the cerebellar and brainstem structures in subjects without meningomyelocele.[38-40] Furthermore, myeloschisis has been demonstrated in 5- to 7-mm embryos, i.e., before the appearance of the choroid plexuses, and CSF has been seen to exit through the physiologic foramina of the IVth ventricle even in patients with meningomyelocele.[41,42]

Secondary Hydrocephalus

In a series of articles published between 1971 and 1981, Williams[43-45] suggested that the pressure gradient postulated to justify the descent of the hindbrain could depend on a decrease in the intraspinal pressure rather than on an increase in the intracranial pressure. Consequently, Chiari malformations could occur even in the absence of hydrocephalus. Williams interpreted the impaction of the cerebellar and brainstem structures in the foramen magnum as the result, and at the same time the cause, of the progression of the condition (Fig. 3.2A). In fact, with the Valsalva maneuver (strain, cough, abdominal compression, etc.) the dilation of the vertebral epidural veins (Fig. 3.2B) would cause the spinal CSF to move cephalad into the cranial cavity, pushing the descended cerebellar tonsil and vermis upwards. The reverse movement of CSF from the skull to the spine would be considerably more difficult, as the increase in the intracranial pressure induced by CSF fluid accumulation within the cranial cavity would favor a further impaction of the hindbrain structures at the foramen magnum, separating functionally the intracranial and intraspinal compartments (Fig. 3.2C). Chronically, this type of mechanism, enhanced by secondary adhesions of the membranes limiting the neural structures within the cisterna magna and the prebulbar cistern, would result in the creation of a secondary hydrocephalus, which in turn would determine a further caudal migration of the cerebellar and brainstem structures. In such a situation, the frequently associated hydromyelia and syringomyelia could represent an alternative pathway for dissipating the increased intracranial pressure through the central spinal canal.

It is worth noting that a similar concept can be found in the thesis for the doctorate in medicine published in Leiden in 1932 by van Houweninge Graftdijk.[46] In his dissertation, in fact, the author assumed that the Chiari malformation acts as a valve, which opposes the movement of CSF from the ventricles down

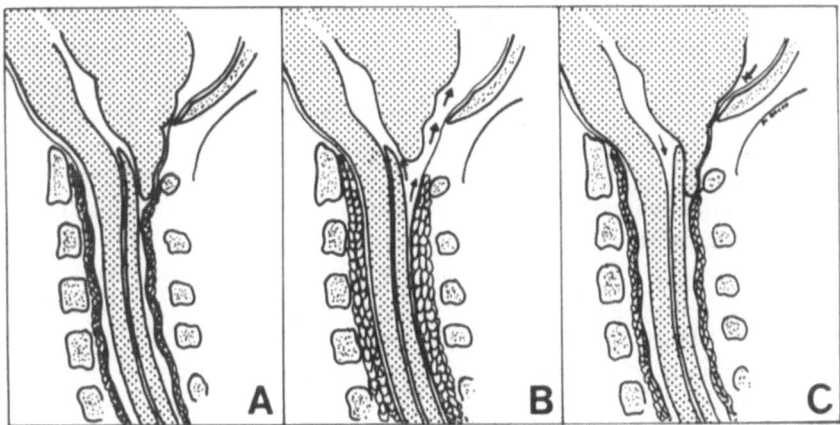

Figure 3.2. Schematic representation of the events accounting for the occurrence of hydrocephalus in Chiari type II malformation, according to Williams. A: Impaction of the cerebellar and brainstem structures at the foramen magnum. B: Cephalad CSF movement into the cranial cavity due to the dilation of the vertebral epidural veins. C: Functional impairment to the caudal movement of CSF from the cranial cavity due to the physical obstacle of the herniated cerebellar and brainstem structures (for further explanation, see text).

into the vertebral canal, while letting the same fluid escape readily in an upward direction from the vertebral canal into the cerebral ventricles or the cerebral subarachnoid spaces.

The explanation proposed by Cameron in 1957,[47] and 9 years later by van Hoytema and van den Berg,[48] is still based on a primary decrease in CSF pressure within the spinal canal, but relatively simpler than the interpretation by Williams. These two authors postulated that a loss of fluid from the IVth ventricle to the amniotic cavity through the defect of the meningomyelocele during fetal life would be responsible for a decrease in pressure within the IVth ventricle, with a series of secondary events: failure in formation of the foramina of Luschka and Magendie; fall of the inferior cerebellar vermis into the roof of the IVth ventricle; caudal displacement of the lower brainstem and cerebellar structures; and global hypoplasia of the whole posterior cranial fossa.

Mechanical Theories

In 1914, the experimental research by Weed and by Dandy and Blackfan led to the recognition of the CSF circulation from the ventricular cavities to the cerebral and spinal subarachnoid spaces, as well as to the identification of the villi and Pacchioni's bodies as the main structures responsible for CSF absorption. Likewise, in clinical practice the internal hydrocephalus was classified into two main types: "communicating" and "noncommunicating," according to the absence or the presence of a block within the CSF circulation preventing a dye, injected into the lateral ventricles, to be recaptured from the lumbar sub-arachnoid spaces.

Based mainly on these new acquisitions and examination techniques, several mechanisms were subsequently proposed to explain the association of Chiari malformations and hydrocephalus on the grounds of a mechanical block in the CSF circulation, within either the aqueduct, the posterior cranial fossa, or the upper cervical canal.

Typical examples of such a mechanical explanation of hydrocephalus may be found in the article published by Russell and Donald in 1935.[49] The authors reported on 10 cases of meningomyelocele and meningocele, all of them charac-terized by Chiari type II malformation. In two instances they observed a noncom-municating hydrocephalus, due to an atresia of the Sylvian aqueduct and the foramina of Lusckha and Magendie, respectively. In two cases hydrocephalus was absent; in both of them the CSF escaped freely through a fistula in the membrane covering the spinal defect. In the remaining infants the hydrocephalus was com-municating, but the authors estimated that a blockage, even though incomplete, occurred at the foramen magnum. In fact, in two cases in which a suspension of India ink had been introduced into the lateral ventricles just before death, they noticed a profuse deposit of pigment throughout the ventricular system and the subarachnoid spaces of the spinal canal below the level of the Chiari malforma-tion, whereas above this level the leptomeninges appeared completely devoid of dye or else they contained only a small amount of it. As Dandy and Blackfan reported that three-fourths to four-fifths of CSF was absorbed at the level of the surface of the brain, Russell and Donald concluded that the partial occlusion at the foramen magnum resulted in a "damming back of CSF in the ventricular sys-tem," with a consequent ventricular dilation. The cause of the occlusion at the foramen magnum was seen as the plugging of the upper cervical spinal canal by the malformed hindbrain which was "likely to hinder any upward flow of fluid into the subarachnoid channels within the posterior fossa, into which it normally passes on its way to escape through the cranial arachnoid villi."

Three years later, Penfield and Coburn[50] performed a decompressive surgical procedure on the posterior cranial fossa in a patient with a meningomyelocele and Chiari type II malformation. They interpreted the caudal migration of the brainstem and cerebellum as well as the secondary block in the CSF outflow from the IVth ventricle as the result of the traction exerted from below by the spinal cord attached to the meningomyelocele at its caudal end.

Unfortunately, Penfield and Coburn did not take into account the anatomic observations by Russell and Donald,[49] which could possibly have prevented them from propounding their hypothesis. The latter authors, in fact, had noticed in their autopsy specimens of Chiari malformation that "the cervical roots always run in a cephalic direction . . . their cephalic direction decreases as successive segments are examined until, in the upper thoracic region, they are either horizontally or caudally inclined" (that is just opposite of what one would expect from a tethering effect occurring first at the lumbar level). However, the Penfield and Coburn explanation of the Chiari malformation was supported by other

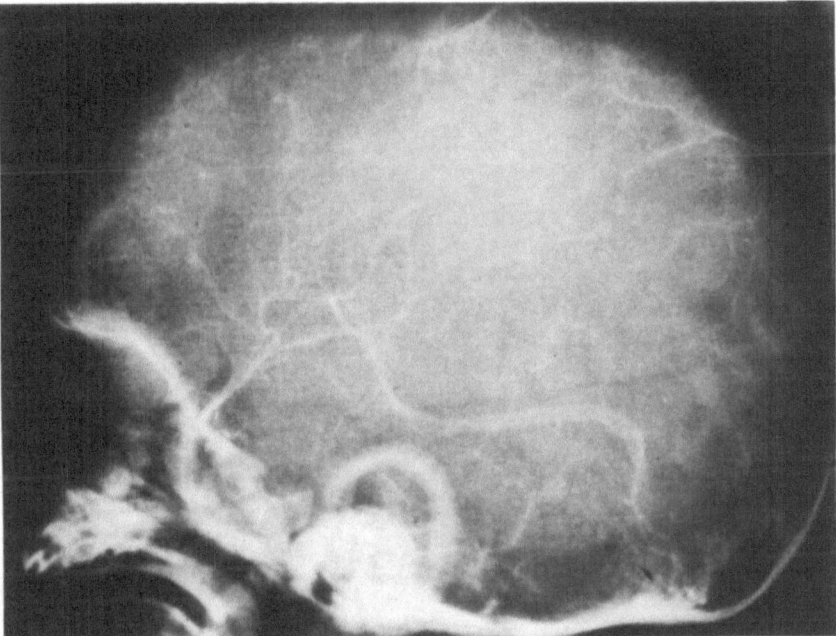

Figure 3.3. Cerebral angiography in a child with Chiari type II malformation showing the characteristically low positioned and elongated great vein of Galen.

authors,[17,51,52] so that it rapidly received wide acceptance. The "traction" theory was then discredited by the demonstration of Chiari malformations in patients without a tethered cord,[53] or in animals in which the bony vertebral canal only minimally outstripped the cord in growth[33] as well as by the observation of the failure in obtaining the caudal dislocation of the brainstem and cerebellar structures in rat and opossum fetuses, by fixing the conus medullaris to the vertebrae.[54] Other examples of physiopathogenic theories aimed at explaining the hydrocephalus accompanying Chiari malformations by the presence of a blockage in the CSF circulation can be found in articles published at the beginning of the second half of this century. These theories, however, were given little attention. Typical is the case of the hypothesis by Megison and co-workers,[55] who identified the anatomo-functional obstacle to the CSF circulation in the venous anomalies occurring in infants with meningomyelocele, such as the elongated great vein of Galen (Fig. 3.3), the shortened straight sinus, and the low positioned transverse sinuses (Fig. 3.4).

"Maldevelopmental" Theories

In the 1950s, several theories were proposed, all of them aimed at identifying a unique pathogenetic mechanism accounting for both the spinal cord and hindbrain anomalies.[56-58] In particular, in 1952 Patten[58] postulated that a noxious

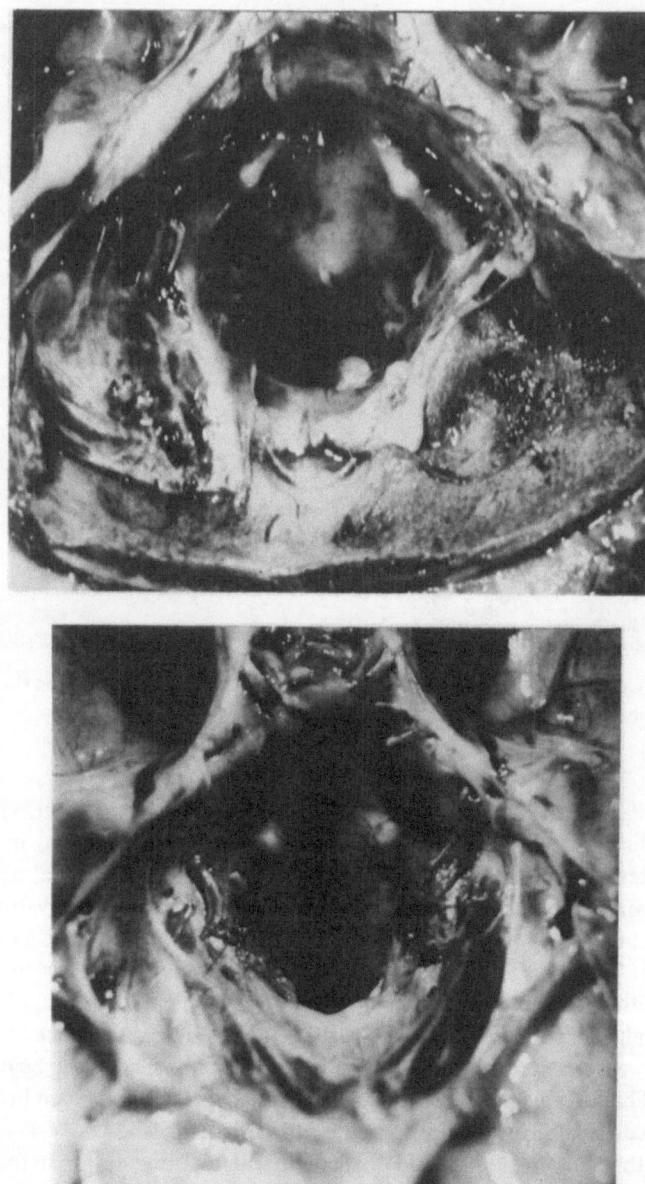

Figure 3.4. Autopsy findings in two cases of Chiari type II malformation: note the hypoplastic cranial fossa and the low positioned venous sinuses.

effect on developing nervous tissue was responsible for its abnormal overgrowth, with a secondary failure of the neural groove to close and subsequent compression of the overdeveloped cerebral and brainstem structures within a relatively small posterior cranial fossa.

The limit of the "overgrowth" theory had to be unequivocally demonstrated when anatomic observations actually showed the total volume of the nervous tissue, including the spinal cord, to be inferior to the norm in infants with meningomyelocele.[24] Also, experimental observations in normal rats and in embryos with trypan blue-induced spinal bifida failed to point out any statistically significant differences between the normal and malformed animals.[59]

In 1958, Daniel and Strich,[56] in reporting on 26 cases of Chiari type II malformation and meningomyelocele, stressed the fact that the anomalies were not confined to the spinal cord and hindbrain, but involved the whole neuraxis and its coverings as well. In particular, the authors drew attention to the bony and dural abnormalities of the posterior cranial fossa, the large foramen magnum, the calvarial changes, the frequent association with hydromyelia and syringomyelia, and the possible occurrence of the other nervous (e.g., double spinal cord) and extranervous (e.g., absence of kidneys) anomalies. Daniel and Strich were particularly impressed by the elongation of the brainstem—especially of the medulla oblongata and IVth ventricle—which, in some of their cases, was twice as long as normal. They interpreted the finding as the result of the failure in formation of the pontine flexure (which, at the 6th week of fetal life, accounts for the shortening of the hindbrain and for the IVth ventricle taking on its characteristic rhomboid shape). In the authors' opinion the excessively long hindbrain could also be responsible for the constant presence of the kink in the lower part of the medulla oblongata, overriding the upper part of the cervical cord. In fact, Daniel and Strich concluded that it was not possible to explain "the S-bend of the lower medulla, the telescoping of the cervical cord, and the wrapping of the cerebellum around the brainstem . . . by traction from a fixed cord or by pressure due to hydrocephalus," but that these anomalies could "only be accounted for by the abnormal growth of the cerebellum and brainstem very early in life."

The "maldevelopmental" theories received significant support in recent years, when several experimental studies were carried out focused on the possibility that Chiari type II malformation accompanying neural tube defects could depend on an alteration of the neural tube/axial skeleton relationship, or on a degradation of the embryonic extracellular matrix.[60-62]

In 1981, Marin-Padilla and Marin-Padilla[63] postulated, for example, that the Chiari malformation in animals with spina bifida experimentally induced by administering vitamin A orally was due to a mesodermal insufficiency resulting in an abnormally short posterior cranial fossa. The authors were convinced that the decrease in size of the posterior cranial fossa would in turn be responsible for a disturbance in the CSF circulation and the secondary hydrocephalus.

Also Richardson[64] believed that the malformed basi-occipital bone limiting the development of the CSF spaces and nervous structures contained within the posterior cranial fossa would account for the hydrocephalus that characterizes a strain of recessively inherited hydrocephalic mice. These animals show an overall deficit in glycosaminoglycans (GAGs), an important component of the extracellular matrix necessary for the normal process of chondrification.

In 1985, Di Rocco and Rende[65] obtained the characteristic features of Chiari type II malformation in rat fetuses, with and without spina bifida, born from mothers who had been given trypan blue subcutaneously once daily from the 7th to the 9th day of pregnancy. Besides the usual explanation of an incompetent posterior cranial fossa accounting for a mechanical distortion and compression of the CSF pathways with secondary hydrocephalus, the latter authors hypothesized that the hydrocephalus accompanying the Chiari type II malformation in their animals (Fig. 3.5) could depend on the same GAGs alteration responsible for the nervous and osseous abnormalities. They noted, in fact, that the malformed fetuses with hydrocephalus showed a characteristic lack in GAGs on the ependymal ventricular surface when compared with the normal animals; at this level, the GAGs are actually involved in the exchange of fluids between the cerebral ventricles and the parenchymal cerebral tissue.[66]

Clinical Features

Clinical signs and symptoms of both Chiari type I and type II malformations are regarded as being related to three main factors: (1) the impact of nervous and vascular structures at the foramen magnum and within the upper cervical canal which predisposes the subject to mechanic, ischemic, and hemorrhagic lesions; (2) the concomitant hydrocephalus; and (3) the frequently associated syringomyelia and hydromyelia. However, the clinical manifestations of Chiari type I and type II malformations differ considerably even with regard to period of life in which they usually become manifest.

Chiari Type I Malformation

It is typical of Chiari type I malformation to become symptomatic in adulthood, though it may be clinically apparent in adolescents and older teenagers as well. Symptomatic Chiari type I malformation in infancy is exceptionally rare. Headache and pain, the latter almost exclusively confined to the neck, shoulder, or proximal arm, are the most common presenting symptoms.[22,29,67] Though in

▶

Figure 3.5. Trypan blue-induced Chiari type II malformation and hydrocephalus in rat fetuses. *A:* Macroscopic sagittal section showing the hydrocephalus, the caudal displacement of the hindbrain, and the abnormal spheno-basilar and basi-occipital angle. *B, C:* The lateral cerebral ventricles are enlarged and the diameter of the axis is increased in a rat fetus with Chiari type II malformation (*left*) as compared with a normal animal (*right*). *D:* Glycosaminoglycans in the malformed fetus (*left*) do not form the characteristic dark film present in the normal animal (*right*) on the ependymal ventricular wall (*arrows*).

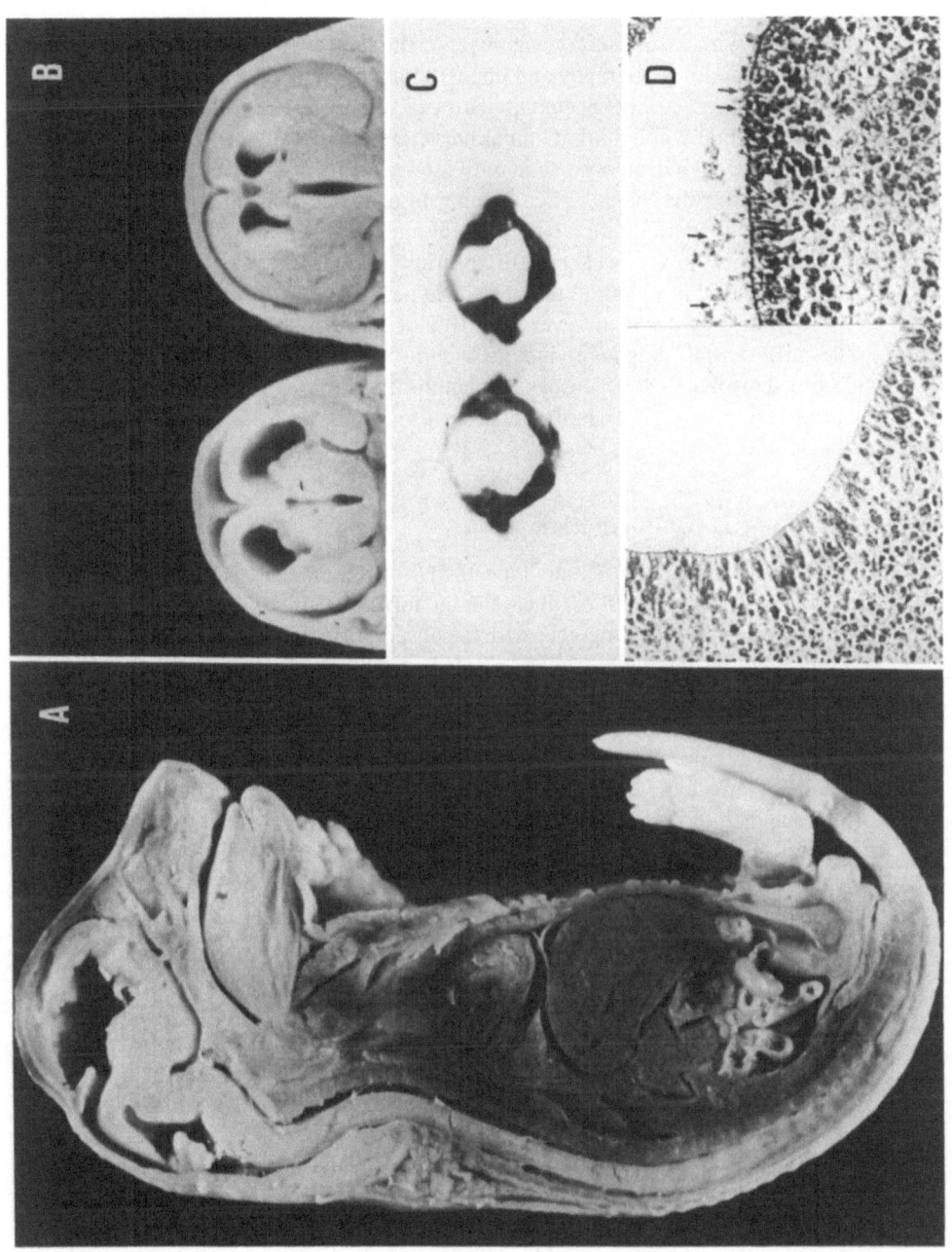

most instances there is no dermatomal distribution, the pain may be dermatomal in cases with an associated syringomyelia; if this is so, the symptom usually carries a poor prognosis.[67]

In patients with associated syringomyelia, the pain may be distributed to the face, mimicking for topography and intensity that of trigeminal neuralgia.[68] The headache is almost always occipital, with exacerbations due to straining, exertion, and especially coughing. Cranial nerve deficits usually correspond to the progress of the cavitation process in untreated subjects with syringobulbia; they cause dysarthria; dysphagia, often leading to aspiration pneumonia; or diplopia.[29,44,69] Motor deficits may be unilateral and localized in the upper arm; in some patients, however, weakness or spasticity of the legs may be prominent. Signs of increased intracranial pressure or hypertensive hydrocephalus are relatively rare, as they occur in fewer than 10% of symptomatic subjects.[34]

The differential diagnosis includes demyelinating diseases in cases of widespread involvement of sensorial and motor functions, and intermittent clinical progression as well as motor neuron diseases in cases with predominant motor deficits.[34]

Chiari Type II Malformation

Clinical manifestations of Chiari type II malformation most commonly occur already in early infancy, almost always in the form of respiratory and swallowing disturbances. Such a fact, together with the observation that the majority of cases is represented by infants born with meningomyelocele, has suggested that the symptomatology is related to congenital anomalies of the brainstem and cerebellar and upper spinal cord structures.[69] In 1986, Gilbert and co-workers,[70] on the grounds of a detailed neuropathologic investigation of 25 children who had died with meningomyelocele, demonstrated indeed a large spectrum of cerebral malformations including hypoplasia or aplasia of cranial nerve nuclei, disorders of the migration of cortical neurons, and cerebellar dysplasia. In particular, marked hypoplasia or aplasia of cranial nerves, especially the hypoglossal and dorsal vagal nuclei, was found in about a fifth of the cases, an incidence similar to that previously reported by other authors.[69,71]

However, as infants with meningomyelocele and Chiari type II malformation do not usually exhibit signs of brainstem, cerebellar, or upper spinal cord dysfunction in the first few days after birth, a causative role in the appearance of clinical symptomatology of other events, such as development of hydrocephalus or the scarring processes due to caseous or infectious meningitis, has been suggested.[72,73]

Further support for this hypothesis has been provided by the observations on the regression of clinical manifestations following surgical procedures for posterior cranial fossa and upper cervical canal decompression.[74-76] In fact, hydrocephalus is almost invariably present and signs of increased intracranial pressure are common in infants with symptomatic Chiari type II malformation, though the syndrome may develop also in subjects whose hydrocephalus has been treated since birth.

The percentage of infants with meningomyelocele and Chiari type II malformation who becomes symptomatic ranges from 5 to 34% of cases; there is an obvious age-related incidence as infants appear to develop symptoms and signs more frequently than toddlers, children, and teenagers.[11,73] Although in a few cases symptoms, especially respiratory and swallowing disturbances, may progress until reaching life-threatening condition or death, in most symptomatic infants the neurologic deficits appear to stabilize or actually improve over time, starting at the end of the first year of life. The anatomic location of the spinal defects seems not to have any significant effect on the frequency with which patients with Chiari type II malformation become symptomatic; also, the favoring role of CNS infections has not been confirmed in recent studies.[11,77]

Respiratory disturbances are the most common symptoms in infants, about 70 to 90% of the cases. They are introduced in the majority of subjects by episodes of stridor, which are easily elicited by the infant's anger, feeding, or agitation. Generally transient and disappearing when the subject is quiet, stridor may, however, evolve into apneic spells or respiratory distress, and, rarely, into periods of prolonged apnea. During apneic spells or episodes of persisting apnea, cyanosis may develop, with possible anoxic seizures; bradycardia is frequent. On such occasion death may ensue. In some patients the severity of respiratory disturbances may be enhanced by the presence of spinal alterations, such as scoliosis and kyphosis.

In about a third of the subjects with respiratory disturbances, it is possible to demonstrate a complete abductor vocal cord paralysis through laryngoscopy; in a minority of patients, the paralysis is unilateral or only a paresis of the vocal cords can be detected.[11,71] In most cases the gag reflex is decreased or even abolished.

Swallowing disturbances may be observed in a large number of infants, with reported figures ranging from 25% to 75% of cases. In most infants, they are clinically apparent because of episodes of regurgitation ("milk in the nostril") and failure to thrive. Episodes of bronchial aspiration, often leading to radiologically evident pneumonia, are frequently encountered. Pharyngo-esophageal dysfunction, incorrectly defined as "achalasia," may be radiologically demonstrated in a significant percentage of patients. Deficits of the other cranial nerves, excluding those controlling respiration and swallowing, are rare even though cranial nerves VI, VII, and even V occasionally can be involved.[37]

Pyramidal tract deficits in this age group are uncommon. When present, they are confined to the upper limbs and clinically evident through weakness, paresis, or increased muscle tone and hyperreflexia. Nystagmus is a relatively frequent early sign, but it usually is not associated with ataxia and cerebellar dysmetria. Finally, a significant percentage of infants show opisthotonos, which may vary from simple retroflexion of the head to severe arching of the spine.

Although most infants with clinical manifestations of Chiari type II malformation actually survive, there is not a recognized degree of severity or a set pattern of evolution apt to anticipate the natural history of the condition in any single subject. Indeed, in about a third of the patients the symptomatology may deteriorate dramatically in a few days with cardiorespiratory arrest, vocal cord paralysis requiring tracheostomy, severe aspiration pneumonia, or seizure disorder.[75] After the first year of life, however, brainstem dysfunction is relatively rare and its evolution is generally considerably less acute. Thus, clinical manifestations in childhood are more commonly characterized by nystagmus, either horizontal or vertical, weakness or spasticity of the upper limbs, and appendicular or trunkal ataxia. Mirror movements of the arms have also been described.[74]

Neuroimaging

Prior to the advent of the current techniques of neuroimaging, such as computed tomography (CT) and magnetic resonance imaging (MRI), the radiologic diagnosis of Chiari malformation was mainly based on the standard x-ray examination supplemented by contrast x-ray studies, namely ventriculography, pneumoencephalography, myelography, and more rarely, cerebral angiography. From among the above-mentioned diagnostic procedures, only the plain x-ray films are still currently used in the preliminary phases of the diagnostic work-up. This type of investigation allows the demonstration of an abnormality of the skull or the spine in only a minority (fewer than 10%) of patients with Chiari type I malformation, but reveals typical anomalies in a large proportion of subjects with Chiari type II malformation. The anomalies include enlargement of the neurocranium in cases with associated hypertensive hydrocephalus, craniolacuniae

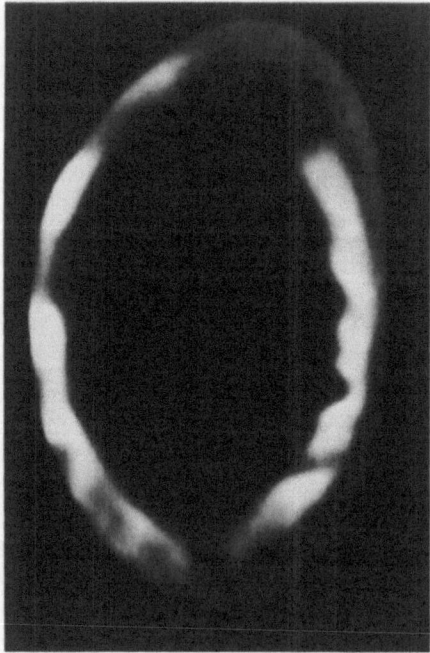

Figure 3.6. CT scan examination in a newborn with Chiari type II malformation revealing the typical craniolacuniae.

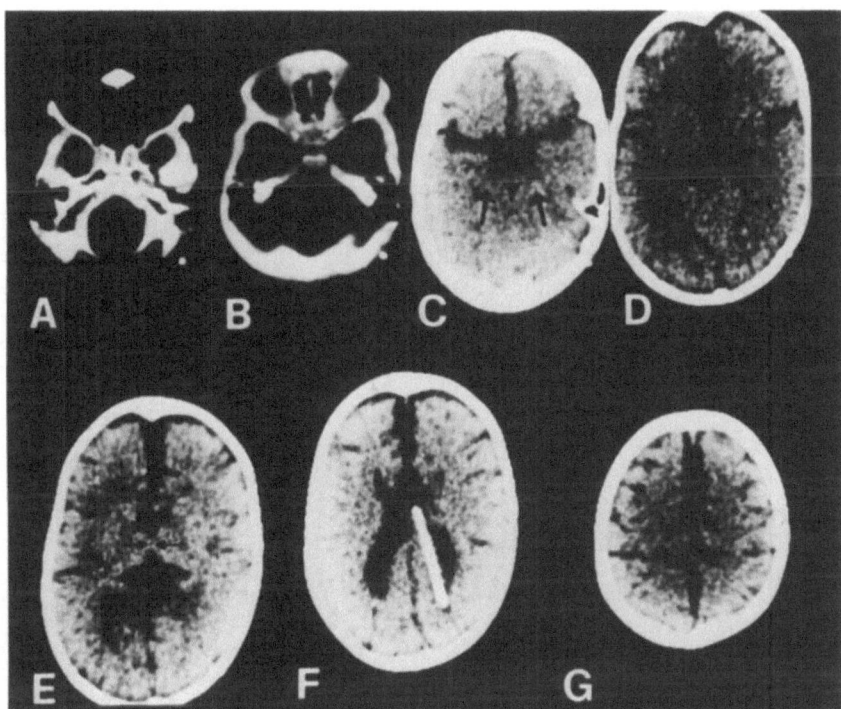

Figure 3.7. CT scan findings in Chiari type II malformation (status post CSF-shunting). A: Enlarged foramen magnum. B: Posterior scalloping of the petrous bone. C: Mesencephalic beaking and "triple peak" appearance (according to Naidich, 1983). D: Towering cerebellum. E: Thick massa intermedia (*arrows*). F: Shunted lateral cerebral ventricles, in which the occipital disproportion is maintained. G: large interhemispheric fissure.

(Luckenschädel) in about 85% of infants with meningomyelocele,[78] an almost constant reduction in size of the posterior fossa, erosion of the postero-medial aspect of the petrous pyramids,[79] enlargement in diameter of the foramen magnum and atlas,[79] and occasionally platybasia, basilar impression, assimilation of the atlas, Klippel–Feil deformity, and malformations of the vertebrae.

Most of the anomalies detected through plain x-ray films may be demonstrated also by using the CT scan examination. For example, the craniolacuniae are easily documented as localized areas of pits and thinnings, especially evident in the upper parietal region, by using the bone window (Fig. 3.6). The lesions may involve both the inner and the outer layers of the skull, even though they may be better observed on the interior aspect of the calvarium. Occurring in the large majority of infants with meningomyelocele at birth, craniolacuniae tend to disappear by 6 months of age, whether or not the associated hydrocephalus is controlled.[30] The enlarged foramen magnum can also be well demonstrated using an appropriate plane of scanning (Fig. 3.7).

Some of the findings provided by plain x-ray films are better evaluated with CT; such is the case, for instance, of the erosion of the postero-medial aspects of the petrous pyramids, which can be noticed in about two-thirds of the patients with meningomyelocele in the submento-vertex radiographs. The findings (Fig. 3.7) have been explained as the result of the pressure exerted by the growing cerebellum on the petrous bone, which induces a posterior scalloping. The severity of the lesion may increase with the age of the patient, but the petrous ridges and the jugular tubercle are constantly spared; the acoustic canal is shortened.[30] The great advantage provided by the CT scan is, however, to be identified in the possibility of demonstrating not only the bone abnormalities but also the anomalies of the dura mater, the parenchymal cerebral and cerebellar tissue, and the CSF spaces, all with only one examination.[80,81]

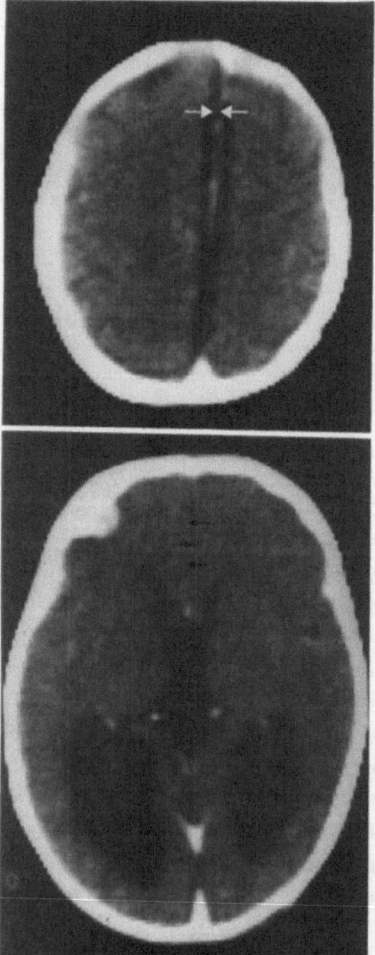

Figure 3.8. CT scan findings in Chiari type II malformation: note the fenestration of the cerebral falx (*white arrows*) and resulting interdigitation of the mesial surface of the frontal lobes (*black arrows*).

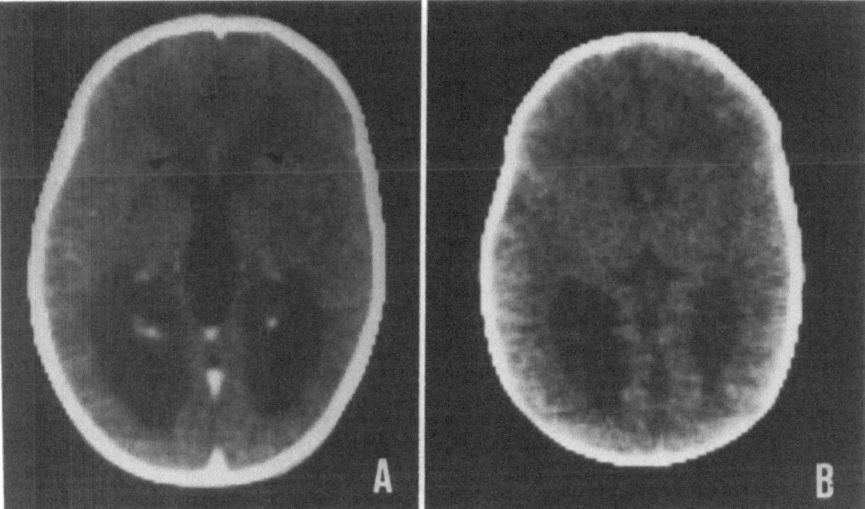

Figure 3.9. CT scan findings in two cases of Chiari type II malformation: note the characteristic dilation of the occipital horns of the lateral cerebral ventricles, the impression exerted by the caudate nucl₍ ₌ on the ventricular contours at the level of the frontal horns (*arrowheads*), and the interdigitations of the frontal lobes (*arrows*) due to the hypoplasia of the cerebral falx. The IIIrd ventricle is dilated in A, and scarcely recognizable in B, because of the hyperplastic massa intermedia.

The identifiable dural anomalies consist of focal deficits in development of the falx and in the hypoplasia and abnormal insertion of the tentorium. Falx fenestration (Figs. 3.8 and 3.9) appears as localized interruptions in the linear falx blush on axial section contrast-enhanced CT; interdigitation of the apposed mesial surfaces of the cerebral hemispheres through the fenestrated or hypoplastic falx modify the linear image of the interhemispheric fissure; tentorial hypoplasia is revealed by the abnormal distance between the tentorial leaves and its low insertion may be appreciated on the axial scans (Fig. 3.10).

The cerebral and cerebellar abnormalities, typical of Chiari type II malformation, such as the abnormal architecture of the cerebral cortex, the large massa intermedia, and the deformed midbrain and cerebellum, are appropriately identified by the CT scan and MRI. To these abnormalities should be added those dynamic modifications induced by the restricted nervous growth within a tiny posterior cranial fossa and abnormally enlarged tentorial incisura, as well as those modifications depending on the mechanical effects of an enlarged supratentorial ventricular system under pressure in untreated subjects, or secondary to the reduction in ventricular volume and pressure in shunted patients. As the presence and severity of the parenchymal changes vary with time from patient to patient, and also in the single subject, the CT and MRI diagnoses of Chiari type II malformation should not be based on the identification of a single specific pathognomonic change, but rather on the combination of several findings.

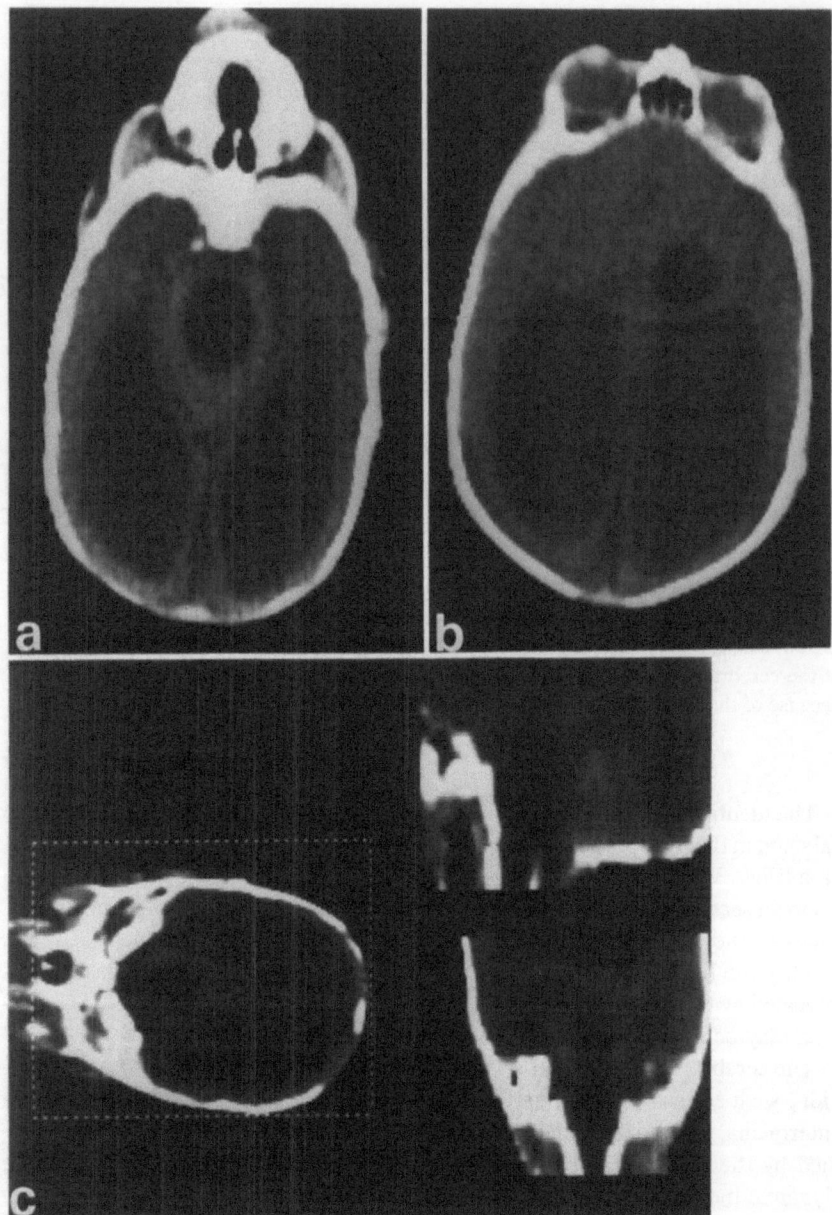

Figure 3.10. CT scan findings in a child with Chiari type II malformation and syringobulbia. Note the following. a: The cystic cavity in the brainstem, the hypoplastic posterior cranial fossa, the caudal dislocation of the markedly dilated occipital horns of the lateral cerebral ventricles, the enlarged interhemispheric occipital fissure. b: Cyst in the right deep nuclei region. The multiplanar image reformation (c) demonstrates the cystic cavity within the brainstem and its possible communication with the IIIrd ventricle as well as the cyst in the basal nuclei; also evident is the low insertion of the tentorium. [From

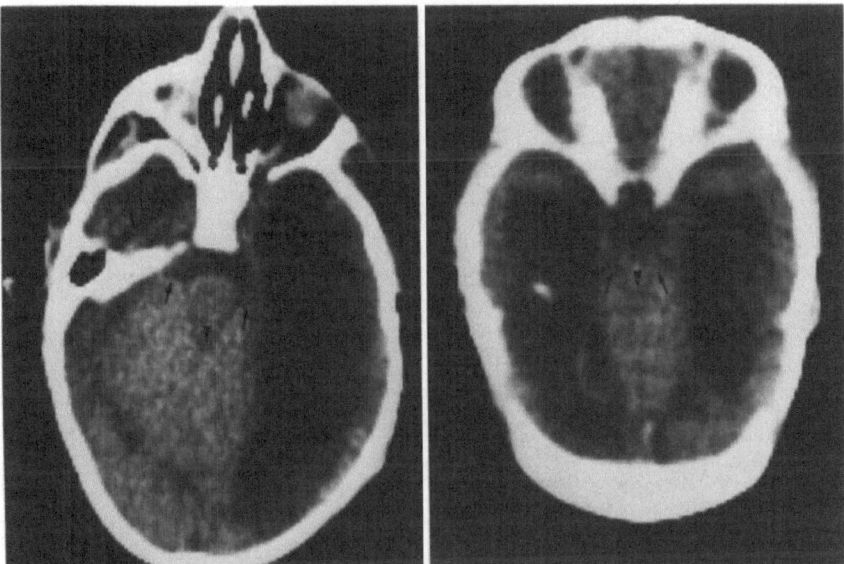

Figure 3.11. CT scan findings in two cases of Chiari type II malformation: note the mesencephalic beaking (*arrowheads*) and the prolongation of the cerebellar lobes (*arrows*) in the cisterns of the cerebellar-pontine angle.

The most interesting identifiable modifications occur at the level of the incisura. A mesencephalic beaking, due to the fusion of the quadrigeminal plate into a unique beak-like structure, is detected in nearly all subjects (Fig. 3.7).[80] The cerebellum becomes invaginated to accommodate the posteriorly "beaked" midbrain; the anterior portions of the cerebellar lobes grow forward between the brainstem and the free edges of the tentorium to wrap the brainstem itself around its lateral surfaces, partially filling out the ponto-cerebellar cisterns (Fig. 3.11). On axial scans (Fig. 3.11) the prolongation of the cerebellar lobes into the cerebello-pontine angle cisterns together with the beaked image of the midbrain at the midline form a "triple-beaked" image, which constitutes one of the most typical findings of the condition.[80] In more than half the cases the CT, or MRI examination, demonstrate a cerebellar upgrowth through the enlarged tentorial incisura, a movement that is enhanced in shunted patients (Fig. 3.7D). The resulting "towering" cerebellum[69] appears to elevate and displace the atria of the lateral cerebral ventricles laterally, acting as a cerebellar pseudotumor.

A second important region for the diagnosis of Chiari type II malformation is that of the cranio-vertebral junction. Though the CT scan may allow the identification of the cerebellar tonsils, the IVth ventricle and the eventual kink of the medulla oblongata (after opacification of the subarachnoid space by water-

C. Colosimo Jr., A. Puca, C. Di Rocco: "Valutazione neuroradiologica dell'idrocefalo e delle alterazioni cranio-encefaliche associate al mielomeningocele." In: C. Di Rocco, M. Caldarelli (Eds) "Mielomeningocele," Casa del Libro, Roma 1983, with permission.]

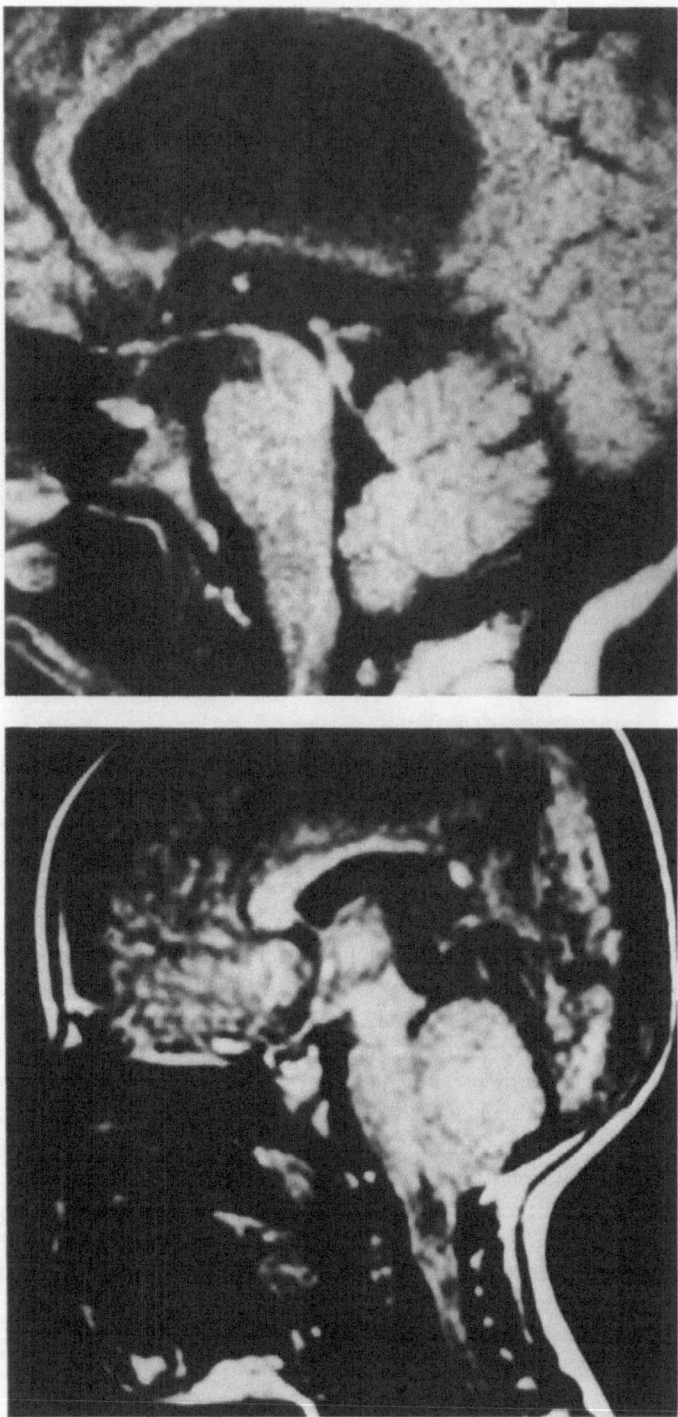

Figure 3.12.

Figure 3.13. Two-dimensional saturation recovery image in the sagittal plane of the cranio-vertebral junction in a child with Chiari type II malformation. Note the elongated IVth ventricle and the herniation of the cerebellar tonsils.

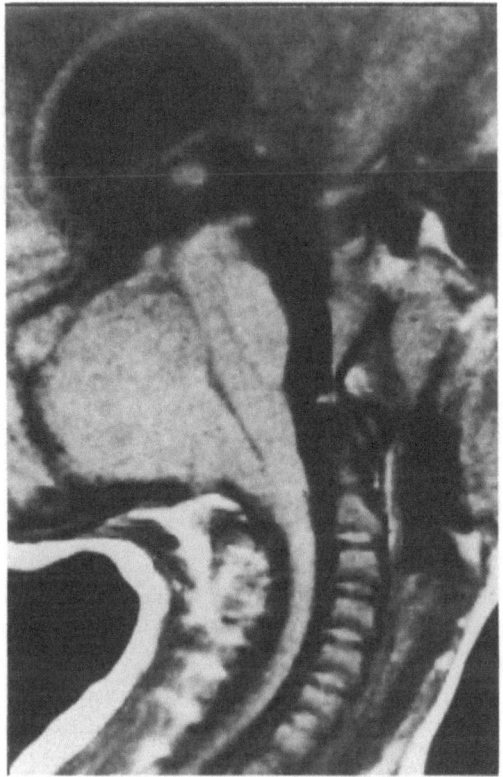

soluble contrast medium, introduced generally through a lumbar puncture), the brainstem–spinal cord passage is better investigated using MRI.[82,83] MRI allows, in fact, the accurate documentation of the different degrees of caudal displacement of the brainstem, IVth ventricle, and cerebellar structures; the visualization of the cerebellar peg; and, when present, the identification of cavitations within the brainstem and spinal cord (Figs. 3.12 and 3.13).

The modifications of the cerebral ventricles and peripheral CSF spaces may be evaluated by both CT and MRI techniques; again, the use of CT often requires the intrathecal injection of a water-soluble contrast medium. The lateral cerebral ventricles are generally enlarged, with a dilation that is characteristically predominant at the level of the atria and occipital horns (Figs. 3.8, 3.9, and 3.14).

◄

Figure 3.12. Two-dimensional saturation recovery image in the sagittal plane of the cranio-vertebral junction in a patient with occult chronic triventricular hydrocephalus (*top*) and in a patient with Chiari type I malformation (*bottom*). Note: (*top*) the marked dilation of the lateral and third cerebral ventricles as well as the stenosis of the aqueduct; the brainstem, the IVth ventricle and the cerebellum maintain their normal position, in spite of the supratentorial hypertensive hydrocephalus; (*bottom*) caudal displacement of the deformed cerebellum.

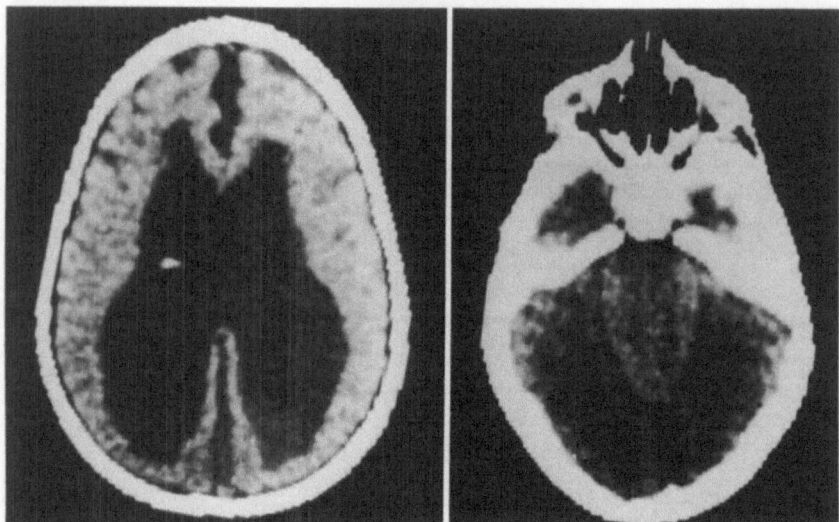

Figure 3.14. CT findings in Chiari type II malformation (status post-CSF-shunting): note the dilation of the lateral cerebral ventricles, particularly evident at the level of the occipital horns. The frontal horns maintain a sharp configuration. The cerebellum is displaced upward (towering cerebellum).

The enlarged occipital horns may be seen to lie within the posterior cranial fossa, as a result of the hypoplastic tentorium (Fig. 3.10). The basal nuclei may induce a significant impression of the ventricular contour at the frontal horns which usually maintain their relatively sharp antero-superior angles (Fig. 3.9). The IIIrd ventricle may also enlarge; however, its dilation is often opposed by a hyperplastic massa intermedia (Fig. 3.7). The IVth ventricle is elongated and displaced craniocaudally, its transverse diameter is narrowed, and the lateral recesses are absent. Finally, the cisternal spaces of the region appear deeply compressed or scarcely recognizable because of the downward displacement of the spinal cord, medulla oblongata, IVth ventricle, vermis, and cerebellar tonsils, which form an overlapping series of hernias. The resulting mass is compressed by the posterior rim of the foramen magnum and by the posterior arch of the atlas, in spite of the relatively large size of these latter structures. The central canal may appear dilated, especially in unshunted subjects; true syringomyelia may be evident in about one-fifth of the cases.

Treatment

At the present time there is no medical therapy for Chiari malformations, though some palliative supportive measures may be adopted according to the patient's need. These are aimed at reducing the intracranial pressure, favoring the respiratory function, and in cases with epilepsy at controlling seizures. Therefore, the current treatment of subjects with symptomatic Chiari type I and type II malformations is essentially represented by surgical procedures directed either at reducing the increased intracranial pressure, or decompressing the nervous structures of the posterior cranial fossa and upper cervical spinal canal.

The surgical indication in Chiari malformations remains a very controversial topic in pediatric neurosurgery, as it is often doubtful as to whether the operation will change the outcome of the condition. In fact, mortality rates generally vary directly with the severity of the neurologic symptoms and the rapidity of clinical deterioration. In a significant percentage of cases, death may even ensue some months or years after an apparently successful decompressive operation. As the large majority of subjects with the anatomopathologic features of a Chiari malformation may long remain asymptomatic,[11] *the mere radiologic diagnosis of the condition is not regarded as a sufficient indicator for surgical treatment.* Therefore, the therapeutic decisions rest on the clinical signs and symptoms. Unfortunately, however, there are no recognized patterns of clinical manifestations unequivocally leading to a surgical indication. Consequently, the operative decision is mainly based on the personal experience of the surgeon and his attitude toward the disease.

Thus, the significant differences in the incidence of patients with Chiari malformation requiring decompressive procedures, as reported in literature, may be readily understood.[11,28,75] Clinical manifestations prompting surgical treatment are different in infants and older children. Swallowing difficulty, vocal cord paralysis, and respiratory disturbances with apnea are the most typical symptoms regarded as indicators for surgical therapy in infants.[28,73,75] However, to make a decision in favor of surgery, these symptoms should show a clear tendency to becoming stabilized.[28,75] For some authors, a failure to thrive due either to early respiratory and swallowing dysfunction, progressive spasticity, or upper-extremity weakness should also be regarded as an indication for surgery.[76]

In children, the clinical manifestations that are considered to indicate the need for surgical treatment include cerebellar syndromes, repeated attacks of torticollis, lower cranial nerve dysfunction, progressive hypotonia, and pyramidal signs.[28] As several patients with Chiari type I and type II malformations show clinical evidence of hydrocephalus and intracranial hypertension, there is general agreement that in these circumstances the treatment should be first to normalize the intracranial pressure. Indeed, the prompt insertion of a ventricular valve-regulated shunt is sufficient to reverse the clinical symptoms in a considerable percentage of these subjects.[11,28,34,73,75,84,85]

Nevertheless, some patients with symptomatic Chiari malformation do not have hydrocephalus or have an apparently satisfactorily functioning CSF shunt. In these cases, the procedure of choice is a posterior fossa decompression with removal of the occipital squama, and a laminectomy of the first cervical vertebra. The rationale of the procedure is to decompress the nervous structures within the posterior cranial fossa and upper cervical canal, as the damage this compression causes is thought to account for the clinical manifestations. Indeed, recent hemorrhages, as well as organized infarcts involving the cerebellum, pons, medulla oblongata, and spinal cord, were demonstrated in all the 14 autopsy cases reported by Pasozomenos and Roessman in 1981.[76] The findings have been explained as depending on a disturbed angioarchitecture of the brainstem, especially evident at the lower medulla which is supplied by arterioles branching at sharp angles from the vertebral arteries, and running caudally. These small caliber arteriolar branches feeding the brainstem would become elongated and eventually rupture because of the progressive extension of the herniated brainstem.

Shrunken and atrophic neurons in the nuclei ambiguous, hypoglossal, gracilis, and cuneatus, observed at autopsy in patients with Chiari type II malformation, have been interpreted to be the result of damage to the cranial nerves.[69,86] However, it has also been hypothesized that these pathologic changes may be secondary to brainstem compression and occur because of pathologic processes that take place after birth.[75]

Basically, the procedure for posterior fossa decompression in Chiari malformation includes a suboccipital craniectomy and a cervical laminectomy, as proposed by D'Errico in 1939.[87] However, controversy still exists among experts on several points such as the extent to which the occipital bone should be removed, and the laminectomy carried out, the opening of the underlying dura mater, and the additional manipulation that may be required to remove portions of the herniated cerebellar structures to establish the free flow of CSF from the IVth ventricle. In neonates and infants, for example, the removal of the occipital squama has been felt to be unnecessary, because of the large diameter of the foramen magnum and the evidence of a brainstem compression confined exclusively to a level below the rim of the foramen magnum itself.[74] In the same population, even the opening of the dura mater above the foramen magnum has been discouraged, because of the risk of disastrous hemorrhage due to the presence of the transverse, occipital, and marginal sinuses packed together in the dura of a hypoplastic posterior fossa.[75]

Although some authors believe that the bone removal without opening the dura mater ensures a sufficient decompression, others advocate not only the dural opening, but also the utilization of a dural graft to increase relatively the space available for the expansion and eventual growth of the underlying nervous structures.[71,75,76]

Finally, the necessity to reestablish the CSF circulation at the level of the exit foramina of the IVth ventricle has been evaluated differently in cases of Chiari type I malformation, where both the decompression of the cerebellar tonsils and the outflow of CSF from the IVth ventricle have been indicated as objectives of surgical treatment,[36] and in subjects with Chiari type II malformation, in which surgery aims only at decompressing the nervous structures by bone removal and dural grafting.[88] The removal of the occipital rim is generally extended to the level of the transverse sinus with careful attention being given to the possible extremely low position of this structure in this type of pathology. The cervical laminectomy should be carried out until the caudally displaced cerebellum and

Figure 3.15. Intra-operative view in Chiari type II malformation: note the transverse dural band (*arrowheads*) that indentates the underlying nervous structures at the level of C1.

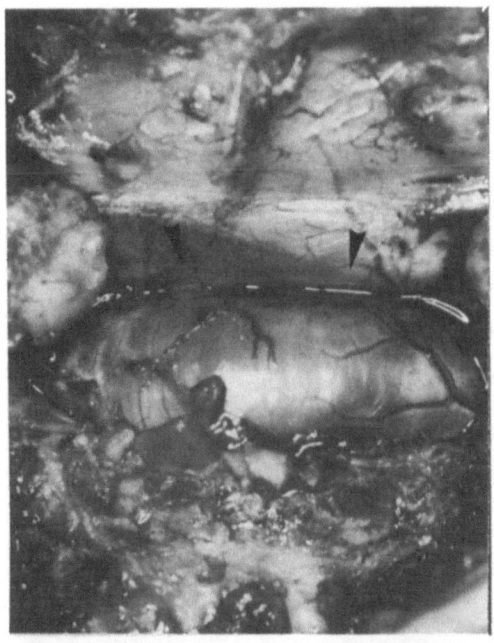

brainstem are completely exposed. In about half the cases, both in Chiari type I and type II malformations, a transverse dural band (Fig. 3.15) is found which constricts, and eventually indentates the underlying nervous structures.[68,75] The release of this dural band is followed by the immediate expansion of the dural sac. In neonates and infants, the opening of the dura may be a critical step in the surgical procedure because of the low position of the venous sinuses, and the presence of an abundant vascular network between the dural leaves, which might become the source of a significant blood loss. A hemorrhage may be prevented to a certain extent by presuturing the dura in the direction of the incision, or applying temporary clips to the membrane before extending the incision itself.

The opening of the dura may also be difficult in older children because of dense subarachnoid adhesions, extending from the nervous structures to the inner face of the dura mater. On the other hand, in some cases the separation of the dura from the underlying cerebellar, brainstem, and spinal cord structures appears relatively easier to perform, but the herniated nervous structures appear intimately packed together in nearly all subjects (Fig. 3.16). By laterally displacing the brainstem, the lower cranial and first cervical nerves can be seen to run abnormally upwards (Fig. 3.17). The lowermost extension of the cerebellar tail or medullary kink varies in different patients, from the C1 to T1 levels.[75,76] The herniated cerebellar tissue usually shows obvious changes in its macroscopic appearance, due to chronic gliosis and the presence of abnormally fine vessels (Fig. 3.16). As a rule, it can be easily distinguished from the normal medullary and spinal cord structures. A direct surgical attack on the herniated cerebellar

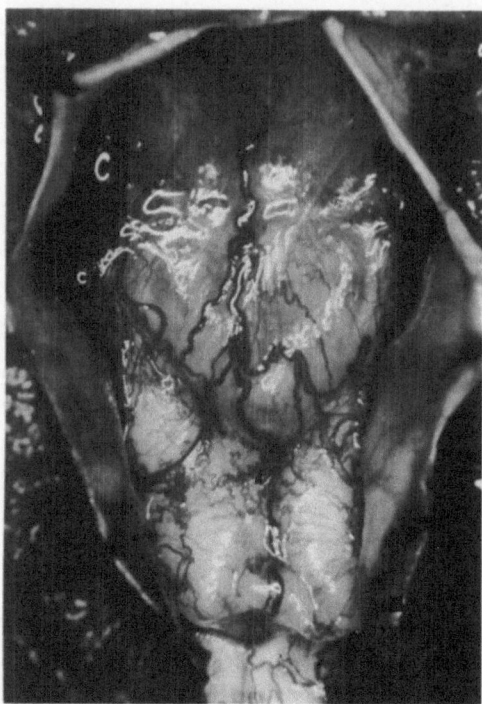

Figure 3.16. Intra-operative view in Chiari type II malformation: the small arrowhead indicates the caudal pole of the inferior cerebellar vermis; the large arrowhead corresponds to the lower level of the medullary kink.

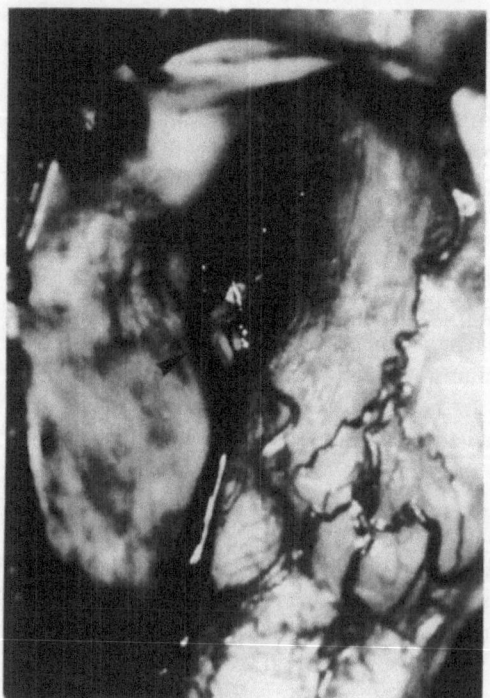

Figure 3.17. Intra-operative view in Chiari type II malformation (same case as Fig. 3.16): the lateral dislocation of the medulla oblongata allows the visualization of the C1 nerve root running upward toward its exit foramen (*arrowhead*).

tissue obstructing the CSF flow and its dissection from the posterior medullary surface was first advocated by Crosby and co-workers.[89] In fact, the subpial resection of the tonsils and the accurate lysis of the arachnoid adhesions, especially at the level of the foramen of Magendie, ensure an optimal outlet of the CSF from the ventricular system. Particular care should be taken when manipulating the herniated tissue as the dorsal displacement of the cerebellar tonsils and vermis may cause damage to the small branches of the posterior cerebellar arteries feeding the dorsal brainstem. There is such a high risk of damaging vital neural and vascular structures, even with the aid of the operating microscope, that some authors have recommended not to dissect the intradural content at all.[22]

It is worth pointing out that in difficult cases intra-operative ultrasound may constitute a useful adjunct in the localization of the IVth ventricle within the dense subarachnoid scar.[76] When the exploration and eventual partial resection of the herniated neural tissues is believed to endanger the patient, the CSF circulation from the IVth ventricle may be achieved by using a stent between this cavity and the spinal subarachnoid space through the foramen of Magendie,[34] or along the aqueduct[28] between and the IIIrd and IVth ventricles. Optional surgical maneuvers are plugging the opening of the central canal at the obex, or performing a myelotomy in case of an associated syringomyelia.[14,68]

Results

The rate with which the decompression of the posterior cranial fossa and upper cervical canal is followed by regression or stabilization of the clinical symptomatology varies greatly in the series reported in literature. In subjects with Chiari type I malformation, the surgical results are much influenced by the eventually associated syringomyelia. Whereas 70–80% of subjects with headache, simple pain in the neck, or cerebellar symptoms are actually cured or improved by the operation,[36,90] subjects with rapidly progressing neurologic deterioration or lower cranial nerve deficits due to the cavitation process of the spinal cord benefit from surgical treatment only in a third to a half of cases.[36,67] In infants with Chiari type II malformation, posterior fossa decompression carries high mortality and morbidity, even when performed by expert hands.[28,75] In the series of 45 subjects described by Park and co-workers in 1983,[75] for example, 17 infants (37.8%) died in a period ranging from 2 days to 2 years and 4 months (mean survival: 2 months) after the operation. It is worth noting that the mortality rate was 71.4% among 14 infants who had developed cardiorespiratory arrest, vocal cord paralysis, or arm weakness within 2 weeks after the onset of symptomatology, in contrast with the 22.6% mortality rate observed in the remaining 31 patients who had shown a more gradual neurologic deterioration. The current mortality rates in series including older children, and in some instances adolescents, range from 5 to 10%[50] and these are significantly lower values than those recorded in the past when deaths burdened the procedure in more than a third of the cases.[87,91]

Respiratory complications represent the major cause of death in operated patients, followed in turn by postoperative infection.[28,75] Considerably better results, however, are reported in a recently published paper,[76] suggesting the favorable role of more refined surgical technique as well as more accurate diagnostic tools, namely, preoperative MRI and intraoperative ultrasound. Surgical mortality should also be evaluated in light of the natural outcome of untreated subjects, as 71% of deaths have been observed in unoperated infants with symptomatic Chiari type II malformation.[75] Morbidity includes transient nocturnal respiratory distress[90] and persistent vomiting, especially in cases where the aqueduct is plugged at the obex,[34] as well as abrupt neurologic deterioration such as, for instance, tetraplegia, often due to excessive head flexion when the child is positioned for operation.[31]

References

1. Chiari H: Ueber Veränderungen des Kleinhirns infolge von Hydrocephalies des Grosshirns. Dtsch med Wochenschr 17:1172–1175, 1891.
2. Chiari H: Ueber Veränderungen des Kleinhirns, Pons und der Medulla Oblongata infolge von kongenitaler Hydrocephalus des Grosshirns. Denkschr Akad Wiss Wien 63:71–116, 1896.
3. Cleland J: Contribution to the study of spina bifida, encephalocele, and anencephalus. J Anat Physiol 17:257–291, 1883.
4. Lebedeff A: Ueber die Entstehung der Anencephalie und Spina bifida bei Vögel und Menschen. Virchows Arch Pathol Anat 8:263–268, 1881.
5. Förster Missbildungen des Menschen. Jena, 1861 (quoted by Cleland).
6. Ahlfeld O: Missbildungen des Menschen, Leipzig, 1882 (quoted by Cleland).
7. Arnold J: Myelocyste, Transposition von Gewebskeinem und Sympodie. Beitr Pathol Anat Allg Pathol 16:1–28, 1984.
8. Schwalbe E, Gredig M: Ueber Entwicklungsstörungen des Kleinhirns, Hirnstamms und Halsmarks bei Spina Bifida (Arnold'sche und Chiari'sche Missbildung). Beitr Pathol Anat Allg Pathol 40:132–194, 1907.
9. Barry A, Patten BM, Stewart BH: Possible factors in the development of Arnold–Chiari malformation. J Neurosurg 14:285–301, 1957.
10. Bucy PC, Lichtenstein BW: Arnold–Chiari deformity in an adult without obvious cause. J Neurosurg 2:245–250, 1945.
11. Caldarelli M, Di Rocco C, Mclone DG: Chiari type II malformation: clinical manifestations and indications for decompression. In: McLaurin B (ed): Spina Bifida, Praeger, New York, 1987, pp 174–181.
12. Emery JL, Levick RK: The movement of the brain stem and vessels around the brain stem in children with hydrocephalus and the Arnold–Chiari deformity. Dev Med Child Neurol (Suppl 11):49–60, 1966.
13. Feigin I: Arnold–Chiari malformation with associated analogous malformation of the midbrain. Neurology 6:22–31, 1956.
14. Gardner WJ, Goodall RJ: The surgical treatment of Arnold–Chiari malformation in adults. J Neurosurg 7:199–206, 1950.
15. Ingraham FD, Scott HW Jr: Spina bifida and cranium bifidum. V. The Arnold–Chiari malformation: a study of 20 cases. N Engl J Med 229:108–114, 1943.

16. Jacobs EB, Landing BH, Thomas W: Vernicomyelia. Its bearing on theories of genesis of the Arnold–Chiari complex. Am J Pathol 39:345–353, 1961.
17. Lichtenstein BW: Distant neuro-anatomic complications of spina bifida (spinal dysraphism). Hydrocephalus, Arnold–Chiari deformity, stenosis of the aqueduct of Sylvius, etc.: pathogenesis and pathology. Arch Neurol Psychiatry 47:195–214, 1942.
18. Lichtenstein BW: Atresia stenosis of the aqueduct of Sylvius, with comments on the Arnold–Chiari complex. J Neuropathol Exp Neurol 18:3–, 1959.
19. MacFarlane A, Maloney AFJ: The appearance of the aqueduct and its relationship to hydrocephalus in the Arnold–Chiari malformation. Brain 80:479–491, 1957.
20. Malis LI, Cohen I, Gross SW: Arnold–Chiari malformation. Arch Surg 63:783–798, 1951.
21. Peach B: Arnold–Chiari malformation. Morphogenesis. Arch Neurol 12:527–535, 1965.
22. Appleby A, Foster JB, Hankinson J, Hudgson P: The Chiari anomalies in adult life. Brain 91:131–139, 1968.
23. Banerji NK, Millar JHD: Chiari malformation presenting in adult life. Its relationship to syringomyelia. Brain 97:157–168, 1974.
24. Brocklehurst G: The pathogenesis of spina bifida; a study of the relationship between observation, hypothesis, and surgical incentive. Dev Med Child Neurol 13:147–, 1971.
25. Caviness VS Jr: The Chiari malformations of the posterior fossa and their relation to hydrocephalus. Dev Med Child Neurol 18:103–116, 1976.
26. Di Rocco C, Caldarelli M: Mielomeningocele. Casa del Libro Editrice, Roma, 1983, p 372.
27. Di Rocco C, Caldarelli M, Velardi F: Idrocefalo e mielomeningocele. Riv Ital Pediatr 7:109–114, 1981.
28. Lapras C, Lofti M: Surgical management of Chiari II malformation in children. Mod Prob Paediatr 18:142–145, 1977.
29. Mohr PD, Strang FA, Sambrook MA, et al.: The clinical and surgical features in 40 patients with primary cerebellar ectopia (adult Chiari malformation). Q J Med 181:85–96, 1977.
30. Naidich TP, Pudlowski RM, Naidich JB, Gornish M, Rodriguez FJ: Computed tomographic signs of the Chiari II malformation. Part 1: Skull and dural partitions. Radiology 134:65–71, 1980.
31. Carmel PW: The Arnold–Chiari malformation. In: Pediatric Neurosurgery. Grune & Stratton, New York, 1982, pp 61–77.
32. Gardner WJ: The Dysraphic States. Excerpta Medica, Amsterdam, 1973.
33. Franchinger E, Fankhauser R: Arnold–Chiari Hirnmissbildung mit Spina Bifida und Hydrozephalus beim Kalb. Schweiz Arch Tierheilk 94:145–149, 1952.
34. Oakes WJ: Chiari malformations, hydromyelia, syringomyelia. In: Wilkins RH, Rengachary SS (eds): Neurosurgery. McGraw-Hill, New York, 1985, pp 2102–2124.
35. Gardner WJ: Anatomic features common to Arnold–Chiari and Dandy–Walker malformation suggest a common origin. Cleve Clin Quart 26:206–222, 1959.
36. Rhoton AL Jr: Microsurgery of Arnold–Chiari malformations in adults with and without hydromyelia. J Neurosurg 45:473–483, 1976.
37. Peach B: Arnold–Chiari malformation with normal spine. Arch Neurol 10:497–501, 1964.
38. Carmel PW, Markesbery WR: Arnold–Chiari malformation in an elderly woman. Arch Neurol 21:258–262, 1969.

39. Teng P, Papatheodorou G: Arnold–Chiari malformation with normal spine and cranium. Arch Neurol 12:622–624, 1965.
40. Verbiest H: The Arnold–Chiari malformation. J Neurol Neurosurg Psychiatry 16: 227–233, 1953.
41. O'Rahilly R, Müller F: The normal and abnormal development of the nervous system in the early human embryo. Riv Neurosci Pediatr (J Pediatr Neurosci) 2:89–94, 1986.
42. Osaka K, Matsumoto S, Tanimura T: Myeloschisis in early human embryos. Child's Brain 4:347–359, 1978.
43. Williams B: Further thoughts on the valvular action of the Arnold–Chiari malformation. Dev Med Child Neurol 13 (Suppl.25):105–, 1974.
44. Williams B: Chronic herniation of the hindbrain. Ann R Coll Surg Engl 63:9–17, 1981.
45. Williams B: Simultaneous cerebral and spinal fluid pressure recordings: II. Cerebrospinal dissociation with lesions at the foramen magnum. Acta Neurochir 59: 123–142, 1981.
46. Van Houweninge Grafdijk CJ: Over Hydrocephalus. Dissertation, Leiden, 1932.
47. Cameron AH: The Arnold–Chiari and other neuro-anatomical malformations associated with spina bifida. J Pathol Bacteriol 73:195–211, 1957.
48. Van Hoytema GJ, van den Berg R: Embryological studies of the posterior fossa in connection with Arnold–Chiari malformation. Dev Med Child Neurol (Suppl 11):61–76, 1966.
49. Russell DS, Donald C: The mechanism of internal hydrocephalus in spina bifida. Brain 53:203–215, 1935.
50. Calliauw L, Dehaene I: The surgical risk in the treatment of Arnold–Chiari malformations. Acta Neurochir 39:173–179, 1977.
51. Ogryzlo MA: Arnold–Chiari malformation. Arch Neurol Psychiatry 48:30–46, 1942.
52. Swanson HS, Fincher EF: Arnold–Chiari deformity without bone anomalies. J Neurosurg 6:314–319, 1949.
53. McConnell AA, Parker HL: Deformity of hind-brain associated with internal hydrocephalus: its relation to Arnold–Chiari malformation. Brain 61:415–429, 1938.
54. Goldstein F, Kepes JJ: The role of traction in the development of the Arnold–Chiari malformation. An experimental study. J Neuropathol Exp Neurol 25:654–, 1966.
55. Megison L, Norrell HA, Wilson CB: Cephalic venous hypertension in the pathogenesis of infantile hydrocephalus. Surg Forum 18:451–, 1967.
56. Daniel PM, Strich SJ: Some observations on the congenital deformity of the central nervous system known as the Arnold–Chiari malformation. J Neuropathol Exp Neurol 17:255–266, 1958.
57. Kapsenberg JC, van Lookerem Campagne JA: A case of spina bifida combined with diastematomyely, the anomaly of Chiari and hydrocephalus. Acta Anat 7:366–388, 1949.
58. Patten BM: Overgrowth of the neural tube in young human embryos. Anat Rec 113:381–393, 1952.
59. Lendon RG: An autoradiographic study of induced myelomeningocele. Dev Med Child Neurol 14 (Suppl 27):80–85, 1972.
60. Caldarelli M, McLone DG, Collins JA, Suwa J, Knepper PA: Vitamin A induced neural tube defects in the mouse. Concepts Pediatr Neurosurg 6:161–171, 1985.
61. Di Rocco C, Rende M: Neural tube defects: some remarks on the possible role of glucosoaminoglycans in the genesis of the spinal malformation, the anomaly in the

configuration of the posterior cranial fossa and hydrocephalus. Childs Nerv Syst 3:334–371, 1987.

62. McLone DG, Knepper PA: Role of complex carbohydrates and neurulation. Pediatr Neurosci 12:2–9, 1985–1986.

63. Marin-Padilla M, Marin-Padilla MT: Morphogenesis of experimentally induced Arnold–Chiari malformation. J Neurol Sci 50:29–55, 1981.

64. Richardson RR: Congenital genetic murine (ch) hydrocephalus. 3: Childs Nerv Syst 1:87–99, 1985.

65. Di Rocco C, Rende M: Congenital hydrocephalus and mucopolysaccharides. Riv Neurosci Pediatr (J Pediatr Neurosci) 1:61–67, 1985.

66. Torack RM, Grave L: Subependymal glycosaminoglycan networks in adult and developing rat brain. Histochemistry 68:55–65, 1980.

67. Saez RJ, Onofrio BM, Yanagihara T: Experience with Arnold–Chiari malformation, 1960 to 1970. J Neurosurg 45:416–422, 1976.

68. Barnett HJM, Foster JB, Hudgson P: Syringomyelia. WB Saunders, Philadelphia, 1973, p 318.

69. Sieben RL, Hamida MB, Shulman K: Multiple cranial nerve deficits associated with the Arnold–Chiari malformation. Neurology 21:673–681, 1971.

70. Gilbert JN, Jones KL, Rorke LB, Chernoff GF, James HF: Central nervous system anomalies associated with meningomyelocele, hydrocephalus, and the Arnold–Chiari malformation: reappraisal of theories regarding the pathogenesis of posterior neural tube closure defects. Neurosurgery 18:559–564, 1986.

71. Schut L, Bruce DA: The Arnold–Chiari malformation. Orthoped Clin North Am 9:913–921, 1978.

72. Correa-Restrepo A, Robertson C, Rozdilsky B: Vernix caseosa meningitis and laryngeal stridor in an infant with myelomeningocele: case report. J Neurosurg 42:718–722, 1975.

73. Hoffman HJ, Park TS, Hendrick EP, Humphreys RP: Manifestazioni e trattamento della malformazione di Arnold–Chiari nel bambino con mielomeningocele. In: Di Rocco C, Caldarelli M (eds): Mielomeningocele. Casa del Libro Roma, 1983, pp 251–260.

74. Hoffman HJ, Hendrick EB, Humphreys RP: Manifestations and management of the Arnold–Chiari malformation in patients with myelomeningocele. Child's Brain 1:255–259, 1975.

75. Park TS, Hoffman HJ, Hendrick EB, Humphreys RP: Experience with surgical decompression of the Arnold–Chiari malformation in young infants with myelomeningocele. Neurosurgery 13:147–152, 1983.

76. Venes JL, Black KL, Latack JT: Preoperative evaluation and surgical management of the Arnold-Chiari II malformation. J Neurosurg 64:363–370, 1986.

77. Wealthall SR, Whittaker GE, Greenwood N: The relationship of apnoea and stridor in spina bifida to other unexplained infant deaths. Dev Med Child Neurol (Suppl) 32:107–116, 1974.

78. Peach B: Arnold–Chiari malformation. Anatomic features of 20 cases. Arch Neurol 12:613–621, 1965.

79. Kruiff E, Jeff R: Skull abnormalities associated with the Arnold–Chiari malformation. Acta Radiol (Diagn) 5:9–24, 1966.

80. Naidich TP, Pudlowski RM, Naidich JB: Computed tomographic signs of Chiari II malformation. II: Midbrain and cerebellum. Radiology 134:391–398, 1980.

81. Naidich TP, McLone DG, Fulling KH: The Chiari II malformation. Part IV. The hind-brain deformity. Neuroradiology 25:179–197, 1983.
82. De La Paz RL, Brady TJ, Buonanno FS, New PFJ, Kistler JP, McGinnis BD, Pykett IL, Taveras JM: Nuclear magnetic resonance (NMR) imaging of Arnold–Chiari type I malformation with hydromyelia. J Comput Assist Tomogr 7:126–129, 1983.
83. Modic MT, Weinstein MA, Pavlicek W, Starnes DL, Duchesneau PM, Boumphrey F, Hardy RJ: Nuclear magnetic resonance imaging of the spine. Radiology 148:755–762, 1983.
84. Fitzsimmons JS: Laryngeal stridor and respiratory obstruction associated with myelomeningocele. Dev Med Child Neurol 15:533–536, 1973.
85. Krayenbühl H: Evaluation of the different surgical approaches in the treatment of syringomyelia. Clin Neurol Neurosurg 77:110–128, 1974.
86. Holinger PC, Holinger LD, Reichert TJ, Holinger PH: Respiratory obstruction and apnea in infants with bilateral abductor vocal cord paralysis, meningomyelocele, hydrocephalus, and Arnold–Chiari malformation. J Pediatr 92:368–373, 1978.
87. D'Errico A: The surgical treatment of hydrocephalus associated with spina bifida. Yale J Biol Med 11:425–430, 1939.
88. Carmel PW: Management of the Chiari malformations in childhood. Clin Neurosurg 30:385–406, 1983.
89. Crosby RMN, Paul RL, Kosnik EJ: Surgical treatment of hydrocephalus caused by Arnold–Chiari malformation in infants and young children. Surg 38:377–379, 1972.
90. Paul KS, Lye RH, Strang FA, Dutton J: Arnold–Chiari malformation: review of 71 cases. J Neurosurg 58:183–187, 1983.
91. Wickramasinghe SF, Eckstein H-B, Nixon HH: Posterior fossa decompression in shunt-treated hydrocephalic children. Dev Med Child Neurol (Suppl 15):11–13, 1968.
92. Adams RD, Schatzki R, Scoville WB: Arnold–Chiari malformation: diagnosis, demonstration by intraspinal lipiodol and successful surgical treatment. N Engl J Med 225:125–131, 1941.
93. Lemire RL, Shepard TH, Alvord EC: Caudal myeloschisis (lumbosacral spina bifida cystica) in a five millimeter (horizon XIV) human embryo. Anat Rec 152:9–16, 1965.
94. Papasozomenos S, Roessman U: Respiratory distress and Arnold–Chiari malformation. Neurology 31:97–100, 1981.
95. Penfield W, Coburn DF: Arnold–Chiari malformation and its operative treatment. Arch Neurol Psychiatry 40:328–336, 1938.

CHAPTER 4

Diastematomyelia and Diplomyelia

P. Bret, J.D. Patet, and C. Lapras

The word diastematomyelia was first introduced in 1837 by Ollivier[1] to delineate a congenital malformation of the spinal cord and spinal column. It is characterized by a splitting of the spinal cord associated with a bony or a cartilaginous septum transfixing the neural tissue, and with other vertebral abnormalities. Such anatomic criteria are widely adopted to define diastematomyelia which represents an extreme degree of the occult spinal dysraphism according to the hypothesis postulated by Lichtenstein[2] in 1940. Diastematomyelia basically differs from diplomyelia by the fact that the former is a sagittal division of a single cord into two "half-cords" by a septum, while the later is a true duplication of the cord into two "twin cords" with no bony transfixion. Since intermediate varieties do exist, these two conditions will be described together in this section, along with those involving the cauda equina.

Although adult cases have been reported occasionally, a majority of cases are encountered in infancy and childhood. The symptomatic features of diastematomyelia are well known and the advent of computerized tomography (CT) evaluation of spinal cord malformations has made its diagnosis easier today. Nevertheless, as acknowledged by recent contributions to this subject, physiopathology of symptoms and indication for operative removal of the spur or for conservative therapy are still controversial matters.

Review of Literature

Up to 1950, very little was known about clinical and radiographic features of diastematomyelia, although a few reports, mainly based on autopsy findings or short clinical series, were analyzed in 1940 (in the earliest review of Herren and Edwards).[3] In 1950, Matson[4] provided the most comprehensive study based on a clinical experience of 11 cases, seven of those with myelographic evaluation. On this occasion, he pointed out the improvement in the neurologic picture following surgical removal of the spur, and detailed the operative technique. In 1952, Bremer[5] formulated his theory of the persistent neuroenteric canal, which later was accepted by general agreement. From this period to the mid-1970s, there is abundant literature on this subject, with various reports including review of large series (quoted in a further section of this study), with special mention reserved for the associated orthopaedic and spinal anomalies,[6,7] the radiographic evaluation,[8] and the questionable relationships between the clinical picture and the presence of a spur.[9]

Prior to Matson's review, the radiographic diagnosis was limited to plain x-ray films. In 1950, Neuhauser[10] pointed out the value of opaque myelography. In 1966, Liliequist[11] reported a case studied by air myelography. In the most recent contributions, the need for early recognition of diastematomyelia in patients with congenital spine anomalies,[12-15] has been pointed out as well as the use of CT scan, which has gained widespread acceptance for use in the diagnosis.[16-32] The routine use of CT has led to recognition of previously unknown varieties (adult cases, cervical diastematomyelia). Despite recent progress in diagnostic procedures, the most debatable point remains today: what is the beneficial effect that can be expected from the operative removal of the spur, especially in asymptomatic or fixed forms?

Pathologic Anatomy

Diastematomyelia

Although a few cases of cervical diastematomyelia have recently been reported[16,18,22,26,27,33,34] as a result of a routine use of CT in the evaluation of the disease, in the typical form, diastematomyelia occurs in the spinal areas from the mid-thoracic to the low lumbar segments. The spinal canal is widened over several segments and its maximal dilatation is at the level of the cord splitting. The canal is duplicated by a sagittal bony or cartilaginous process. The canal duplication may be partial (spur), total (septum), or manifested only by a fibrous band.

The half-cords are separated from each other by a vertical cleft and usually show notable asymmetry. The side of the hypoplastic cord is usually, but not always, consistent with the lateralization of the neurologic signs or of the "orthopaedic syndrome." The two half-cords are almost always positioned lateral to each other, despite the description given by Rokos[35] of a "frontal diastematomyelia," an anatomic case in which the two half-cords were positioned in the sagittal plane. Each portion of the half-cord harbors one pair of roots and is invested by its own pial, arachnoidal, and dural covering. The resulting dural cleft usually lies over a distance of several segments, while the bony spur involves a single vertebral segment. The transfixing spike is located at the lower end of the cleft, close to the area where the two half-cords re-unite caudally (Figs. 4.1A and B, 4.3A and B). Other pathologic patterns have been reported. These variations are summarized in Fig. 4.2A–F and include: incomplete diastematomyelia, diastematomyelia with a single cleft including two spurs located at different segments,[36] double diastematomyelia,[37] and involvement of the low conus medullaris or of the cauda equina. Rarely, the two half-cords may remain split caudally to the bony septum and end in two prominent fila terminale (Fig. 4.2D). The low

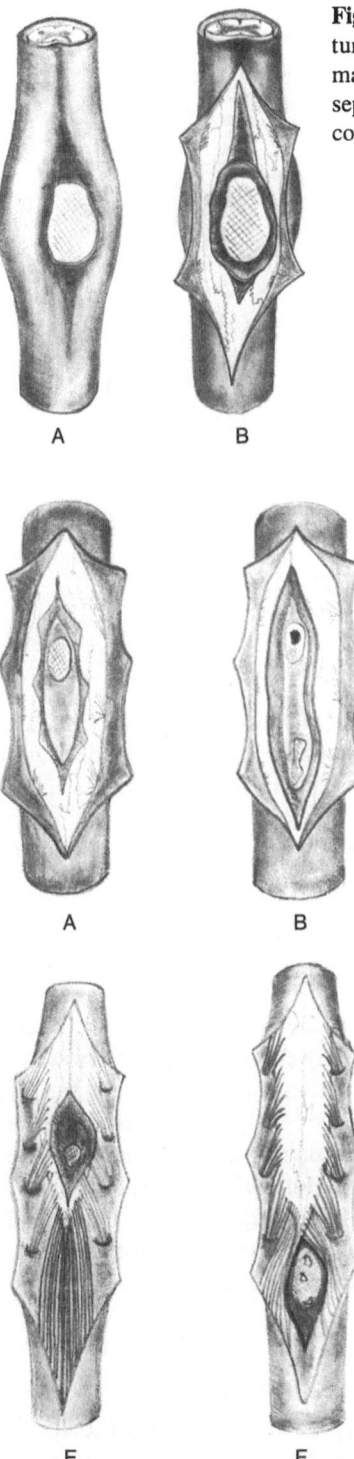

Figure 4.1. A: Diastematomyelia with a bony septum. Two dural sacs are present. B: Incision of dura mater shows a sheath of dura accompanying the bony septum. The cord is split in two asymmetric half-cords.

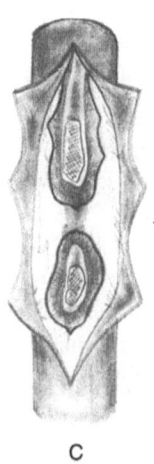

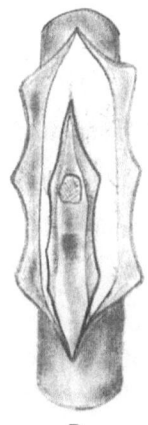

Figure 4.2. Anatomic variations.
A: Diastematomyelia with a spur located at the upper end of the cleft. B: Diastematomyelia with two bony spurs and one cleft. C: Double diastematomyelia. D: Diastematomyelia with half-cords remaining split caudal to the spur. E: Diastematomyelia of the low conus medullaris. F: Diastematomyelia involving the cauda equina.

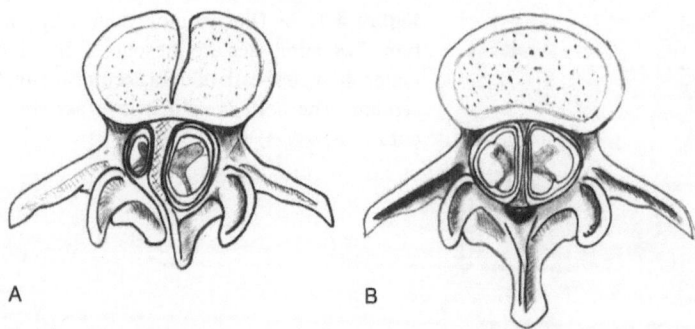

Figure 4.3. A: Dorsal diastematomyelia with a bony spur. The half-cords are asymmetric. A spina bifida (occult form) and a partial splitting of the vertebral body are present. B: Diastematomyelia with a sagittal fibrous band.

situation of the conus medullaris in diastematomyelia is acknowledged by both anatomic and myelographic studies.

Associated Malformations

Dorsal to the Cord Splitting

Spina bifida occulta is very common in diastematomyelia, involving multiple adjacent levels in most cases. Fusion of the laminae is also a common feature, with variable combinations with spina bifida. Cutaneous abnormalities are also commonly associated and include various conditions: nevoid changes, dermal sinus, hypertrichosis, lipoma, meningocele, and in its most severe degree meningomyelocele.

Ventral to the Cord Splitting

Different dysraphic types of vertebral body deformities may be encountered with diastematomyelia: hypoplastic hemivertebra, vertebral agenesis, butterfly vertebra, vertebral fusion, and sagittal splitting of the vertebral bodies. Narrowing of the vertebral body in the antero-posterior direction is usually noted at the level of the spur, while the other malformations may be encountered remote to the diastematomyelic segment. The most pronounced anomalies are noted in individuals with severe scoliosis. Other ventral malformations are consistent with the development of aberrant endodermal or ectodermal material between the neural crests: intestinal fistula, intrathecal enteroid cyst, dermoid cysts, epidermoid cysts, extradural teratomas, lipomas, aberrant renal tissue, or intrathecal Wilms' tumor.[21,38]

Associated Rostral Malformations

The simultaneous occurrence of diastematomyelia and of a Chiari II deformity has been reported in a few articles.[39-43] In 1891, Chiari reported his first type II anatomic case. On this occasion, he provided an accurate description of an associated diastematomyelia located in the upper lumbar column: "...at the upper lumbar level, the cord was split in two along the midline. Below the fifth lumbar segment, the half-cords joined together into a single tube."[44] Hydrocephalus due to aqueduct stenosis without underlying hindbrain deformity, hydromyelia, posterior fossa dermoid cysts and Klippel–Feil syndromes have also in few occasions been reported in association with diastematomyelia. It seems reasonble to assume that, due to the usual lack of extensive radiographic or CT evaluation, their actual incidence is likely underestimated.

Associated Caudal Malformations

Both anatomic and surgical explorations have shown that the conus medullaris in these patients ends below the L2–L3 disk and that a prominent film, or several fibrous bands, suggest an associated tethered cord syndrome. The active role of these anomalies in spinal cord dysfunction is questionable.

Sacral agenesis has been reported, isolated or in association with other severe malformations (sirenomelia, urinary tract anomalies, renofacial dysplasia), usually in postmortem descriptions.[38,45–48]

Diplomyelia

Early descriptions obviously showed that some confusion existed between diplomyelia and diastematomyelia, before Lichtenstein's[2] statement that diasteatomyelia resulted from the splitting of a single spinal cord while diplomyelia represented a true duplication of the cord. Accordingly, diplomyelia anatomically shows two neural tubes, each of these with four gray columns and two pairs of roots. The "twin-cords" are invested with their own pial covering but share a common arachnoidal and dural sac. Each cord is rotated approximately 90° so that the ventral columns face each other. Diplomyelia is basically characterized by the absence of a sagittal spur (Fig. 4.4D).

Definite opposition between diastematomyelia and diplomyelia seems somewhat artificial. Many variations can occur, several patients simultaneously showing features belonging to both conditions, diplomyelia with dural compartmentalization or with median septum, or diastematomyelia with additional roots

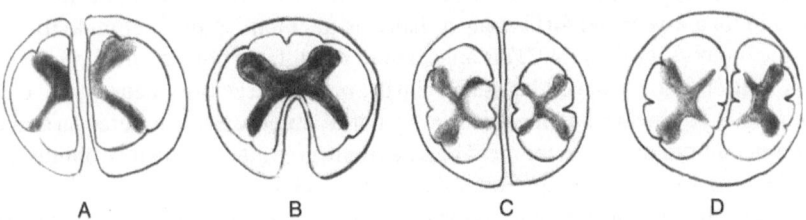

Figure 4.4. A: Diastematomyelia. B: Intermediate type: partial diastematomyelia. C: Intermediate type: diplomyelia with two separate dural sacs. D: Diplomyelia.

arising from the inner cord (Fig. 4.4A–D). Furthermore, a great majority of the reported cases are morphologically described by means of radiographic and operative findings. Very little information is, therefore, available from the literature regarding the only definite criterion distinguishing the two conditions, that is, the existence or not of four gray columns within the separated neural elements.

Embryology

The embryonic pathogenesis of diastematomyelia remains today a matter of controversy in the same manner that there is no complete agreement as to the pathogenesis of other types of neuro-ectodermal defects. Our knowledge is based on few autopsy cases and animal experimental studies undertaken in the late 19th century. These experiments have documented the ability of various agents (namely hyperthermia) to induce the duplication of the dorsal surface of the embryo.

Three groups of embryogenic hypotheses have been considered.

1. *Hypothesis*: arrested development of the spinal cord. This possibility has been ruled out by authors following statement of Herren and Edwards that splitting or duplication of the cord could not be explained on this basis. There is no corresponding developmental stage during which the cord is double.[3]

2. *Hypothesis*: reopening of a previously closed neural tube was initially introduced by Morgagni in 1761 (cited by Blocklehurst[49]) in an attempt to explain spina bifida with meningomyelocele. Regarding diastematomyelia, this hypothesis was considered further by Gardner.[50] He postulated that the neural tissue division originally resulted from rupture of the neural tube due to hydromyelia, with delayed interposition of fibrous or bony tissue. Gardner's theory has received little support from further studies, although it provides an attractive explanation in cases where diastematomyelia is associated with anomalies of the rostral neural axis.

3. *Hypothesis*: deficient closure of the embryonic neural groove. This is generally assumed as the most likely embryologic hypothesis. The high frequency of diastematomyelia showing both posterior and anterior vertebral malformations suggests a mechanism inducing the persistence of ectasic mesenchymal tissue protruding into the normal neural tissue in the early stages of the neural tube differentiation. In 1950, Bremer[5] proposed the theory of the persistence of a neurenteric canal. It was based on the observation made in 1906, by Keen and Koplin, of a 2-year-old girl having a fistulous tract joining the rectum to the skin of the lumbo-sacral region. This appeared to result from nonclosure of the primitive neurenteric canal (Lieberkuhn's canal), or of an accessory neurenteric canal connecting the primitive intestinal cavity to the amnios. He postulated an aberration in embryologic development of a neurenteric canal completely obliterating and giving rise to many abnormalities of the spinal cord, vertebral defects, and fistulous tracts. Herren and Edwards[3] questioned whether the spinal cord anomaly had to be regarded as the primary disorder or if it developed secon-

dary to abnormal spinal development. Because during embryonic life the cord develops long before the spinal column, they considered diastematomyelia as the primary malformation. They observed that in chick embryos the lateral extremities of the plate, prior to fusing, may migrate ventrally for a short distance and later retreat dorsally, resulting in fusion of the tube. However, if their migration should continue ventrally, the lateral extremities of the neural plate may finally fuse with the ventral portion of the plate and induce the completion of two separate tubes. If the cleft between the two half-cords should be wide enough, mesenchymal tissue might develop therein together with arachnoidal, dural, and bony elements.

Physiopathology

In the authors' opinion, complete agreement has not been reached regarding the definite relationships between vertebral and spinal cord anomalies of diastematomyelia, and the symptomatic features noted in involved patients. This is an important question, since the conclusion that surgical removal of the bony spur is the proper treatment of diastematomyelia has to be predicated on the actual mechanism of spinal cord dysfunction.

Mechanical Factors

They include traction, tearing, and compression phenomena of the cord at the splitting area and are the most commonly advocated hypotheses. The hypothesis suggested by Marr and Uihlein[51] that the spur could cause tumor-like compression to the spinal cord has not been confirmed. However, it could be reasonably assumed in patients in whom a large bony spike filling the whole cleft is disclosed at operation. Matson[52] and Barson[53] have advocated the theory of the differential rate of growth of the spinal column and of the spinal cord. Matson's statement that preventive surgery was rational was based on this view. Accordingly, in diastematomyelia, the relative "ascent" of the cord in the spinal canal during growth is supposed to result in lengthening of the cord cleft due to progressive tearing by the bony septum or spur, the latter being firmly attached to the spinal canal. This differential growth theory, though attractive, remains unsatisfactory. As mentioned by Guthkelch,[9] it is not in accordance with the facts and fails to explain several clinico-anatomic features of the disease: the normal "ascent" of the cord within the canal in terms of vertebral levels of its termination is complete at the age of 2 months. Therefore, the maximal damage would be achieved in early infancy and presenting symptoms of diastematomyelia would theoretically be evident at this age. Obviously, this is not in accordance with the usual clinical picture, the average age of patients in large series ranging from 5 to 10. This age incidence challenges Matson's statement that the maximal risk of neurologic deterioration in diastematomyelia is during the periods of spurts of growth of the vertebral column, because the periods during which the spine is elongating most rapidly are during infancy and adolescence. Occasionally presenting symptoms may occur in adult life. Furthermore, after removal of the spur, there is neither radiologic nor operative documentation of upward movement of the "liberated" cord relative to the bony landmarks. For these reasons, and also to explain the usually good response of the neurologic syndrome to the operative removal of the septum, Guthkelch has advocated the possible role of repeated head and neck flexion causing traction and neuronal damage in the split cord by the trans-fixing septum. In this view, the pathogenesis of symptoms remains unclear in patients harboring a spur remote from each end of the cleft or no cord fusion cau-dal to the spur.

Among other mechanical factors possibly responsible for increasing neuro-logic deficits, the role of the associated scoliosis or of other congenital malforma-tions (fibrous bands, teratomas, enteroid cysts) exerting a compressive or stretching effect on the spinal cord is questionable. In this view, the contribution of an associated tethered cord syndrome due to a shortened filum terminale deserves special mention.[54]

"Non-Mechanical" Factors

Anatomic studies and operative data suggest that unilateral hypoplasia of one of the two half-cords may play an important role in the pathogenesis of symptoms. Especially, the orthopaedic syndrome detailed by James and Lassman[6,55] acknowledges the existence of long-lasting cord dysfunction even if it becomes evident in late childhood or early adolescence. The orthopaedic syndrome seems unlikely to be due to a mechanical compression by the spur and was thought to be compatible with a prenatal anomaly of the neural mesodermal junction.[9] Little information is available regarding possible anomalies of the vascular sup-ply of the cord in diastematomyelia. Vandresse and Cornelis have raised the feasibility of ischemic damage due to a compression of the main arterial spinal axes, or to an unequal distribution of the anterior vascular network between the two half-cords.[54]

It seems reasonable to consider the pathogenesis of symptoms noted in diastematomyelia as a various combination of compressive and stretching mechanical factors together with primary spinal cord anomalies. The importance of the latter might have been overlooked, and it may be true that the bony septum dividing the cord actually has very little effect on the symptoms.

Signs and Symptoms

Many clinical descriptions of diastematomyelia based upon few cases or larger series are available in the literature.* A great majority of these studies deal with

---

*Refs 3, 4, 7–9, 11–15, 23, 29, 42, 43, 47, 51, 54, 56–79.

pediatric cases and point out the prominent female incidence among patients. However, in addition to the Freeman[61] and English[80] cases, published in 1961 and 1967, the possible occurrence of diastematomyelia in the adult age is acknowledged by recent contributions,[16,18,26,31,33,37,81-84] with a high proportion of cervical cord diastematomyelia. Late recognition of diastematomyelia is undoubtedly explained by the recent advent of the new radiologic evaluation procedures of CT and magnetic resonance imaging.

The clinical features of diastematomyelia are well known today. The occasional variations noted in the age of patients and in the clinical patterns at first referral reflect the fact that a wide range of medical and surgical specialties are concerned. Diastematomyelia may come to the clinician's attention under several circumstances. Usually, the clinical pattern exhibits a variable combination of cutaneous anomalies, and orthopaedic and neurologic impairment.

Cutaneous Anomalies

These are always present and should raise the possibility of an underlying spinal dysraphism. The most common abnormality is localized hypertrichosis with, in its most suggestive form, a long patch of hair surrounding the dysraphic area. Palpation in the hypertrichosis area may reveal a deformed spinous process or a spina bifida occulta. Nevoid changes, dermal sinus, or a simple dimple may be noted in the thoraco-lumbar midline area, as well as a fatty subcutaneous mass, a lipoma, or a meningocele. Occasionally, associated meningoceles at other spinal levels have been reported. These cutaneous anomalies are overlooked in most cases, the diagnosis of diastematomyelia usually not being considered, except when there is evidence of an underlying dysraphic condition, such as spina bifida with meningomyelocele.

The Orthopaedic Syndrome

This term was introduced in 1960 by James and Lassman,[6] who detailed the characteristic morphologic deformities of the vertebral spine and the lower limbs. They are rarely evident at birth, although they are likely to be present from this period of life, at least in a minor degree. In more than 50% of cases, patients are referred because morphologic abnormalities (or their consequences) have become obvious during later growth. Walking retardation is the most common presenting feature in early childhood, whereas in late childhood and in early adolescence patients usually exhibit anomalies of gait or poor posture. A hypoplastic lower limb with definite length discrepancy and unilateral weakness is strongly suggestive of diastematomyelia, especially if signs of external spinal dysraphism are disclosed at examination. The calf and the foot are predominantly hypoplastic, although in few cases the thigh, the buttock, and the lumbar muscles may be unilaterally involved. A wide variety of foot deformities has been described, either isolated or in association with a hypoplastic limb. They include pes planus, pes equinovarus, calcaneovalgus, and vertical talus. The most frequently noted anomaly is a reducible or fixed internal club-foot deformity. Ankle-jerk is invariably absent.

Patients having a hypoplastic lower limb commonly show significant spinal curvature, mainly thoraco-lumbar but also lumbar scoliosis. In some authors' experience,[7,12,23,85,86] congenital scoliosis was found to be the primary complaint in a majority of cases. This fact is not consistent with most neurosurgeons' opinion, which is that symptomatic spine deformities may be absent or disclosed only by physical or x-ray evaluation revealing a mild scoliosis. This is likely attributable to a difference in patient selection from one series to another. Nevertheless, it is generally agreed that in congenital scoliosis, there is a high percentage (estimated from 5% to 18% overall) of patients presumably having a spinal bony septum. Authors usually claim that in this patient group the removal of the septum should be done primarily if the surgical correction of scoliosis is planned.

Neurologic Symptoms

The significance of the neurologic status of patients with diastematomyelia is debatable. Some patients show minimal impairment or fixed anomalies, such as the absence of a reflex in the hypoplastic area. These do not carry any clear correlation with the extent of spinal cord damage. Conversely, some patients may show signs of increasing neurologic deterioration. Physical examination may disclose pyramidal tract signs, complete absence of tendon reflexes or of the anal reflex, and sensory changes in the area supplied by the lower lumbar or sacral roots. Even with such physical findings, patients may suffer only minimal disability. However, patients may suffer sphincter disturbances or, infrequently, complete paraplegia. Deteriorating neurologic status is thought to respond well to spur removal. Many observers have claimed that prompt improvement of progressive paraplegia and of incontinence may be expected from operation, provided it is accomplished as soon as deterioration is noted.

Infrequent and Atypical Presentations

Acute paraplegia has been reported as a complication of corrective surgery for kyphoscoliosis.[78,86,87] These circumstances accentuate the importance of early detection of diastematomyelia in congenital scoliosis by proper x-ray or CT evaluation. Recurrent meningitis may also result from repeated infections via a fistulous tract (dermal sinus). Acute backaches were well described in two cases by Guthkelch[9] as sudden painful spasms in the back legs, occurring after physical activity and lasting a few minutes. A case presenting with a perforating ulceration of the toes was reported in 1982.[88] In our institution, we observed a similar case with a big toe ulcer and underlying osteitis.[89]

Neuro-Imaging

Diagnosis of diastematomyelia includes traditional procedures (plain x-ray films, tomograms, myelography), computed tomography (CT), and magnetic resonance imaging (MRI).

Figure 4.5. Frontal tomogram of the dorsal spine showing a calcified diastematomyelic septum at the level of **T7–T11**. There is incomplete fusion of the right and left halves of the vertebral bodies.

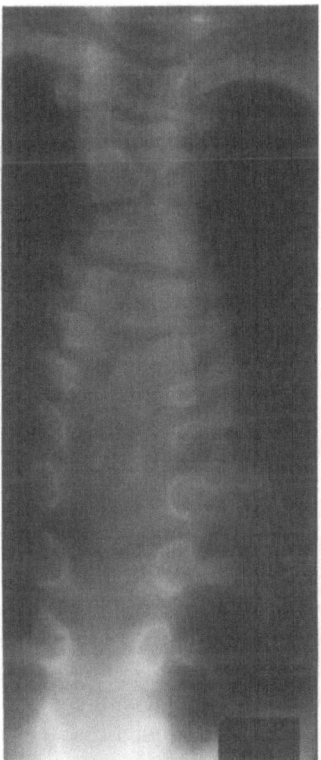

X-ray Findings

Plain x-ray films and tomograms show the bony spur and associated vertebral abnormalities.[8] The near-midline bony spur is pathognomonic. It is best seen on frontal projections, and its length measured over the number of vertebral bodies involved: the longest spur may involve four adjacent vertebral levels, while the shortest may be less than 1 mm. Along the spinal axis, the most rostral spur reported in the literature was located at the level of C2–C3.[18] In 34 children, Hilal[8] reported nine dorsal and 25 lumbar septa. The rostral septae are longer than the caudal ones, and they are associated with severe scoliosis.

Tomography is essential for the diagnosis of small or partially calcified spurs (Fig. 4.5). Usually, the dorsal part of the spur is larger than the ventral one, and reaches the fused laminae of one or two vertebrae. A single vertebral body attachment of the spur without connections with the posterior arch is observed in 11% of patients.[8] A defect or a clear line near the ventral part of the bony spur, close to the vertebral body, is sometimes apparent on tomography. This finding, as well as the presence of the bony spur on radiographs taken during the first months of life, suggest that ossification of the spur is independent of the vertebra. Anomalies of vertebral bodies range from simple narrowing to complete or incomplete fusion of multiple segments. Narrowing of the vertebral body in the antero-posterior direction occurs only at the level of the spur. Other anomalies include partial or complete splitting of the body in the sagittal plane, hemivertebral hypoplasia, and agenesis. Generally, the severity of scoliosis is correlated with the degree of anomalies of the vertebral bodies. Anomalies of the posterior arches are often described in diastematomyelia. Fused laminae are frequently associated with spina bifida. This combination is reason for a very strong suspicion of diastematomyelia. In most cases, the defect involves multiple levels, the affected vertebrae being contiguous. These anomalies are a better indication of the spur's location than the skin pigmented area or vertebral body anomalies. Interpedicular distance is widened in the majority of cases and the pedicles are flattened. The largest widening is observed at the level of the spur and a few segments above and below it.

Myelography

Diastematomyelia refers to the split spinal cord, and not to either a bony spur or vertebral anomaly (Figs. 4.6 and 4.7). In case of a fibrous band or cartilaginous septum, the anomaly cannot be demonstrated by plain x-ray films or tomography. Myelography, using metrizamide, is necessary[2,37,90,91] (Fig. 4.8). The spur appears as a defect in the contrast column extending over one or several segments. But such an aspect is also simulated by simple artifacts. Therefore, it is important to identify spinal cord anatomy. The space between the two halves of the cord, and the split around the spur, are usually well seen. Nerve roots arise laterally

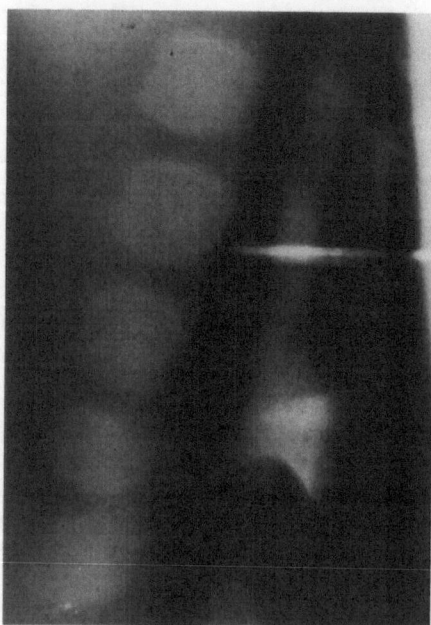

Figure 4.6. Gas myelography. Lateral tomogram showing a lumbar calcified septum.

Figure 4.7. Gas myelography. Frontal tomogram: the septum is at the lower end of the intermedullary space.

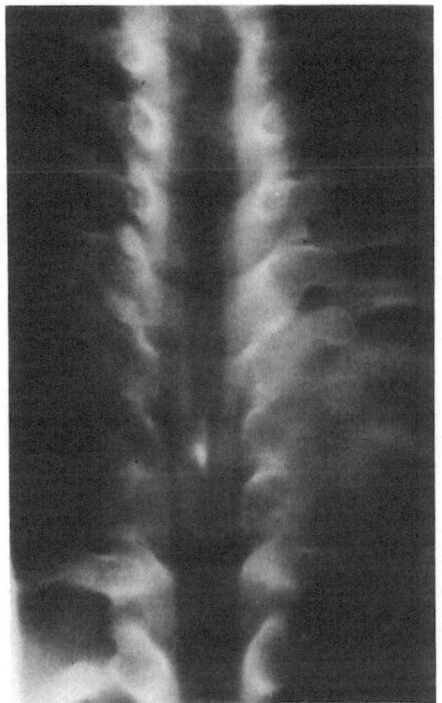

from the cord and aberrant nerve roots are sometimes observed, even at a level other than of the vertebral anomalies.[91]

CT Scan

The most accurate radiologic evaluation of diastematomyelia is obtained by metrizamide CT (Fig. 4.9A and B). A fibrous septum, or a spur calcified slightly, may be seen. Vertebral body abnormalities (cross-sectional shape of the vertebral body, interpedicular distance) are accurately studied.[17,23,92]

The diagnosis of spinal cord cleft, even small, is possible, and, by the study of nerve roots and arachnoid, difference is made between diastematomyelia and diplomyelia. Other abnormalities are well studied[17,20,30,32] such as dural bands, spinal adhesions, or associated intra- or extradural lipomas. For caudal diastematomyelia, the conus is especially studied, looking for either a thick or a short and lipomatous filum.

MRI

While scoliosis is a cause of difficulties, MRI permits one to identify alterations of the spinal cord, such as dysplasia or lipoma. MRI is of help for the differential diagnosis between diastematomyelia and pseudodiastematomyelia.[24]

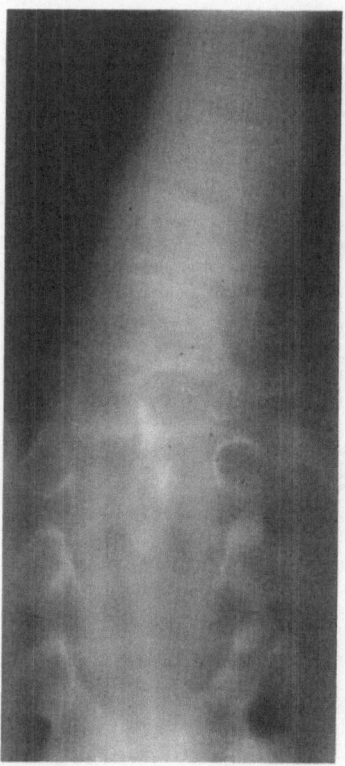

Figure 4.8. Meterizamide myelography of a diastematomyelia with scoliosis. On this frontal tomogram, the spur is at the upper end of the cleft. The maximum interpedicular distance is at the level of the spur.

Treatment

Surgery

Surgical technic has been extensively studied.[72,93,94] The aim of surgery is to decrease the strain sustained by the cord. For this purpose, the bony spur has to be removed, all adhesions between cord and dura divided, the dural funnel transfixing the cord resected, an associated narrow canal enlarged, and, if present, a tethering band released. At the end of the procedure, the dura is closed to obtain a normal dural sac, trying to prevent cerebrospinal fluid leakage and secondary adherences.

The patient is placed in the prone position. Incision is performed in the midline and widely extended above and below the lesion, beyond the pigmented and hairy skin area. Dissection is difficult at the level of the malformation because of lack of unmistakable landmarks. It could be dangerous when spina bifida is associated, or the frontal plane rotated by kyphoscoliosis, or the spinal canal narrowed. The best landmark is the normal dural sac near the malformation. Muscles are separated from laminae, beginning near normal spinous processes at both extremities. From each extremity, muscle dissection proceeds until all the enlarged spinal area is exposed.

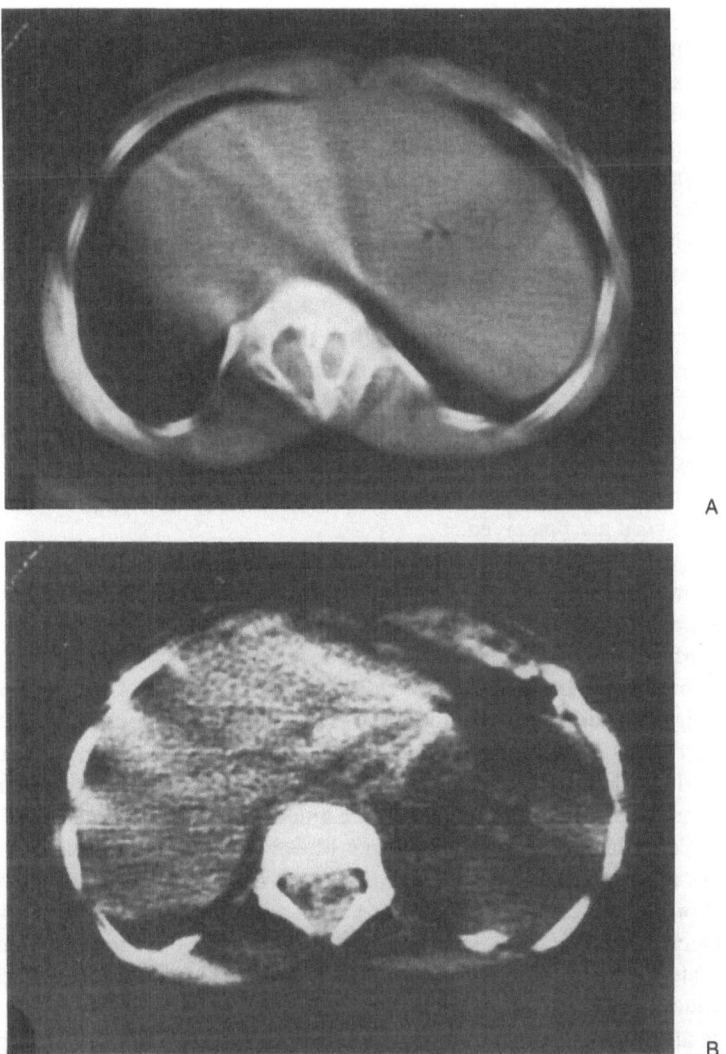

Figure 4.9. A: CT with metrizamide of a diastematomyelia showing a calcified septum. B: CT of the same patient as in A. Septum is no more visible, but the two half-cords are well documented by metrizamide. An occult spina bifida is noted at this level.

In the same manner, bone removal is begun in a normal area, the nearest possible to the malformation, at the level where the canal begins to enlarge. However, laminectomy of normal areas must not be extended too far because of the risk of producing or aggravating kyphoscoliosis and because of difficulties encountered by secondary orthopaedic surgery. Piecemeal bone removal is performed from the normal to the pathologic laminae, as far lateral as possible on each side, avoiding beginning in the midline because the real spur's width is unknown. The two dural sacs are progressively exposed, and the last pieces of bone in the midline are finally resected, uncovering the dural cleft. Frequently, the bony spicule fills only a part of the cleft, near its lower extremity. Spur removal is performed easily while it is superficial; going deeper into the narrow cleft it becomes more difficult, hampered by numerous veins. Rarely, a small spur is removed in one piece after twisting it; most commonly, it has to be removed by progressive resection with a small tipped rongeur. It is necessary to remove all the spur because regrowth has been reported.[94] When the veins in the cleft are much developed, it is not safe to perform hemostasis by blind pressure. Rather, it is recommended to stop extradural dissection in the cleft, better to work intradurally after opening the posterior dura by an incision encircling the dural cleft and extended toward each extremity. The two halves of the cord and their connections with the dural funnel are examined. The half-cords are frequently asymmetrical and connected to the midline by dense fibrous adhesions and some venous branches. All medial adhesions are divided until the two half-cords are freed, and slightly retracted to each side by a blunt spatula. The few nerve roots emerging from the medial part of the half-cord are preserved.

Diplomyelia is recognizable because the roots from the medial part are well shaped, and because the medial cleft generally contains neither a bony spur nor a dural funnel. After the cord is freed, achieving the spur's total removal is easy, until its base has been made flush with the anterior wall of the spinal canal. This goal is not always possible, because the entire anterior wall of the canal sometimes bulges posteriorly in the midline from a large base. It is useful to preserve some part of the dural funnel and cut it conveniently to obtain a flap closing the anterior dural defect. It is better to use a biologic glue to fasten this dural flap than to use stitches, because separating the anterior dura from the vertebral body could be complicated by extradural venous bleeding. Lateral adhesions of the half cords are not divided because they contain arterial pedicles and nerve roots. At the end of the procedure, the posterior dura is tightly closed, directly or with a dural patch. When the bony spur is located in the conus or in the cauda equina, diastematomyelia is frequently associated with a tethered cord by a thick and short filum. After extending laminectomy in a caudal direction, this abnormal filum is also divided. It is not recommended to perform at the end of surgery a skin resection followed by a skin graft, to treat the cosmetic problem at the same time. One may work with an orthopaedic team to perform the surgical treatment of kyphoscoliosis, but the added time necessary to do the fusion also may be excessive.

Surgical Indications

Indication for surgery is widely accepted when the patients show a deteriorating neurologic status (pain, motor deficit, sphincter disturbances, trophic ulceration of the feet), presenting themselves in a patient heretofore intact and without muscle atrophy, hypoplastic segment of a lower limb, absence of reflex, sensory loss.

When diastematomyelia is discovered in association with scoliosis, the surgical indications depend on evolution of the spinal deformity. Early treatment of progressive curves is emphasized, using plates or rods and wires, and bone grafts.[7,12,13,63,69] Before orthopaedic surgery, prophylactic treatment of the diastematomyelia is advisable, whether done in a single session or in two stages.[12,63,73,85] If straightening the spine is performed while the spinal cord is still fixed by the spur or still tethered, neurologic deficit or sphincter disturbances not previously observed may complicate the orthopaedic procedure.[85] When scoliosis is stable and not severe and orthopaedic surgery is to be delayed, indications for surgical treatment of the anomaly is controversial because the scoliosis may be progressive after the laminectomy. Winter[7] reported 21 cases requiring further vertebral fusion after laminectomy.

In asymptomatic patients, diastematomyelia is disclosed only if it is associated with skin anomalies. Kennedy[67] reported 65 cases and recommended withholding surgery unless symptoms develop. Conversely, James and Lassman,[64] and Guthkelch,[9] advocated prophylactic surgery since natural evolution is usually complicated by neurologic symptoms, as shown by long follow-up; since when neurologic complications occur, results of surgery are uncertain. Guthkelch reported 15 initially asymptomatic cases: in eight cases prophylactic surgery was performed and the patients remained symptom free. In seven cases, children were treated conservatively, and only one remained asymptomatic for 10 years; the others needed late surgery because evolution was complicated.

Results

Results of surgery on secondary neurologic complications are uncertain. Of 40 patients reported by James and Lassman,[64] 25 were unchanged after surgery, 6 were clinically improved, and 2 were worse. Seven remaining individuals were still asymptomatic after surgery, as they had been before. Results for secondary sphincter disturbances are quite different. Surgical treatment seems to provide complete recuperation in a majority of cases.[9,95] Trophic ulcerations respond well to surgery, as we observed.[68]

For associated scoliosis and diastematomyelia, 13 cases of laminectomy performed by orthopaedic surgeons were reported by Lassale;[69] as seven postoperative neurologic deteriorations were observed, a double anterior and posterior graft without laminectomy was recommended. On the other hand, Frerebeau[13] reported 21 cases of diastematomyelia associated with scoliosis in 16 cases. Patients were treated by neurosurgical and orthopaedic teams during the same session, the laminectomy being performed before orthopaedic treatment. Stabilization of scoliosis was achieved in all cases (two cases needed an additional anterior graft); two cases with pre-operative neurologic complications improved. No case was worsened. Our experience (68) was comparable.

In conclusion, prophylactic surgery for diastematomyelia seems wise because long-lasting follow-up may show neurologic deterioration and because delayed surgery is not always able to cure a complicated evolution.

References

1. Ollivier CP: Traité des Maladies de la Moëlle Épinière, Third edition, Vol. I. Mequignon-Marvis, Paris, 1837.
2. Lichtenstein BW: "Spinal dysraphysm". Spina bifida and myelodysplasia. Arch Neurol Psychiatry 44:792–810, 1940.
3. Herren RX, Edwards JE: Diplomyelia (duplication of the spinal cord). Arch Pathol 30:1203–1214, 1940.
4. Matson DD, Woods RP, Campbell JB, Ingraham FD: Diastematomyelia (congenital clefts of the spinal cord). Diagnosis and surgical treatment. Pediatrics 6:98–112, 1950.
5. Bremer JL: Dorsal intestinal fistula, accessory neurenteric canal, diastematomyelia. Arch Pathol 54:132–138, 1952.
6. James CCM, Lassman LP: Spinal dysraphism: an orthopaedic syndrome in children accompanying occult forms. Arch Dis Child 35:315–327, 1960.
7. Winter RB, Haven JJ, Moe JH, Lagaard SM: Diastematomyelia and congenital spine deformities. J Bone Joint Surg 56:27–39, 1974.
8. Hilal SK, Marton D, Pollack E: Diastematomyelia in children. Radiology 112:609–621, 1974.
9. Guthkelch AN: Diastematomyelia with median septum. Brain 4:729–742, 1974.
10. Neuhauser EB, Wittenborg MH, Delhinger K: Diastematomyelia transfixation of the cord or cauda equina with congenital anomalies of the spine. Radiology 54:659–664, 1950.
11. Liliequist B: Diastematomyelia: report of a case examined by gas myelography. Acta Radiol (Diagn) 3:497–502, 1965.
12. Banniza von Bazan UK, Rompe G, Krastel A, Martin K: Diastematomyelie ihre Bedeutung für die behandlung von MiBildungsskoliosen. Z Orthop 114:881–889, 1976.
13. Frerebeau P, Dimeglio A, Gras A, Harbi H: Diastematomyelia. Report of 21 cases surgically treated by a neurological and orthopedic team. Childs Brain 10:328–339, 1983.
14. James CCM, Lassman LP: Diastematomyelia with median septum in spina bifida occulta. Indications for surgery. Z Kinderchir Grenzgeb 22:460–464, 1977.
15. McMaster MJ: Occult intraspinal anomalies and congenital scoliosis. J Bone Joint Surg 66:588–601, 1984.
16. Anand AK, Kuchner EF, James R: Cervical diastematomyelia: uncommon presentation of a rare congenital disorder. Comput Radiol 9:45–49, 1985.
17. Arredondo F, Haughton VM, Hemmy DC, Zelaya B, Williams AL: The computed tomographic appearance of the spinal cord in diastematomyelia Radiology 136:685–688, 1980.
18. Beyerl BD, Ojemann RG, Davis KR, Hedley Whyte ET, Mayberg MR: Cervical diastematomyelia presenting in adulthood. Case report. J Neurosurg 62:449–453, 1985.
19. Claussen CD, Lohkamp FW, von Bazan UB: The diagnosis of congenital spinal disorders in computed tomography (C.T.) Neuropaediatrie 8:405–417, 1977.
20. Claussen C, Banniza von Bazan U, Jaschke W, Schilling V: Die Bedeutung der Computertomographie in der Diagnostik Kongenitales Spinaler Missbildungen, Insbesondere der Diastematomyelie. Roefo Fortschr Geb Roentgenstr Nuklearmed 133:520–527, 1980.

21. Fernbach SK, Naidich TP, McLone DG, Leestma JE: Computed tomography of primary intrathecal Wilms tumor with diastematomyelia. J Comput Assist Tomogr 8:523–528, 1984.

22. Giordano GB, Davidovits P, Cerisoli M, Giulioni M: Cervical diplomyelia revealed by computed tomography (C.T.). Neuropediatrics 13:93–94, 1982.

23. Gras M, Dimeglio A, Frerebeau P, Rolin B, Bourbotte G, Castan P: Diastematomyelie: exploration neuroradiologique moderne et corrélations anatomo-cliniques. A propos de vingt observations. Rev Int Pediatr 144:35–36, 1984.

24. Han JS, Benson JE, Kaufman B, Rekate HL, Alfidi RJ, Bohlman HH: Demonstration of diastematomyelia and associated abnormalities with MR imaging. Am J Neuroradiol 6:215–219, 1985.

25. Haughton VM: Present status of C.T. in the lumbar spine examination. Eur Neurol 21:198–203, 1982.

26. Kuchner EF, Anand AK, Kaufman BM: Cervical diastematomyelia: a case report with operative management. Neurosurgery 16:538–542, 1985.

27. Levine RS, Geremia GK, McNeill TW: C.T. demonstration of cervical diastematomyelia. J Comput Assist Tomogr 9:592–594, 1985.

28. Lohkamp F, Claussen C, Schuhmacher G: C.T. demonstration of pathologic changes of the spinal cord accompanying spina bifida and diastematomyelia. Prog Pediatr Radiol 6:200–227, 1978.

29. Scatliff JH, Bidgood WD, Killebrew K, Staab EV: Computed tomography and spinal dysraphism: clinical and phantom studies. Neuroradiology 17:71–75, 1979.

30. Scotti G, Musgrave MA, Harwood-Nash DC, Fitz CR, Chuang SH: Diastematomyelia in children. Metrizamide and CT metrizamide myelograph. Am J Roengenol 135:1225–1232, 1980.

31. Tadmor R, Davis KR, Roberson GM, Chapman PH: The diagnosis of diastematomyelia by computed tomography. Surg Neurol 8:434–436, 1977.

32. Whittle IR, Besser M: Congenital neural abnormalities presenting with mirror movements in a patient with Klippel–Feil syndrome. J Neurosurg 59:891–894, 1983.

33. Roosen N, De Moor J: Cervicobrachialgia with congenital vertebral anomalies and diastematomyelia. Surg Neurol 21:493–496, 1984.

34. Schiffer J, Till K: Spinal dysraphism in the cervical and dorsal regions in childhood. Childs Brain 9:73–84, 1982.

35. Rokos J: Pathogenesis of diastematomyelia and spina bifida. J Pathol 117:155–161, 1975.

36. Lourie H, Biemy JP: Diastematomyelia with two spurs and intradural neural crest elements. J Neurosurg 32:248, 1970.

37. McClelland RR, Marsh DG: Double diastematomyelia. Radiology 123:378, 1977.

38. Abraham E: Sacral agenesis with associated anomalies (caudal regression syndrome): autopsy case report. Clin Orthop Relat Res 145:168–171, 1979.

39. Cameron AH: The Arnold–Chiari and other neuro-anatomical malformations associated with spina bifida. J Pathol Bacteriol 73:195–211, 1957.

40. Davis ED: Diastematomyelia with early Arnold–Chiari syndrome and congenital dysplasic hip. Clin Orthop 52:179–184, 1968.

41. Kapsenberg JG, Vanlookeren-Campagne JA: A case of spina bifida combined with diastematomyelia, the anomaly of Chiari and hydrocephalus. Acta Anat 7:366–388, 1949.

42. Messimy R, Metzger J, Bar D: Diastematomyelie et malformation d'Arnold–Chiari associées. A propos de 3 cas. Livre Jubilaire du Pr P.F. Girard, Lyon, 1976.

43. Moes CA, Hendrick EB: Diastematomyelia. J Pediatr 63:238–248, 1963.
44. Chiari H: Veber veränderungen des kleinhirns infolge von hydrocephalie des Grosshirns. Dtsch Med Wochenschr 42:1172–1175, 1891.
45. Banniza von Bazan U: Kaudales Regressionssyndrom und Diastematomyelie. Was Enthaelt Hohls Erstbeschreibung Einer Kreuzbe indysgenesie. Z Orthop Grenzgeb 1:65–72, 1977.
46. Noeldge G, Billmann P, Boehm N: Kaudale Regression mit Sirenomelie und Dysplasia Renofacialis (Potter-syndrom). Roefoe Fortschr Geb Roentgenstr Nuklearmed 136:587–591, 1982.
47. Schwartz W, Poulsen HK, Andersen PE: Sirenomelia: das Kaudale Regressionsyndrom. Monatsschr Kinderheilkd 130:565–566, 1982.
48. Talamo TS, Macpherson TA, Dominguez R: Sirenomelia. Angiographic demonstration of vascular anomalies. Arch Pathol Lab Med 106:347–348, 1982.
49. Blocklehurst G: The pathogenesis of spina bifida: a study of the relationship between observations, hypothesis and surgical incentive. Dev Med Child Neurol 13:148, 1971.
50. Gardner WJ: Diastematomyelia and Kliffel–Feil syndrome. Relationship to hydrocephalus, syringomyelia, meningocela, myelomeningocele and anencephalus. Cleve Clin Quart 31:19–44, 1964.
51. Marr GE, Uihlein A: Diplomyelia and compression of spinal cord and not of cauda equina, by congenital anomaly of third lumbar vertebra. Surg Clin North Am 24:963–968, 1944.
52. Matson DD: Neurosurgery of Infancy and Childhood, Second edition. Charles C Thomas, Springfield, IL, 1969.
53. Barson AJ: The vertebral level of termination of the spinal cord during normal and abnormal development. J Anat 106:487–497, 1970.
54. Vandresse JH, Cornelis G: Diastematomyelia: report of eight observations. Neuroradiology 10:87–93, 1975.
55. James CCM, Lassman LP: Diastematomyelia. Arch Dis Child 33:356, 1958.
56. Anderson FM: Diastematomyelia. Report of 2 case submitted to laminectomy. Acta Orthop Scand 36:257–264, 1966.
57. Arcomano JP, Sengstacken RL, Wunderlich HO: Diastematomyelia. J Dis Child 104:393, 1962.
58. Basauri L, Palma A, Zuleta A, Holzer F, Poblete R: Diastematomyelia. Report of 18 cases. Acta Neurochir 51:91–96, 1979.
59. Benstead JC: A case of diastematomyelia. J Pathol Bacteriol 6:553–557, 1954.
60. Chambers WR: Diastematomyelia case diagnosed pre-operatively. J Paediatr 45:668–671, 1954.
61. Freenan LW: Late symptoms from diastematomyelia. J Neurosurg 18:538–541, 1961.
62. Holman CB, Svien HJ, Bickel WH: Diastematomyelia. Pediatrics 15:191–194, 1955.
63. Hood RW, Riseborough EJ, Nehme AM, Micheli LJ, Strand RD, Neuhauser EBD: Diastematomyelia and structural spinal deformities. J Bone Joint Surg 64:520–528, 1980.
64. James CCM, Lassman LP: Diastematomyelia. A critical survey of 24 cases submitted to laminectomy. Arch Dis Child 39:125–130, 1964.
65. Jones JB: Diastematomyelia. Clin Orthop 21:164–168, 1962.
66. Kapsalakis Z: Diastematomyelia in 2 sisters. J Neurosurg 21:66–67, 1964.

67. Kennedy PR: New data on diastematomyelia. J Neurosurg 51:355–361, 1979.
68. Lapras C, Bret P, Capdeville J: La diastématomyélie. Réflexion à propos d'une série de 6 observations. Neurochirurgie 24:381–389, 1978.
69. Lassale B, Rigault P, Pouliquen JC, Padovani JP, Guyonvarch G: La diatematomyelie (ou syndrome de la double chorde). Etude de 21 cas. Rev Chir Orthoped 66:123–139, 1980.
70. Lefevre J, Klein MR, Faure C: Diastematomyélie. Rev Neurol 94:357–362, 1956.
71. McCann P: Diastematomyelia. Irish J Med Sci 6:155–160, 1966.
72. Maroun FB, Jacob JC, Heneghan WD: La diastematomyélie, ses manifestations cliniques et son traitement chirurgical. Neurochirurgie 18:285–316, 1972.
73. Mathieu JP, Decarie M, Dube J, Marton D: La diastematomyélie. Etude de 69 cas. Chir Pediatr 23:29–35, 1982.
74. Perret G: Symptoms and diagnosis of diastematomyelia. Neurology 10:51–60, 1960.
75. Rigault P, Pouliquen JC, Guyonvarch G, Durand Y: Quatre cas de diastematomyélie. Rev Chir Orthop 58:33–50, 1972.
76. Ritchie GW, Flanagan MN: Diastematomyélia. CMAJ 100:, 1969.
77. Seaman WB, Schwartz HG: Diastematomyelia in adults. Radiology 70:692, 1958.
78. Shorey WD: Diastematomyelia associated with dorsal kyphosis producing paraplegia J Neurosurg 12:300–305, 1955.
79. Ugarte N, Gonzalez-Crussi F, Sotelo-Avila C: Diastematomyelia associated with teratomas. J Neurosurg 53:720–725, 1980.
80. English WJ, Maltby GL: Diastematomyelia in adults. J Neurosurg 27:260–264, 1967.
81. Albert-Jay L: La diastematomyélie. Rapport d'un cas chez l'adulte. Revue de la littérature. Thèse Méd Paris, 1979, 144 pp.
82. Chehrazi B, Haldeman S: Adult onset of tethered spinal cord syndrome due to fibrous diastematomyelia: case report. Neurosurgery 16:681–685, 1985.
83. Garcia FA, Kranzler LI, Siqueira EB, Weinberg PE, Kranzler KJ: Diastematomyelia in an adult. Surg Neurol 14:93–94, 1980.
84. Garza-Mercado R: Diastematomyelia and intramedullary epidermoïd spinal cord tumor combined with extradural teratoma in an adult: case report. J Neurosurg 58:954–958, 1983.
85. Kuhner A, Hame J, Krastell A, Banniza UK, Martin R: Rôle de la diastematomyélie dans le diagnostic différentiel et le traitement des paraplégies cypho-scoliotiques. Neurochirurgie 22:755–759, 1976.
86. McEwen GD, Bunnel WP, Sriram K: Acute neurological complications in the treatment of scoliosis. A report of the scoliosis research society. J Bone Joint Surg 57A:404, 1975.
87. Faithfull DK: Diastematomyelia complicating congenital scoliosis. J Neurosurg 18:538–541, 1961.
88. Tax HR, Person V, Tuccio M: A podiatric presentation of diastematomyelia. J Am Podiatry Assoc 72:337–341, 1982.
89. Claudy AL, Thivolet J, Meyer F: La diastematomyelie: une cause rare de mal perforant plantaire. Lyon Méd 6:503–509, 1976.
90. Mann KS, Khosla VK, Gulati DR, Malik AK: Spinal neurenteric cyst. Association with vertebral anomalies, diastematomyelia, dorsal fistula and lipoma. Surg Neurol 21:358–362, 1984.
91. Scatliff JH, Till K, Hoare RD: Incomplete, false and true diastematomyelia. Radiological evaluation by air myelography and tomography. Neuroradiology 116:349–354, 1975.

92. Weinstein MA, Rothner AD, Duchesnau P, Dohn DF: Computed tomography in diastematomyelia. Radiology 118:609–611, 1975.
93. Meacham WF: Surgical treatment of diastematomyelia. J Neurosurg 27:78–85, 1967.
94. Pang D, Parrish RG: Regrowth of diastematomyelic bone spur after extradural resection. J Neurosurg 59:887–890, 1983.
95. Gunasekera WSL, Richardson AE, Seneviratne KN, Eversden ID: Clinical correlation of urodynamic findings in patients with localized partial lesions of the spinal cord and cauda equina. Surg Neurol 21:148–154, 1984.

CHAPTER 5

Spondylolisthesis

L. Aulisa and F. Serra

History

Anterior displacement of the fifth lumbar vertebral body (L5) over the sacrum was first described in 1782 by the Belgian obstetrician Herbinaux,[1] but not until 1854 did Kilian[2,3] first use the term "spondylolisthesis" (from *spondylos*, meaning vertebra and *olisthesis*, meaning slippage) to refer to this condition. He noted that the displacement occurs progressively and hypothesized a slow subluxation of the facets as its cause.

In 1855 Robert,[4] using experimental models, concluded that an interruption of the posterior vertebral arch (and, in particular, of the pars interarticularis, i.e., spondylolysis) is necessary for the onset of spondylolisthesis. Subsequent anatomopathologic studies demonstrated that spondylolisthesis is not always associated with spondylolysis. Neugebauer,[5] in 1888, for example, reported that displacement of the vertebra could be caused by an elongation of the pars interarticularis rather than by its actual lysis.

Classification

Recently, radiologic data obtained from extensive case studies have allowed a more accurate description of the various conditions from which spondylolisthesis may arise. Most authors use the pathogenic classification proposed by Wiltse et al.[6] and approved by the International Society for the Study of the Lumbar Spine. Other very valid classification systems have, however, been proposed by Taillard in 1957,[7] Pipino in 1970,[8] and Marchetti and Bartolozzi in 1984.[9] According to Wiltse et al., there exist five types of spondylolisthesis.

Dysplastic Spondylolisthesis

According to Newman,[10] 25% of all cases of spondylolisthesis occurring in children fall into this category. Dysplastic spondylolisthesis develops due to the presence of congenital malformations of the sacrum and of the posterior verte-

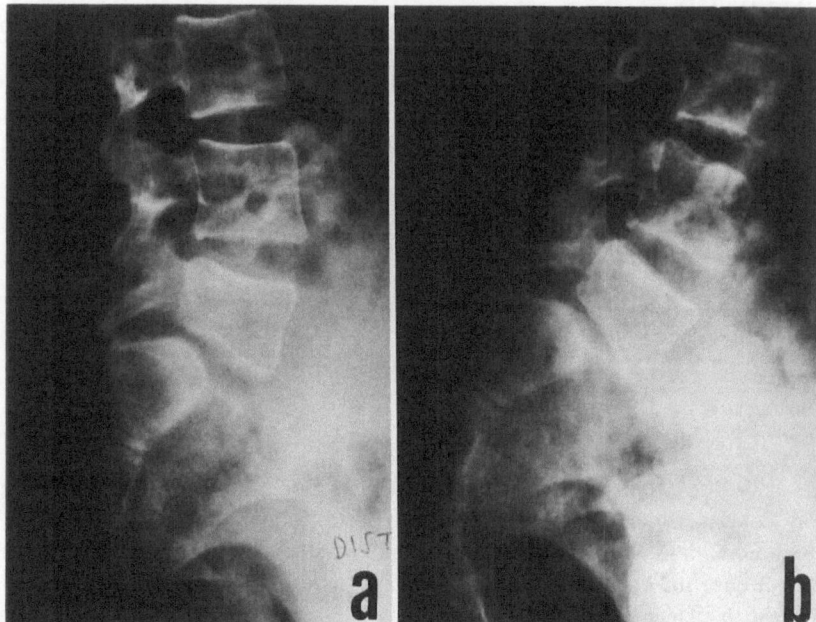

Figure 5.1. a: A 12-year-old female with dysplastic spondylolisthesis. True lumbo-sacral subluxation is represented by articular aplasia plus hypoplasia of the pars interarticularis and of the upper surface of the sacrum. **b**: The same patient after 1 year: the displacement has worsened considerably and luxation of the articular facets is now present.

bral arch of L5. This represents a true lumbo-sacral subluxation (Fig. 5.1). Malformations such as hypoplasia of the upper surface of the body of the first sacral vertebra, hypoplasia or aplasia of the facets, elongation of the pars interarticularis, and spina bifida all reduce the efficiency of the stabilizing system represented by the posterior articular complex. Displacement may be quite severe, and when it exceeds 25%, the patient may be affected by a cauda equina syndrome or by a compression radiculopathy. The neurologic syndrome is less severe and may even be absent when lysis of the pars interarticularis, a not uncommon event, occurs (Fig. 5.2).

Isthmic Spondylolisthesis

This is the most frequent type of spondylolisthesis in patients under 50 years of age. The cause is always a lesion of the pars interarticularis. Two main subgroups can be distinguished: in the first, the condition develops because of an interruption of the pars interarticularis (spondylolysis), whereas in the second type, the pathogenic factor is an elongation, rather than an actual break, in this structure. This elongation may be congenital, or it may be the result of microfractures of the

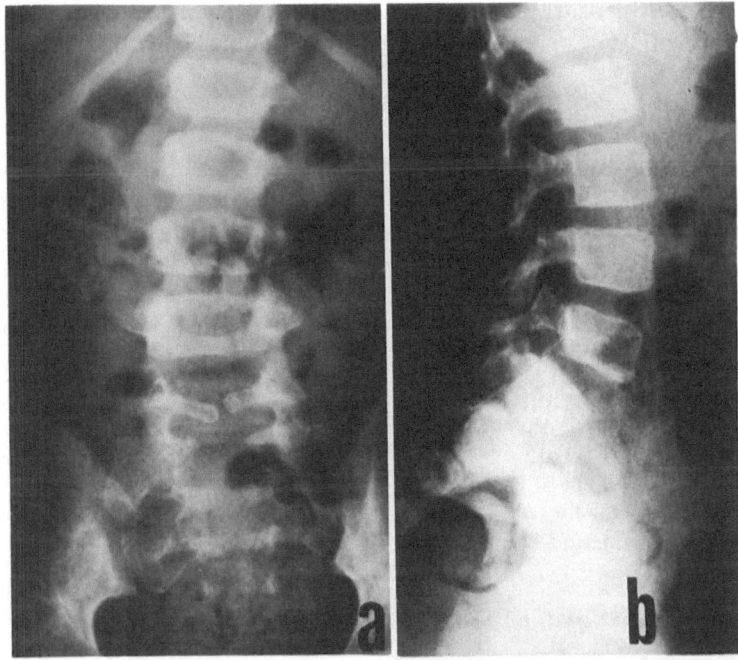

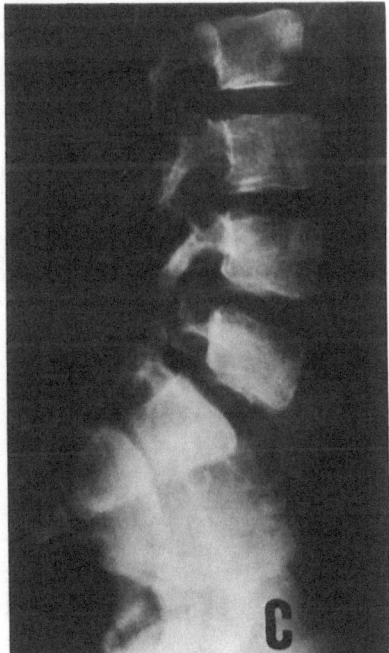

Figure 5.2. A 9-year-old female with dysplastic spondylolisthesis characterized by (**a** and **b**) hypoplasia of the articular facets, hypoplasia and elongation of the pars interarticularis, and spina bifida. **c**: The same patient 2 years later: lysis of the pars interarticularis has occurred, rendering the situation less dramatic.

pars interarticularis. If the vertebra is subjected to significant tangential forces while these fractures are healing, an elongation of the bony callus will result.

Degenerative Spondylolisthesis

Some moderate cases of spondylolisthesis may be provoked by degenerative alterations associated with spondylolisthesis, such as structural destruction of the capsule and ligaments of the posterior joints and the consequent hypermobility of the affected spinal segment. Degenerative spondylolisthesis is typically found in patients over 50 years of age and affects females more frequently than males. Junghann's pseudospondylolisthesis is to be included in this category.[11]

Traumatic Spondylolisthesis

This form is fairly rare because an extremely violent trauma is necessary to fracture the posterior arch. It is usually associated with other bone or soft tissue lesions. Rather than a true spondylolisthesis, this condition is more accurately described as a fracture-luxation.

Pathologic Spondylolisthesis

Slippage of the vertebral body, in this case, is due to the destruction of the posterior arch by infectious diseases, neoplasia, or malacic diseases, such as Paget's disease or Albers–Schoenberg's disease. Modification of the structure and reduced mechanical resistance of the bone lead to an elongation of the pars interarticularis.

This chapter will deal primarily with isthmic spondylolisthesis, which is by far the most commonly seen form in children and young adults. The term "spondylolisthesis," then, will hereafter refer to that anatomic pathology in which the most important feature is a lysis of the pars interarticularis with an anterior displacement of the vertebral body, pedicles, superior facets, and transverse processes. The inferior facets, laminae, and spinous process remain in place.

Pathogenesis and Natural History

Four theories on the pathogenesis of spondylolisthesis currently exist:

Congenital Theory

The spondylolysis is believed to be caused by a defect in the fusion of the two separate centers of ossification of the posterior arch.

Traumatic Theory

The lysis is actually a fracture caused by trauma undergone in either the position of flexion or that of extension.

Trophostatic Theory

Lysis of the pars interarticularis is thought to be caused by bony necrosis which results from compression of the arteries nourishing the area by facets that are subluxated in response to hyperlordosis.[12] Nathan[13] completed this theory with his statement that the lysis is actually a result of a slow lysis of the pars interarticularis provoked not only by the mechanical overload brought on by hyperlordosis, but also by a pinching of the pars interarticularis by the facets which are often hypertrophic.

Dysplastic Theory

The lysis is believed to be the result of normal mechanical forces applied in the erect position to a congenitally dysplastic area caused by a disturbance in ossification.[7,14] This dysplasia may be characterized by hypoplasia and elongation of the pars interarticularis or by cystic formations, cracks, areas of bone reabsorption, or sclerosis involving the entire posterior arch.

There are appealing elements in all of these theories, and each of them can be at least partially supported by clinical and experimental observations. The high incidence of spondylolisthesis observed in certain ethnic groups and the hereditary nature of the lesion lend credence to the first theory. While many authors estimate the incidence of spondylolisthesis in the Caucasian race to be approximately 5% (Neugebauer, 5%[15] Willis, 5.19%;[16] Rowe and Roche, 4.2%[17]), the rate observed among the Japanese, Bantus, and Eskimoes is considerably higher. Stewart[18] found that, among the Eskimoes of the northern Yukon, a population in which consanguineous mating is common, the incidence of spondylolisthesis was 40% among males and 37% among females.

The hereditability of the lesion has been confirmed by various studies conducted on family members of patients affected by spondylolysis: Baker,[19] for example, found that 28% of the parents of 18 children with spondylolysis had lesions themselves. Friberg[20] found lesions in seven out of nine children whose parents both suffered from spondylolisthesis.

In spite of these facts, there are two incontrovertible objections that can be raised against the congenital theory: (1) the pars interarticularis does not contain two separate centers of ossification and (2) lysis of the pars interarticularis has never been described in either a fetus or in a neonate. The youngest patient reported to have had such a lesion was 4 months old.[21]

The traumatic theory is based on the fact that many patients with spondylolisthesis have recent histories of trauma. In addition, there are a number of documented cases of spondylolysis that were found to have occurred following violent trauma in persons in whom the pars interarticularis was structurally normal (Fig. 5.3). However, experimental studies,[22] as well as extensive case studies on vertebral trauma, have demonstrated that an isolated fracture of the pars interarticularis provoked by trauma is extremely rare. Many authors, on the basis of evidence from large case studies, believe that the lysis should be considered to be a stress fracture rather than the result of a single traumatic event. The most

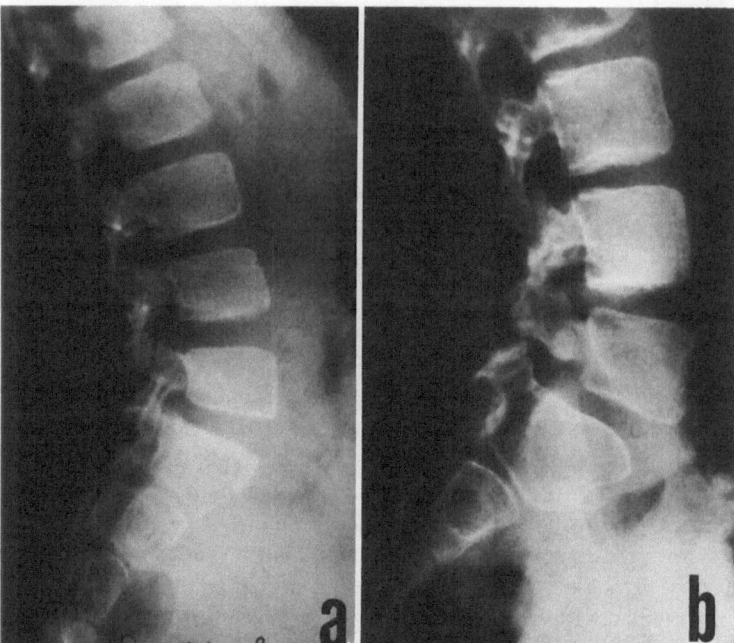

Figure 5.3. A 16-year-old male with isthmic spondylolisthesis thought to have occurred following trauma to a normally formed pars interarticularis. **a**: A lateral view of the spine obtained at age 9 for urologic complaints reveals no anatomic alterations whatsoever in the lumbo-sacral spine. **b**: A second film taken 7 years later following complaints of chronic lumbago shows lysis of the pars interarticularis and early anterior displacement of L5. The patient attributed his pain to a violent trauma undergone 1 year prior to the second film.

indicative studies have been carried out on athletes. A high incidence of spondylolysis, often involving more than one vertebra, has in fact been noted among those professional athletes (52% among gymnasts and 49% among weight lifters) whose spines, and in particular, the pars interarticularis, undergo severe and repeated dynamic stress.[23-25] The microtraumatic theory alone, however, fails to account for the hereditary nature of most cases of spondylolysis.

The dysplastic theory offers a valid contribution to the resolution of this apparent contradiction: the dysplasia would represent a congenital factor that predisposes the patient to the occurrence of lysis, the actual onset of which would be triggered by the mechanical stresses described above. This pathogenetic chain of events would seem to be confirmed by the fact that spondylolysis occurs neither in quadripeds nor in patients who have never walked.[26] Moreover, the lesion is found predominantly at the level of L5, which is the portion of the vertebral column that is subjected to the greatest amount of static and dynamic stress associated with daily activities.

Interaction between the biologic component and the mechanical one is confirmed further by the natural histories of both spondylolysis and spondylolisthesis. Spondylolysis is, in fact, rare in patients less than 5 years of age, frequent in those between 7 and 10 years of age, and appears very rarely after the age of 20. Not all cases of spondylolysis evolve into spondylolisthesis. There is some degree of conflict in the results of the various case studies concerning this latter point: estimates range from 2 to 3% by Delpierre[27] to 50% by Nachemson.[28] The latter author points out, however, that only a small percentage of these patients suffered displacements exceeding 30%.

The evolution is, in any case, a gradual process and generally occurs between the 10th and 15th year of life during the period of rapid growth. These data demonstrate that, similar to that which occurs in scoliosis, mechanical stresses are capable of bringing about a significant evolution only when the plasticity of the bony structure is at its maximum as occurs during puberty. In the presence of an evolving lesion, in fact, the severity of the deformity is proportional to the velocity of the growth rate.

Pathologic Features

It is quite difficult to document completely the pathologic features of spondylolysis because observation and study of the lesion at the time of its onset are almost impossible. Studies based on autopsy and/or intra-operative observations deal almost exclusively with late-stage lesions which some authors consider to be invertebrate pseudoarthrosis.

Spondylolysis appears as a defect of the bony substance at the level of the pars interarticularis, just below the superior facets and the transverse processes. The extent of the gap is proportional to the degree of spondylolisthesis. The surfaces of the bone surrounding the defect are smooth, regular, and structurally normal. The lesion is filled with a fibrous tissue, often hypertrophic, which extends on to the normal bone to which it is firmly attached. In younger patients, the surfaces of the bone adjacent to the lesion may be less regular and the borders may be indented. The tissue found in the gap may be fibro-cartilaginous.

The alterations found in spondylolisthesis are all secondary to the spondylolysis, which divides the vertebra into two segments and thus deprives the vertebral body of its posterior anchorage. The pedicles, superior articular, and transverse processes remain attached to the vertebral body, while the lamina and inferior articular and spinous processes are anchored to the superior facets of the vertebra below.

From a lateral direction, the body of the slipped vertebra has a trapezoidal shape with the anterior edge higher than the posterior. Because of the progressive degeneration of the disk, the intervertebral space becomes markedly reduced and may, in the adult, nearly disappear. Friction between the inferior border of the displaced vertebral body and the vertebra below it leads to erosion and sclerosis of the former. An inferior concavity develops and the deformity resembles an

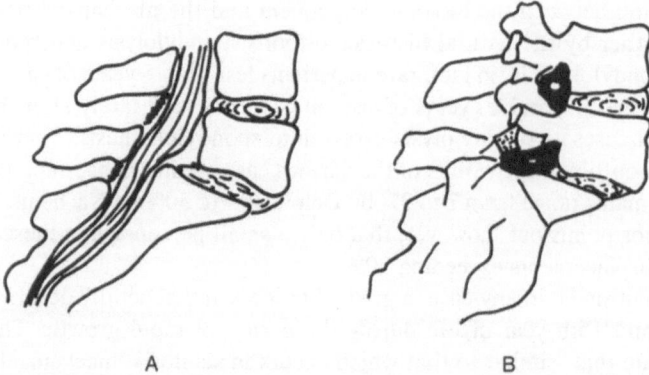

A   B

Figure 5.4. Anatomopathologic alterations of the vertebral canal and of the foramina that occur in spondylolisthesis.

italic letter S. The pathologic contact between these two vertebrae causes deformation of the lower one as well. An anterior osteophyte on the superior surface of the sacrum is found only in adult patients.

Deformities of the spinal canal and of the foramina, as well as alterations that occur in the nerves themselves, are particularly interesting because of their clinical implications. The spinal canal of the displaced vertebra has an ovoid shape because of the increased anterior–posterior diameter which is proportional to the degree of slippage. The relatively posterior position of the vertebra below and the abrupt return to a normal anterior–posterior diameter of the spinal canal causes the "bayonet deformity." This alteration is typical of those cases of spondylolisthesis caused by lysis of the pars interarticularis, which affects only the anterior wall of the spinal canal (Fig. 5.4A). The foramen of the involved vertebra is smaller than normal and angled due to an anterior–inferior displacement of that part of the pedicle that remains attached to the vertebral body. The slippage is caused by forces that are transmitted to the pars interarticularis through the inferior facets of the vertebra above. Degeneration of the disk causes a further narrowing of the intervertebral space and, consequently, of the foramen (Fig. 5.4B).

Alterations of the cauda and of the nerve roots are the direct result of the skeletal changes. Deformity of the cauda is usually minimal because of its position in the posterior part of the spinal canal, which, as has already been noted, is not deformed. When, on the other hand, the posterior arch is not interrupted (pseudospondylolisthesis), damage to the cauda may be more severe. In spondylolisthesis due to spondylolysis, the nerve roots appear very taut because of the narrowing of the foramen and the deformity of the sagittal axis of the spinal canal.

Clinical Manifestations

The clinical manifestations of spondylolysis and spondylolisthesis are extremely variable and may often be so surprising as to obscure the true cause of the patient's pain. Most cases are completely asymptomatic, which means that there are a significant number of patients affected by these two conditions who will be diagnosed only on the basis of x-ray films obtained for other reasons.

In symptomatic patients, moreover, there often exists a notable discrepancy between clinical and radiographic findings. The patient with severe spondylolisthesis or spondylolysis may have few or no complaints, whereas those with spondylolysis in which there is only slight displacement may suffer severe low back pain or sciatica. It is, furthermore, fairly uncommon that symptoms, when present, are reported to have appeared during childhood or early youth. This is the period in which lysis begins and the displacement occurs, and the reason for the delay in the appearance of symptoms is not yet clear. Lafond[29] reported that, of the 415 patients he observed, only 23% experienced problems prior to the age of 20 years. It is difficult, then, to establish with certainty the percentage of symptomatic cases of spondylolysis and spondylolisthesis that occur before bone growth is completed. Most authors agree, however, with Marique's[30] estimate of approximately 20%.

When symptoms do appear in the young patient, their initiation usually coincides with the period of rapid growth experienced during puberty (between 10 and 15 years of age) when slippage of the vertebral body occurs. The patient often complains of lumbago following lower back strain or prolonged periods of sitting. In other instances, no specific factor can be related to the onset of symptoms.

The pain is usually located in the lower portion of the lumbar spine. Lumbosacral pain is seldom reported, and it is quite rare that a patient will complain of pain in the dorso-lumbar region. The pain may become more intense following strenuous activities and may be alleviated or disappear entirely with rest. Very rarely, and only in those cases of severe spondylolisthesis, the lumbar pain radiates to one or both of the gluteal regions and the posterior thighs. Clinical symptoms of nerve root compression, although rare in children, are common in adult patients. The nerve trunks in a subject who is still growing adapt more easily to the forces of traction and compression caused by the displaced vertebra. The cauda equina syndrome may occur in cases of grade IV spondylolisthesis or in spondyloptosis.

Contracture of the ischio-crural muscles, either isolated or associated with other symptoms, may be seen in both spondylolysis and spondylolisthesis. The cause of this hypertonia is not yet clear. Radicular irritation caused by the increased tension applied to the filum terminale by the unstable vertebral segment could be the cause. The contracture, in fact, disappears completely following surgical stabilization or even conservative treatment of the spondylolisthesis. The degree of contracture varies from patient to patient. Severe forms cause typical changes in the posture and gait of the patient. Flexion of the hips and knees, retroversion of the pelvis, and flattening of the lumbar concavity are present in both the erect and supine resting positions. Attempts to extend the hips passively cause pain and usually meet with very limited success.

Ambulation does not usually provoke pain, but the gait of these patients is quite characteristic: the child takes small steps, holding his legs rigid and rotating the pelvis. Often, to maintain the flexed position of the knees, the child walks on his toes.

Clinically, spondylolisthesis of the IVth degree and spondyloptosis are characterized by a progressive shortening of the trunk and postural changes to compensate for the anterior displacement of the center of gravity. As the trunk shortens, a typical transverse cutaneous fold appears at the level of the umbilicus. The pelvis rotates in order to bring the sacrum into a vertical position, resulting in a flattening of the gluteal region, which, due to the sacral prominence, resembles a heart. The hips rotate with the pelvis and assume a flexed position. Active extension is impossible. Exaggerated lordosis is present in that segment of the spine cranial to the displacement (Fig. 5.10).

In the presence of the above-mentioned findings, clinical diagnosis of spondylolisthesis may be easy. In the majority of cases, however, such is not the case. While diagnosis of spondylolysis is impossible solely on the basis of the physical examination, spondylolisthesis should be suspected when a characteristic "stair step" can be palpated between the spinous processes of two adjacent vertebrae.

Radiographic Features

Radiologic examination forms the basis not only for diagnosing spondylolysis and spondylolisthesis, but also for evaluating the etiology, gravity, and evolution of these conditions. Standard radiographic techniques may, in many cases, be sufficient, but there are several complementary exams that may, at times, prove helpful.

Basic Radiologic Examination

Standard radiologic films should include anterior–posterior, lateral, and right and left oblique views.

Anterior–Posterior View

Diagnosis can rarely be made on the basis of this view alone, though indirect signs of spondylolysis or spondylolisthesis may appear. A change in the alignment of the spinous processes, for example, should suggest the presence of either mono- or bilateral lysis. Shifting of the spinous processes is, in fact, a radiographic expression of a relative rotation between two vertebrae due to the instability caused by the defect in the posterior arch. Degenerative arthritic changes in the articular facets, typical of rotatory luxation in the adult, are never seen in

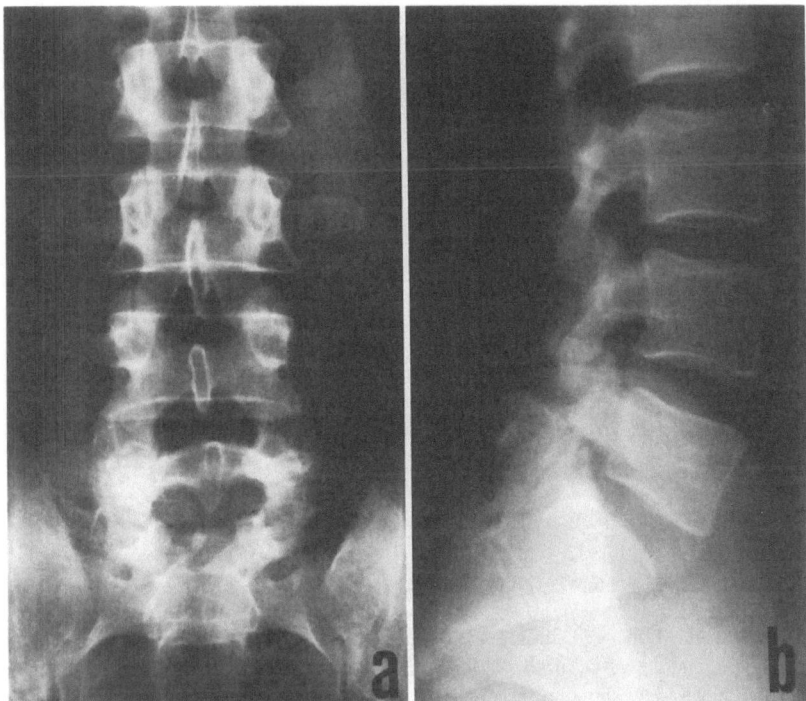

Figure 5.5. A 16-year-old male with isthmic spondylolysis of L5. **a:** The antero-posterior view shows indirect signs of spondylolysis: "shifting" of the spinous processes and "aniso-coria" of the pedicles due to hyperostosis. **b:** The lateral view confirms the diagnosis of spondylolysis.

children. The presence of a disalignment in the spinous processes in a young sub-ject is therefore often an indication of pars interarticularis pathology.

A hyperostosis of one half of the posterior arch, defined by the French as "ver-tebral anisocoria," may be an indirect sign of lysis in the contralateral half of the arch. The hyperostosis is, in these cases, a result of the functional overload placed on the uninvolved half of the arch (Fig. 5.5). The image of an "inverted Napoleon's cap," described by De Seze and Durieu[31] is a characteristic finding in severe spondylolisthesis and spondyloptosis. The image is a projection of the body and transverse processes of L5 on the sacrum (Fig. 5.6).

Lateral View

Lateral views of the spine are the most significant films to consider in this pathol-ogy, though they are not always sufficient to document spondylolysis. The lysis, when visible, appears in these films as a hypo-opaque oblique fissure, slanted antero-inferiorly, which involves the pars interarticularis and separates the

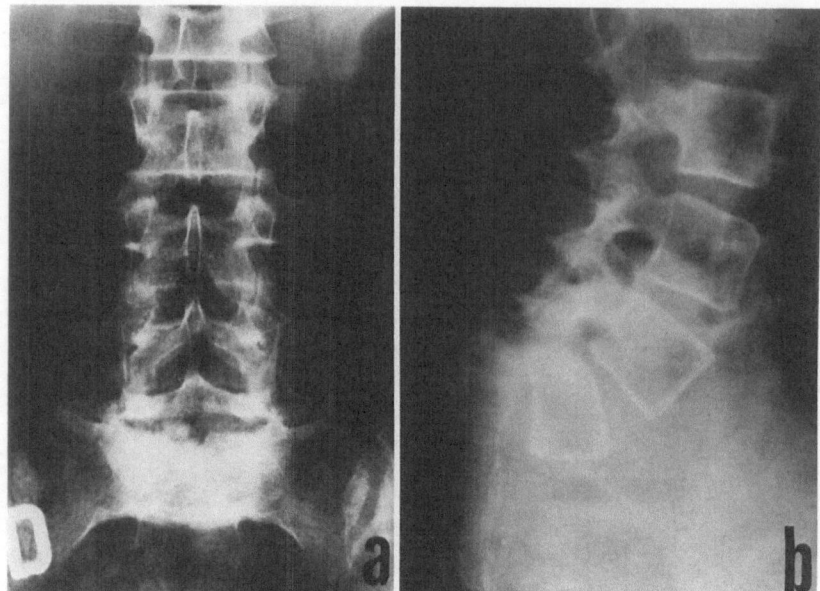

Figure 5.6. A 10-year-old female with spondylolysis of L5. **a**: Antero-posterior view showing the characteristic image described by De Seze as an "upside down Napoleon's cap." **b**: Lateral view showing the ptosis.

vertebral body and superior articular processes from the rest of the posterior arch. The width of the fissure depends on the age of the lysis and on the degree of slippage. The pars interarticularis usually appears elongated and hypoplastic. Particularly when the patient is standing, the lateral view permits the physician to locate and assess alterations, not only in the displaced vertebra, but also in the adjacent vertebrae and intervertebral disks.

Various methods may be used to evaluate the degree of slippage: Meyerding[32] divided the upper surface of the body of the first sacral vertebra (S1) into four sections and, by projecting the intersection of the posterior margin of the displaced vertebra with each of these sections, defined four degrees of displacement (Fig. 5.7). Grade I describes displacements of 0 to 25%, whereas in grade III the displacement may be up to 75%. Displacement of more than 75% is defined as spondyloptosis.

Marique[30] and Taillard's[7] method, though more complicated, provides a more precise evaluation of the displacement (Fig. 5.8). Two lines are drawn: one tangent to the lower surface of the displaced vertebra and the second tangent to the upper surface of the vertebra below. Using the intersection of these two lines as a center point, three arcs are then traced: arc 1 is drawn tangent to the posterior border of the lower vertebra; arc 2, tangent to the anterior border of the same vertebra; and arc 3, tangent to the posterior border of the olisthetic vertebra. The

Figure 5.7. Meyerding's method for classifying four degrees of displacement in spondylolisthesis.

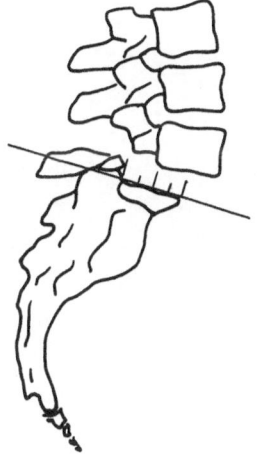

distance between arcs 1 and 2 (B) thus represents the length of the surface of the body of the normal vertebra, whereas the distance between arcs 1 and 3 (A) represents the displacement. Using the ratio A:B :: X:100, one can obtain the percentage of displacement.

Dynamic radiologic studies carried out during maximum flexion and maximum extension may also be helpful in evaluating the stability of the lesion.

45° Oblique Views

Forty-five-degree oblique view from both the right and left allow more detailed study of the posterior arch which appears on x-ray film in the typical image of

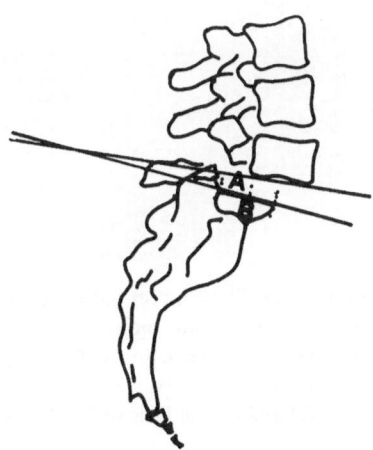

Figure 5.8. Marique–Taillard method for determining the percentage of vertebral displacement.

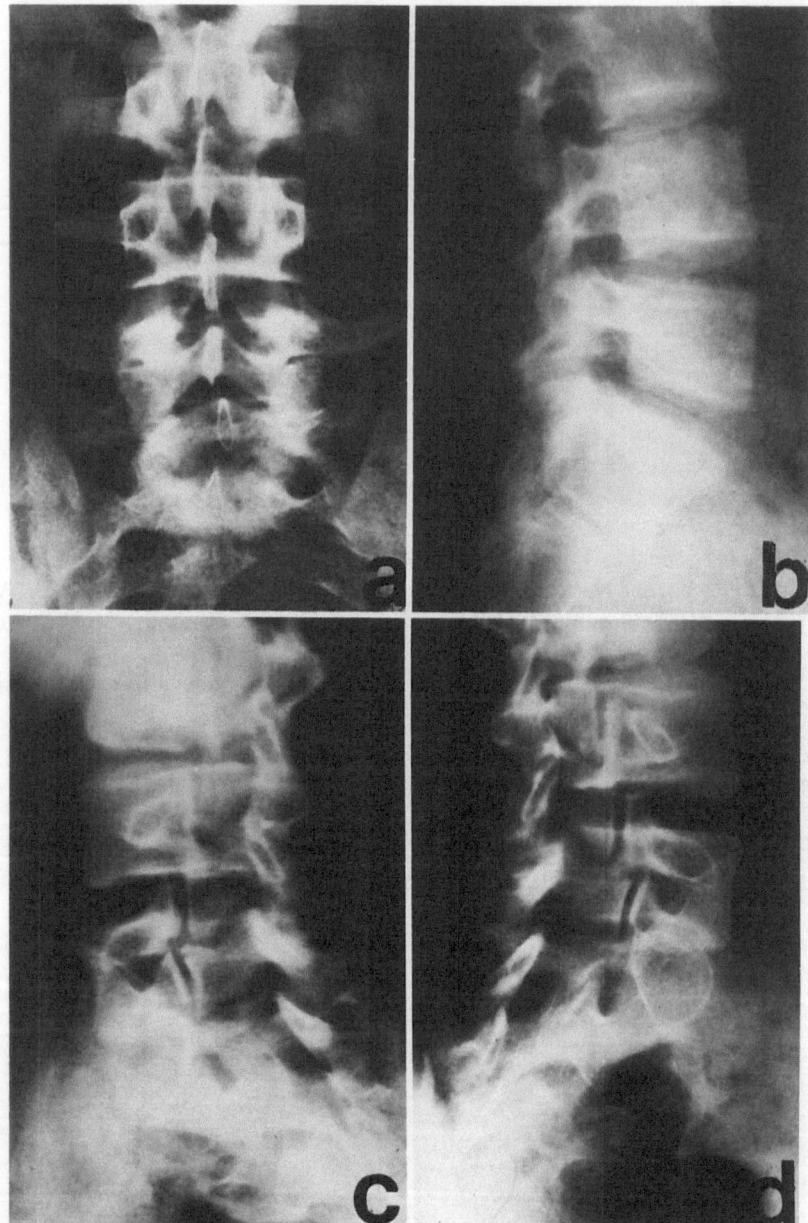

Figure 5.9. Sixteen-year-old male with monoisthmic spondylolysis of L5. **a**: Anterior–posterior view shows indirect signs of spondylolysis, such as disalignment of the spinous processes and "anisocoria vertebrale". **b**: The lateral view is completely negative. **c**, **d**: Oblique views, however, clearly show complete lysis of the pars interarticularis on the right (**c**) and partial lysis on the left (**d**).

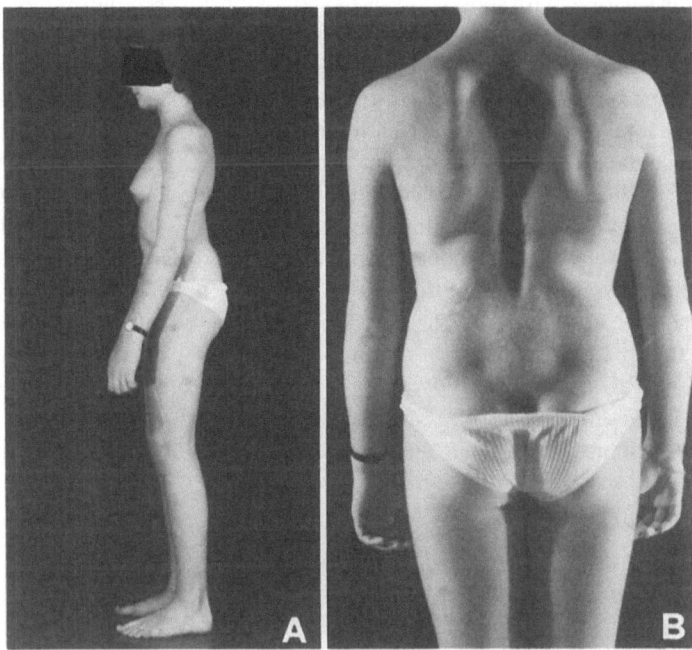

Figure 5.10. Ten-year-old female affected by spondyloptosis involving L5. Her radiologic films can be seen in Fig. 5.6. **A:** Typical posture associated with this condition caused by contracture of the ischio-crural muscles and characterized by flexion of the hips and knees and retroversion of the pelvis. The center of gravity is displaced anteriorly. **B:** Shortening of the trunk and flattening of the gluteal region which, due to the prominence of the sacrum, resembles a heart.

Lachapelle's dog: the pars interarticularis forms the neck of the dog; the transverse process, the snout; and the pedicle, the eye. The body of the dog is formed by the laminae and the superior and inferior articular processes represent respectively the ears and front legs. The pars interarticularis can be clearly seen from both the right and left, permitting the physician to diagnose spondylolysis with certainty. When the pars interarticularis is interrupted, the image previously described changes to that of a decapitated dog (Fig. 5.9). The physician is thus able to diagnose both mono- and bilateral spondylolysis and to evaluate the anatomic characteristics of the lesion itself. Morphologic alterations of the pars interarticularis, such as elongation or hypoplasia, can also be well documented.

Complementary Examinations

Tomography is indicated only in those cases in which an incomplete evolving lysis is suspected. Severe progressive compression radiculopathy that is resistant to therapy in a patient with spondylolysis or spondylolisthesis requires *myelography* to rule out the presence of a non-olisthetic cause for the compression. A concomitant lesion, such as a neoplasm, should be suspected in the presence of other neurologic symptoms, sphincter disturbances, or perineal hypoesthesia. Herniation of the intervertebral disk, rare in the adult patient with spondylolisthesis, has never been documented in children or adolescents with this condition. When it does occur, the herniation involves the disk above the olisthetic vertebra. The myelograms of patients with spondylolysis show no pathologic features. In spondylolisthesis, an impression appears on the anterior surface of the dura made by either the posterior margin of the sacrum or that of the vertebra underlying the displaced one. In some cases, the nerve roots are laterally displaced and seem to adhere tightly to the walls of the foramina without any apparent amputation.

Computed tomography and *nuclear magnetic resonance studies* provide very graphic images of these lesions, but do not offer any real further information that cannot be obtained from other types of studies for the diagnosis or treatment of these conditions.

Therapeutic Approaches

Various therapeutic approaches may be chosen depending on the age of the patient at the time of the initial visit. In the adult patient with spondylolisthesis, the decision of whether or not to begin treatment should be based on the severity of symptoms. The onset of pain, although not an accurate index of the degree of deformity, is a sign of vertebral instability. In children and adolescents, on the other hand, the physician should take into account not only the symptomatology but also the evolutionary characteristics of the lesion itself.

Spondylolysis

Asymptomatic spondylolysis, which represents the great majority of cases, requires no treatment. Radiologic examination should be performed every 6 months during the period of rapid growth to evaluate progression of the lesion. Physical activity should by no means be restricted in these patients. When symptoms do appear, the spinal column should be immobilized in a position of correct lordosis using a plaster or plastic corset. The corset should be worn 24 hours a day for a minimum of 6 months. The patient should also undergo an intensive regimen of physiotherapy aimed principally at maintaining muscle tone. In most cases, this therapeutic approach is capable not only of totally relieving pain and other possible symptoms, but often of bringing about a complete resolution of the lysis itself. When conservative, noninvasive therapy fails, and all other causes of the lumbar pain have been ruled out, surgical stabilization of the lesion is indicated.

Spondylolisthesis

The choice of therapy for the child or adolescent with spondylolisthesis depends on the symptomatology, severity, and progression of the displacement. Patients with grade I asymptomatic spondylolisthesis require only the periodic radiologic evaluation described in the previous discussion of spondylolysis. In these cases, however, it is advisable to restrict those activities and sports that place increased strain on the unstable vertebra. Further limitations are not necessary.

Grade I displacement associated with symptoms requires conservative orthopedic treatment. Most cases respond well to such an approach, and only a few will require surgical stabilization. In grade II spondylolisthesis, surgery is indicated not only when symptoms persist, but also when progression of the displacement has been demonstrated. The presence of risk factors such as spina bifida or hypoplasia of the articular facets are also indications for surgery in the prepubertal or pubertal patient, as are anatomic findings such as verticalization of the sacrum, trapezoidal profile of the displaced vertebra, or convexity of the body of the first sacral vertebra. Surgical intervention is always indicated in cases of grade III and grade IV spondylolisthesis.

The choice of the surgical technique to be used from among the many that have been proposed is often difficult. The large variety of techniques currently being used testifies to the fact that none of them is able to offer the perfect solution for the numerous anatomic varieties of spondylolisthesis, and much less for the most severe forms of this condition. Although it is impossible to describe all of the procedures now in use, we will discuss those most commonly performed.

Removal of the Posterior Arch and Neurolysis

When the surgeon is convinced that the patient's symptoms are secondary to hypermobility of the posterior arch and invasion of the foramina by the fibrocartilaginous tissue from the area of the lysis, removal of the posterior arch and neurolysis is indicated. This technique, proposed by Gill[37] in 1955, involves ablation of the posterior arch, opening of the ligamentum flavum, and neurolysis. The indication for this type of surgery is controversial. Gill himself pointed out that the procedure is unsuitable for the treatment of patients who are not yet fully grown because of the high risk in these patients of aggravating the spondylolisthesis as a result of the destabilization which undoubtedly follows removal of the posterior arch.[38-41]

Arthrodesis

In situ stabilization of the vertebral column by arthrodesis can be performed either postero-laterally or anteriorly.

Postero-Lateral Arthrodesis

Posterior fusion has been found to be associated with numerous treatment failures caused by sequelae such as pseudoarthrosis or plastic deformation of the transplant itself. For these reasons, Watkins,[41] in 1953, proposed that the fusion be extended to the lateral surfaces of the articular and transverse processes. In spondylolysis and grade I spondylolisthesis involving L5, arthrodesis is performed between L5 and the sacrum. In more severe cases, the fusion should be extended to L4 as well. This procedure is relatively simple to perform and produces excellent results with spondylolysis or with spondylolisthesis involving less than 50% displacement.[28,35,36,42-45]

Fusion of Vertebral Bodies

Following diskectomy, arthrodesis is performed between the body of the displaced vertebra and that of the one underneath. Sicard and Tonzard[46] and Freebody et al.[47] describe an anterior transperitoneal approach via subumbilical median laparotomy to gain access to L5. Wiltberger[48] and Cloward,[49] however, prefer a posterior approach, and using Gill's technique, remove the posterior arch prior to fusion of the vertebral bodies. The results obtainable with this interbody fusion are comparable to those that can be seen with the postero-lateral technique. The latter is more popular because of the ease with which it can be performed, as well as because of the lower rate of complications that occur with its use.

Arthrodesis Following Reduction of the Listhesis

Osteosynthesis has made an important contribution to the solution of the problem of obtaining a reduction of the displacement prior to stabilization as well as to that of maintaining the reduction after arthrodesis. In fact, before the introduction of this technique, stabilization attempts by Harris[50] and Neuman[70] among others, had proved unsuccessful because of the impossibility of maintaining the obtained correction during the period of the consolidation of the arthrodesis. Complete reduction is still impossible, but noninvasive techniques such as that of Scaglietti[51,52] and/or surgical procedures, such as those of Harrington et al.,[53,54] Roy-Camille et al.[55] and Louis and Maresca[56] can produce a partial reduction of the displacement. The indication for reduction, either pre- or intra-operatively, of spondylolisthesis of less than 50% is still open for discussion. As was pointed out previously, excellent results can be obtained in these cases using simple in situ arthrodesis. Noninvasive reduction procedures can still be useful in these patients when sciatic neuralgia is present. Several authors[57-59] have observed complete remission of symptoms following even partial reduction of this type, thus avoiding the need to explore the nerve roots and dura surgically.

Persistence of symptoms, on the other hand, requires that other causes for the compression be sought. When displacement exceeds 50%, in situ fusion is no longer capable of arresting the evolution of the deformity,[35,60-63] given the considerable forces that are placed on the arthrodesis itself. In these cases, reduction becomes obligatory.[52,56,59,61,62,65] Following reduction and stabilization using osteosynthesis, arthrodesis can be performed using either the postero-lateral or anterior approach. In extremely severe cases, to obtain greater stability, combined arthrodesis (anterior and postero-lateral) is often necessary.

References

1. Herbinaux G: Troite sur divers accouchments laborieux e sur le polypes de la matrice. JL, De Boubers, Bruxelles, 1782.
2. Kilian HF: De Spondylolisthesi gravissimae pelvangustiae causa nuper detecta, commentatio anatomico-obstetrica. Lit c Georgii, Bonnae, 1854.
3. Kilian HF: Schilderungen neuer Beckenformen und ihres Verholtens in Leven, Mannheim: Verlag von Vassermann 8 Mathy, 1854.
4. Robert L: Monatsschrift fur Geburtskunde und Frauenkrankheiten.
5. Neugebauer Fl: A new contribution to the history and etiology of spondylolisthesis. The New Sydenham Society, London, 121, 1888.
6. Wiltse LL, Newman PH, Macnab I: Classification of spondylolysis and spondylolisthesis. Clin Orthop 117:23–29, 1976.
7. Taillard W: Le spondylolistésis. Masson, Paris, 1957.
8. Pipino F: Le spondylolistesi: classificazione, quadro clinico e radiologico, terapia incruente, valutazione medico-legale. LV Cong SIOT, Napoli, 1970.
9. Marchetti PG, Bartolozzi P: Le spondilolistesi: classificazione ed etiopatogenesi. Prog Pat Vert 6:9–16, 1984.
10. Newman PH: A clinical syndrome associated with severe lumbo-sacral subluxation. J Bone Joint Surg 47B:472–481, 1975.
11. Junghanns H: Spondylolisthesis, pseudo-spondylolisthesis und Wirbelscheibung nach Hinten. Bruns Beitr Klin Chir 151:376–382, 1931.
12. Meyer H, Burgdorff H: Untersuchuhgen uber das Wirbelgleiten. Thieme, Leipzig, 1931.
13. Nathan H: Spondylolysis: its anatomy and mechanism of development. J Bone Joint Surg 41A:303–310, 1959.
14. Brocher I: Die Pathogenese der Spondylolisthesis mit besonderer Berucksichtigung ihrer Beziehung Unfallheilkunde. Langeb Arch u Dtsch Chir 276:329–336, 1953.
15. Neugebauer FL: The classic: a new contribution to the history and etiology of spondylolisthesis. Clin Orthop 117:4–22, 1976.
16. Willis TA: The separate neural arch. J Bone Joint Surg 13:709–721, 1931.
17. Rowe GG, Roche MA: The etiology of separate neural arch. J Bone Joint Surg 35A:102–110, 1953.
18. Stewart TD: The age incidence of neural arch defects in Alaskan natives, considered from the standpoint of etiology. J Bone Joint Surg 35A:937–940, 1953.
19. Baker DR, McHollick W: Spondyloschisis and spondylolisthesis in children. J Bone Joint Surg 38A:933–934, 1956.
20. Friberg S: Studies on spondylolisthesis. Acta Chir Scand 82(suppl 55): 1939.
21. Borkow SE, Kleiger B: Spondylolisthesis in the newborn. A case report. Clin Orthop 81:73–76, 1971.
22. Hitchcock HH: Spondylolisthesis: observations on its development, progression and genesis. J Bone Joint Surg 22:1–7, 1940.
23. Jackson DW, Wiltse LL, Cirincione RJ: Spondylolysis in the female gymnast. Clin Orthop 117:68–73, 1976.
24. Monticelli G, Ascani E: Spondylolysis and spondylolisthesis. Acta Orthop Scand 46:498–506, 1975.
25. Semon LR, Spengler P: Significance of spondylolysis in college football players. Spine 6:172–174, 1981.
26. Rosemberg JN, Barger LW, Freidman B: The incidence of spondylolysis and spondylolisthesis in the non-ambulatory patients. Spine 6:34–37, 1981.

27. Delpierre J: Traitment conservateur de la spondylolyse et du spondylolisthesis Acta Orthop Belg 47:464–467, 1981.
28. Nachemson A: Repair of the spondylolisthetic defect and intertransverse fusion for young patients. Clin Ortho 117:101–105, 1976.
29. Lafond G: Surgical treatment of spondylolisthesis. Clin Orthop 22:175–181, 1962.
30. Marique P: Le spondylolistésis. Acta Chir Bel V. 50 (Suppl 3), 1951.
31. De Seze S, Durieu J: Le spondylolisthesis. Etude clinique et radiologique d'après 70 observations personelles. Semaine Hop Paris 23:1551–1578, 1947.
32. Meyerding HW: Spondylolisthesis. Surg Gynecol Obstet 54:371–377, 1932.
33. Hensinger RN, Lang JR, MacEwen GD: Surgical management of spondylolisthesis in children and adolescents. Spine 1:207–216, 1976.
34. Wiltse LL, Jackson DW: Treatment of spondylolisthesis and spondylolysis in children. Clin Orthop 117:92–100, 1976.
35. Bradford DS: Spondylolysis and spondylolisthesis. In: Chou SN (ed): Spinal Deformity and Neurologic Dysfunction. Raven Press, New York, p 171–200.
36. Moe JH, Winter RB, Bradford DS, Lonstein JE: Scoliosis and other spinal deformities. WB Saunders Philadelphia, 1980.
37. Gill GG, Manning JG, White HL: Surgical treatment of spondylolisthesis without spine fusion. J Bone Joint Surg 37A:493–520, 1958.
38. Laurent LE: Spondylolisthesis. Acta Orthop Scand (Suppl 35), 1958. Vol. 28.
39. Laurent LE, Osterman K: Operative treatment of spondylolisthesis in young patients. Clin Orthop 117:85–91, 1976.
40. Nachemson A, Wiltse LL: Editorial comment: spondylolisthesis. Clin Orthop 117: 2–3, 1976.
41. Watkins MB: Posterolateral fusion pseudoarthrosis and posterior element defects of the lumbosacral spine. Clin Orthop 35:80–85, 1974.
42. Wiltse LL: Spondylolisthesis in children. Clin Orthop 21:156–172, 1961.
43. Turner RH, Bianco AJ: Spondylolysis and spondylolisthesis in children and teenagers. J Bone Joint Surg 53A:1298–1306, 1971.
44. Monticelli G, Costanza G: Spondylolisi e spondilolistesi: il trattamento. Prog Pat Vert 6:91–101, 1984.
45. Savini R, Cervellati S, Cioni A, Palmisani M, Panso L: Il trattamento chirurgico nella spondilolisi e spondilolistesi lievi dell'infanzia e dell'adolescenza. Prog Pat Vert 6:135–142, 1984.
46. Sicard A, Tonzard A: Le traitment chirurgical du spondylolisthesis de la 5° lombaire. Nouv Presse Med 77:1129–1134, 1969.
47. Freebody D, Bendall R, Taylor RD: Anterior transperitoneal lumbar fusion. J Bone Joint Surg 53B:617–621, 1971.
48. Wiltberger BR: Intervertebral body fusion by the posterior bone dowel. Clin Orthop 35:69–79, 1964.
49. Cloward RB: Lesion of the intervertebral disks and their treatment by interbody fusion methods. Clin Orthop 51:27–30, 1963.
50. Harris RI: Spondylolisthesis. Ann R Coll Surg Engl 8:259–264, 1951.
51. Scaglietti O, Frontino G, Bartolozzi P: Tecnica della riduzione della spondilolistesi lombare e sua contenzione definitiva. Atti SIOT: 292–300, 1970.
52. Scaglietti O, Frontino G, Bartolozzi P: Technique of anatomical reduction of lumbar spondylolisthesis and its surgical stabilization. Clin Orthop 117:164–175, 1976.
53. Harrington PR, Tullos HS, Travaglini F: Trattamento chirurgico delle grave spondilolistesi dell'infanzia. Atti 52 Cong SIOT, 1977, pp 371–379.

54. Harrington P, Dickson JH: Spinal instrumentation in the treatment of severe progressive spondylolisthesis. Clin Orthop 117:157–163, 1976.
55. Roy-Camille R, Sailant G, Beurier J, Comarmano G: L5 S1 spondylolisthesis. Etiological factors and therapeutic indications. Rev Chir Orthop 65:83–84, 1979.
56. Louis R, Maresca C: Stabilization chirurgicale avec reduction des spondylolyses et des spondylolisthesis. Int Orthop 1:215–225, 1977.
57. Ascani E: Personal communication, 1976.
58. Padua S, Aulisa L: Risultati preliminari della riduzione e stabilizzazione chirurgica nelle spondilolistesi. Arch Putti 24:113–128, 1976.
59. Marchetti PG, Bartolozzi P: Le spondilolistesi. Aulo Gaggi, Bologna, 1985.
60. Boxall DW, Winter RB, Bradford DS, Moe JH: Management of severe spondylolisthesis (Grade III and Grade IV) in children and adolescents. J Bone Joint Surg 61A: 479–495, 1979.
61. Gui L, Savini R: Il trattamento chirurgico delle spondilolistesi gravi. Prog Pat Vert 6:151–166, 1984.
62. Logroscino CA, Nizegorodcew T, Caporale M: Il trattamento chirurgico della spondilolistesi per via anteriore: luci ed ombre di una tecnica di attualità. Prog Pat Vert 6:183–189, 1984.
63. Marchetti PG, Bartolozzi P: Il trattamento chirurgico della spondilolistesi nell'età dell'adolescenza. Prog Pat Vert 6:119–136, 1984.
64. De Wald RL, Font HM, Taddonio RF, Neuwirth MG: Severe lumbosacral spondylolisthesis in adolescents and children. J Bone Joint Surg 63A:619–626, 1981.
65. Del Torto U: Surgical reduction and stabilization of spondylolisthesis. Clin Orthop 75:281–284, 1971.

CHAPTER 6

Neurenteric Cysts

Jean-François Hirsch and Elizabeth Hoppe-Hirsch

Neurenteric cysts develop mainly at the level of the spinal cord, seldom at that of the cranial cavity. They are defined as cysts that are lined by gastrointestinal mucosa and are in direct contact with the central nervous system. Thus defined, they are rare: no more than 25 intraspinal neurenteric cysts have been described in the literature after the original publication of Puussepp in 1934.[1]

Some confusion has arisen as to the nomenclature of these cysts, reflected in part by the multiplicity of given names. Such terms as foregut cysts, enteric cysts, enterogenous cysts, archenteric cysts, and gastrocystomas reflect the resemblance to intestine of the histologic findings while the terms "teratomatous cyst" and "teratoid tumor" suggest multiplicity of germ-cell layers.

In our opinion, the term "neurenteric cyst" should be reserved to those cysts that histologically resemble the intestine and are in direct contact with the central nervous system. Bronchiogenic cysts are supposedly derived from the bronchi and are therefore lined by a ciliated epithelium resting on a fibrous tissue and eventually containing plates of cartilage. However, except when cartilage is found, it is very difficult to separate the two groups since both intestine and bronchi are derived from the primitive foregut (which is lined by ciliated epithelium). Therefore bronchiogenic cysts should be considered as a variant of enteric cysts.

When cysts are present in the mediastinum, in the abdomen, or behind the spine, they should be called pre- or post-vertebral enteric cysts and considered as related anomalies since their embryologic development is very likely similar, as proven by the frequency in all cases of associated vertebral anomalies.

Pathology

The wall of neurenteric cysts is more often described as thin and translucent than thick. The intracystic liquid has been found clear or milky. The histologic examination usually reveals an avascular fibrous connective tissue with an inner epithelial lining resting on a basement membrane (Fig. 6.1). The epithelial cells vary from flat to cuboidal or columnar. Periodic acid–Schiff stains demonstrate mucin-containing cells which occasionally are characteristic goblet cells similar

Figure 6.1. Monostratified epithelium with enteroid prismatic muciparous cells, limiting the cyst cavity. H&E, × 1,000.

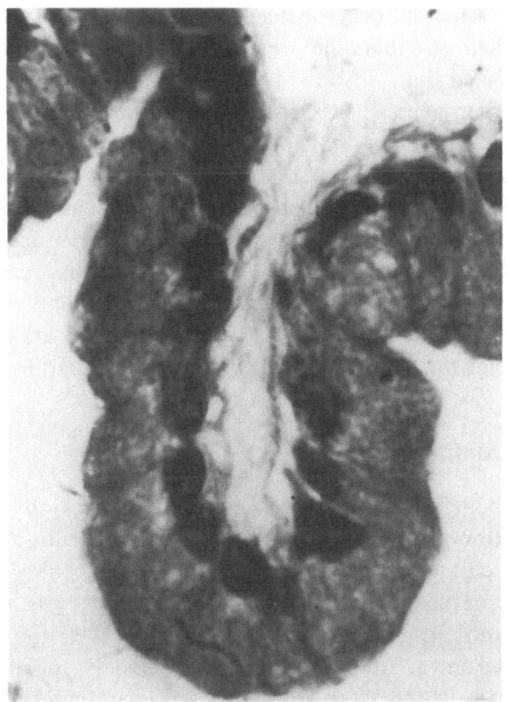

to those seen in the intestinal tract. The epithelium is made of one layer of cells but can also be pseudostratified and ciliated, resembling bronchi, or squamous of esophageal type.

Neurenteric cysts are therefore characterized by the presence of a mucin-secreting columnar enterogenous epithelium; their wall replicates a gastrointestinal wall with an intestinal type of mucosa, submucosa, and even sometimes layers of smooth muscle: nonintestinal tissue components are not seen. On the basis of this description and of the associated vertebral anomalies, neurenteric cysts can be separated from the teratomatous cysts.

Intraspinal Neurenteric Cysts

At the meeting of the Societé de Neurologie de Paris, on the 6th of December, 1934, Puussepp, from Esthonia, described a quadriplegia, occurring in a 27-year-old marine officer, due to "a rare variety of teratoma," an intestinoma. This condition, which had run a slow and irregular course and which was finally cured by surgery, is probably the first description of an intraspinal neurenteric cyst.

Later, 17 other articles[2-18] were published. In 1955 Knight et al.[2] showed in their case that there were associated vertebral anomalies. In 1963 Scoville et al.[6] stated that, in spite of rather sparse publications and confusing nomenclature, enterogenous cysts probably were not too rare: Matson et al. at the Children's Hospital, Boston, in personal communications had stated that they had removed such cysts in some six to eight children. However, Guilburg et al.[18] noticed that in 20 years they had observed only one neurenteric cyst among 502 cases of spinal cord compression. In the Service de Neurochirurgie des Enfants Malades in Paris, among 120 cases of spinal cord compression in children, one intraspinal neurenteric cyst was operated on: reports of two other cysts in adults were added and published in 1971.[11] Neurenteric cysts are certainly rarely reported lesions. This rarity does not allow a precise estimation of their incidence.

Anatomy

By definition, there was an intraspinal cyst in the 26 patients already reported. However, the cyst was communicating with an extraspinal cyst in two cases. Neurenteric cysts are intradural.

In most cases, intraspinal neurenteric cysts are located in front of the spinal cord. In four of the 26 published cases, the precise location of the cyst is unknown. The cyst was located behind the spinal cord in four patients and in front of it in 18. Thus neurenteric cysts are anteriorly situated in 85% of patients. Sometimes the anterior compression of the cord is so heavy that, through the posterior approach, the neurenteric cyst can be misdiagnosed and taken for an intramedullary tumor.

The distribution of the cysts along the vertebral column is shown in Table 6.1. This table demonstrates that, if neurenteric cysts are slightly more frequent in the upper part of the spinal cord, they are actually distributed along its entire length.

Associated vertebral anomalies were present in 14 patients and absent in eight in the 22 case reports in which this information is given. Table 6.2 gives the distribution of these vertebral anomalies.

Except for the enlarged spinal canal which can be due to the development of the cyst, all these anomalies are congenital. Several anomalies are usually associated in the same patient.

Table 6.1. Distribution of neurenteric cysts along the vertebral column in 26 patients[1-18]

	Number	Percent
Cervical	9	35
Cervico-dorsal	4	15
Dorsal	9	35
Dorso-lumbar	4	15

Table 6.2. Associated vertebral anomalies[1-18]

Anterior spina bifida	6
Posterior spina bifida	4
Diastematomyelia	3
Hemivertebrae	4
Fused vertebrae	5
Costal anomalies	2
Enlarged spinal canal	6

Other associated congenital anomalies, such as jejunal diverticulum, have been described in these patients. Ileal reduplication, accessory pancreas, dermal sinus, spina aperta, and cutaneous hemangioma have also been reported.

All these congenital anomalies, whether vertebral or not, contribute to understanding the embryologic development of the neurenteric cysts.

Sex and Age

The sex of the patients is known in 20 of the 26 published cases. A male prevalence is observed since 15 patients are male and only six female; thus approximately three patients out of four are male. However, the number of cases is too small to consider this prevalence as surely established ($p = 7\%$).

The age of the patients is given in 20 cases. It is of great interest to notice that most neurenteric cysts were discovered in children or adults while such a congenital lesion would have been expected to become clinically apparent in infants. Thus these cysts can remain clinically silent for a long period. Sometimes they follow an irregular course with occasionally spontaneous clinical regressions. The clinical picture is certainly closely related to the intracystic pressure.

Clinical Features

The clinical picture is detailed in 17 reports concerning 19 patients. In most cases, the clinical features are those of a spinal cord compression; they associate cervical or back pain and vertebral stiffness together with neurologic signs. These neurologic signs, extremely variable in intensity from one case to another, are determined by the level of the compression. In three out of the 19 cases, a prevertebral cyst was communicating with the intraspinal cyst. In one case with a communication between the cyst and a reduplicated ileum,[14] a severe meningitis was associated. In infants the clinical picture is rarely characteristic so that the diagnosis usually relies on the associated anomalies.

In six out of the 19 cases, an irregular course with spontaneous regressions and later recurrences of the symptoms and signs is reported. Therefore it is quite clear that these neurenteric cysts can remain silent for years. It is also of interest to notice that the beginning or the worsening of the clinical features is preceded by trauma in four cases and a manipulative procedure in two.

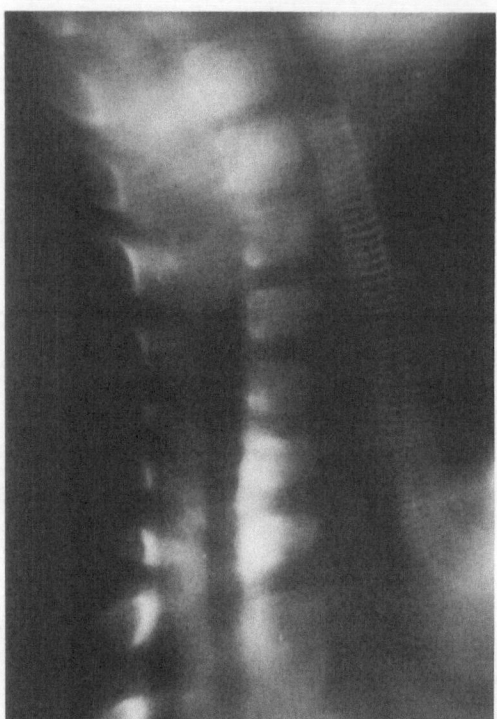

Figure 6.2. Air myelogram in an intraspinal neurenteric cyst.

Radiologic Features

The radiologic investigation of a patient with a neurenteric cyst should always begin with good plain x-ray films and tomograms of the column since vertebral anomalies such as anterior or posterior spina bifida, diastematomyelia, hemivertebrae, fused vertebrae, costal anomalies, or enlarged spinal canal are often found. However, since these anomalies are missing in many cases, a myelogram is indicated whenever there is any suggestion of neurologic abnormality. In 13 out of the 19 cases reported, such a myelogram was performed and easily demonstrated the cyst (Fig. 6.2). In one case[11] the position of the cyst changed slightly with the position of the patient. When a prevertebral cyst is associated, the trachea and the barium-filled esophagus can be seen displaced foreward.

Today magnetic resonance imaging (MRI) studies replace myelograms and demonstrate simultaneously intraspinal neurenteric cysts, associated vertebral anomalies, and eventually prevertebral cysts.

Treatment

All intraspinal neurenteric cysts should be treated by surgical excision. This excision should be as complete as possible, but the surgical procedure should not threaten the spinal cord or its vascular supply.

There were four deaths in the 19 reported cases, due mainly to pre- or postoperative infection in infants (mortality rate: 21%). In the other patients, the results were good since the neurologic signs regressed. In two cases cure was obtained at a second operation, the first operation having been insufficient or inadequate. All other patients were cured at the first operation; no recurrence was observed even though the excision, in some cases, had been incomplete.

In patients with an associated prevertebral cyst, a separate surgical approach should be planned to remove this second lesion in the neck, the mediastinum, or the peritoneal cavity.

Intracranial Neurenteric Cysts

Intracranial neurenteric cysts have been reported exclusively in the posterior fossa, although Matson[19] discussed in one case the possibility of such a cyst in the parapituitary area and although Hirano and Ghatak[20] thought that colloid cysts of the IIIrd ventricle derived from an endodermal structure. Moreover it is very likely that some posterior fossa neuroepithelial cysts reported in the literature[21,22] arise from foldings of the neuroepithelium that lines the ventricular system. However, other cysts, either because they are located in front of the brainstem[4,19,23] or because their epithelium contains mucin-secreting cells,[24,25] should be classified as neurenteric cysts. Thus defined, seven intracranial neurenteric cysts have been reported, five located in front of the pons and two at the level of the IVth ventricle.

Symptoms and signs of intracranial hypertension and of cerebellar involvement, sometimes hydrocephalus, were present. The duration of symptoms ranged from several months to several years. The majority of these intracranial neurenteric cysts were found in adults. Computed tomography (CT) shows these cysts as clearly defined round areas of low attenuation but with no peripheral contrast enhancement.

These intracranial neurenteric cysts should be operated on. No report of recurrence after surgery has ever been published.

It is very likely that these cysts originate from the most cranial portion of the primitive intestine.

Related Anomalies

Several theories have been proposed to explain the development of neurenteric cysts:[26-28] they share the opinion that all individuals bearing such cysts have passed through a stage with a dorsal enteric fistula and a cleft in both neural tube and notochord. However, when such a fistula occurs, growth and processes of repair can result in different types of developmental anomalies which are therefore related by their pathogenesis. Bentley and Smith[29] have suggested classifying these lesions together as manifestations of the "split notochord syndrome."

Besides the spinal and central nervous system malformations, visceral malformations which, on histologic examination, show the presence of smooth muscle and enteric mucosa in their walls, should be included in this syndrome.[30-35]

When obliteration of the enteric fistula fails completely, the track passes back from the gut through the mesentery or mediastinum and traverses a complete spina bifida, to open on the skin in the midline.

When only the dorsal part of the fistula persists, a sinus is formed, passing forward from the midline of the skin of the back. A posterior enteric diverticulum

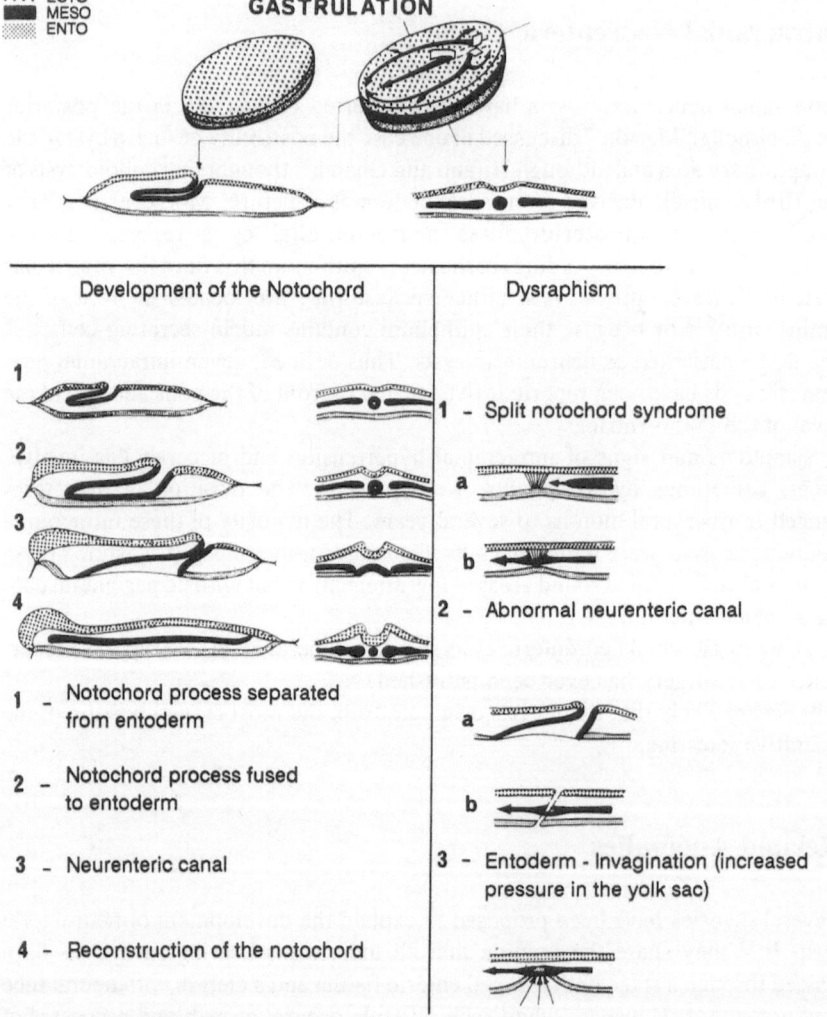

Figure 6.3. Pathogenesis of neurenteric cysts. Right column: normal development of the notochord. Left column: the different theories put forward to explain the function of neurenteric cysts.

is created when the ventral part of the embryonic fistula remains and communicates with the gut. In the case reported by Millis,[14] it was communicating with an intraspinal neurenteric cyst and responsible for an infection.

Posterior enteric cysts are due to the persistence of the intermediate part of the embryonic fistula. The atrophic portions are often represented by fibrous bands which can pass through a vertebral defect and merge with the spinal cord. These cysts are mediastinal or mesenteric; they can also be postvertebral in position.[36,37] The association of a posterior enteric cyst with an intraspinal neurenteric cyst has been observed.[8]

Pathogenesis

Different theories[26-28,30,32,36] have been put forward to explain the presence of normal intestinal tissue in contact with the central nervous system and its association with vertebral anomalies. As already stated they all share the opinion that a split notochord is a necessary stage (Fig. 6.3). Therefore the onset of the anomaly should be dated back as far as the third week of embryonic life.

In Bremer's theory, the yolk sac bulges through a median cleft in the back which is essentially a magnified accessory neurenteric canal.

In Saunder's theory the local cleavage of the notochord is of unknown origin; it results in an endo-ectodermal adherence which is at the origin of the enteric diverticulum. Veeneklaas' theory is also based on an abnormal adherence between the foregut and the spine.

For Beardmore and Wiglesworth a local endo-ectodermal adhesion at a presomite stage partially blocks the invagination of the notochord and causes it to split. The traction exerted at the adhesion during growth will eventually end in an enteric diverticulum.

Whatever be the pathogenesis, the final and major consequence can be the dorsal enteric fistula linking the intestine to the skin of the back through the vertebral column and spinal cord. However, the initial defect can be modified by growth and processes of repair, resulting in such anomalies as neurenteric cysts with or without associated vertebral anomalies.

References

1. Puussepp M: Variété rare de tératome sous-dural de la région cervicale (intestinome). Quadriplegie. Extirpation. Guérison complete. Rev Neurol (Paris) 41:879–886, 1934.
2. Knight G, Griffiths T, Williams I: Gastrocystoma of the spinal cord. Br J Surg 42:635–638, 1955.
3. Neuhauser EBD, Harris GBC, Berrett A: Roentgenographic features of neurenteric cysts. J Roentgenol Radium Ther Nucl Med 79:235–240, 1958.
4. Small JM: Pre-axial enterogenous cysts. Proceedings of the Society of British Neurological Surgeons. 64th (abst). J Neurol Neurosurg Psychiatry 25:184, 1962.

5. Langmaid C, Jones R: Enterogenous cysts of the spinal cord with associated anomalies. Proceedings of the Society of British Neurologic Surgeons: 68th Meeting (abstr). J Neurol Neurosurg Psychiatry 26:559, 1963.
6. Scoville WB, Manlapaz JS, Otis RD, Cabieses F: Intraspinal enterogenous cyst. J Neurosurg 20:704–706, 1963.
7. Nemeth K: Enterogene zyste des Rückenmarks. Zbl Allg Pathol 108:196–200, 1965.
8. Dorsey JF, Tabrisky J: Intraspinal and mediastinal foregut cyst compressing the spinal cord. Report of a case. J Neurosurg 24:562–567, 1966.
9. Brun A, Saldeen T: Intraspinal enterogenous cyst. Acta Pathol Microbiol Scand 73:191–194, 1968.
10. Klump TE: Neuroenteric cyst in the cervical spinal canal of a 10 week-old boy. J Neurosurg 35:472–476, 1971.
11. Kahn AP, Hirsch JF, Da Lage C, Lyon G, Saporta L, Evrard P: Les kystes entériques intrarachidiens. A propos de trois observations. Neurochirurgie 17:33–44, 1971.
12. Silvernail W, Brown RB: Intra-medullary enterogenous cyst. Case report. J Neurosurg 36:235–238, 1972.
13. Bale PM: A congenital intraspinal gastroenterogenous cyst in diastematomyelia. J Neurol Neurosurg Psychiatry 36:1011–1017, 1973.
14. Millis RR, Holmes AE: Enterogenous cyst of the spinal cord with associated intestinal reduplication, vertebral anomalies, and a dorsal dermal sinus. Case report. J Neurosurg 38:73–77, 1973.
15. Yamashita J, Maloney AFI, Harris P: Intradural spinal bronchogenic cyst. Case report. J Neurosurg 339:240–245, 1973.
16. Pilz P, Fischbach R, Brenneis M: Enterogene cyste des Halsmarkes mit mucomyelie. Acta Neuropath (Ber) 40:277–278, 1977.
17. Fabinyi GC, Adams JE: High cervical spinal cord compression by an enterogenous cyst. Case report. J Neurosurg 51:556–559, 1979.
18. Guilburg JN, Arieh YB, Peyser E: Spinal intradural enterogenous cyst. Report of a case. Surg Neurol 14:359–362, 1980.
19. Matson DD: Neurosurgery of infancy and childhood, Second edition. Springefield, IL, Charles C. Thomas, 1969.
20. Hirano A, Ghatak NR: The fine structure of colloid cysts of the third ventricle. J Neuropathol Exp Neurol 33:333–341, 1974.
21. Shuangshoti S, Netsky MG: Neuroepithelial (colloid) cysts of the nervous system. Further observations on pathogenesis, location, incidence and histochemistry. Neurology 16:887–903, 1966.
22. Hasegawa H, Ushio Y, Oku Y, Iwata Y, Kanai N, Kamikawa K: Neuroepithelial cyst of the cerebellar vermis. Surg Neurol 6:181–184, 1976.
23. Hirai O, Kawamura J, Fukimutsu T: Prepontine epithelium-lined cyst. Case report. J Neurosurg 55:312–317, 1981.
24. Afshar F, Scholtz CL: Enterogenous cyst of the fourth ventricle. Case report. J Neurosurg 54:836–838, 1981.
25. Mehta VS, Chowdhury C, Bhatia R: Neuroenteric cyst of the cerebellum. Postgrad Med J 660:287–289, 1984.
26. Bremer JL: Dorsal intestinal fistula: accessory neurenteric canal; diastematomyelia. AMA Arch Pathol 338:132–138, 1952.
27. Saunders RL: Combined anterior and posterior spina bifida in a living neo-natal human female. Anat Rec 87:255–278, 1943.
28. Beardmore HE, Wiglesworth FW. Vertebral anomalies and alimentary duplications. Clinical and embryological aspects. Pediatr Clin North Am 5:457–474, 1958.

29. Bentley JFR, Smith JR: Developmental posterior enteric remnants and spinal malformations. The split notochord syndrome. Arch Dis Child 35:76–86, 1960.
30. Veeneklaas GMH: Pathogenesis of intrathoracic gastrogenic cyst. Am J Dis Child 83:500–507, 1952.
31. Fallon M, Gordon ARG, Lendrum AC: Mediastinal cysts of fore-gut origin associated with vertebral anomalies. Br J Surg 41:520–533, 1953.
32. McLetchie NGB, Purves JK, de ch Saunders RL: The genesis of gastric and certain intestinal diverticula and enterogenous cysts. Surg Gynecol Obstet 99:135–141, 1954.
33. Cameron AH: Malformations of the neuro-spinal axis, urogenital tract and foregut in spina bifida attributable to disturbances of the blastopore. J Pathol Bacteriol 73:213–221, 1957.
34. Rhaney K, Barclay GPT: Enterogenous cysts and congenital diverticula of the alimentary canal with abnormalities of the vertebral column and spinal cord. J Pathol Bacteriol 77:457–471, 1959.
35. Gimeno A, Lopez F, Figuera D, Rodrigo L: Neuroenteric cyst. Neuroradiology 3:167–172, 1972.
36. Prop N, Frensdorf EL, Van de Stadt FR: A postvertebral entodermal cyst associated with axial deformities: a case showing the "entodermal-ectodermal adhesion syndrome." Pediatrics 39:555–562, 1967.
37. Odake G, Yamaki T, Naruse S: Neurenteric cyst with meningomyelocele. Case report. J Neurosurg 45:352–356, 1976.

CHAPTER 7

Sacral and Lumbo-Sacral Agenesis

Gérard Bollini

Sacral agenesis is a rare condition consisting of partial or complete absence of the sacrum. With minimum orthopedic interventions, almost all of the patients with sacral agenesis become community walkers, usually without aid. *Lumbo-sacral* agenesis is a somewhat rarer condition consisting of absence of part or all of the lumbar spine and sacrum, with ilio-lumbar disassociation and instability; "arthogrypotic-like" deformity of the lower limb including hip dislocation, knee contracture, foot deformity; and paraplegia. Orthopedic management of such a patient can include amputation and use of prostheses. Anomalies of the viscera, particularly in the genito-urinary system and in the rectal area, are often seen in these two conditions. Bladder or external sphincter dysfunction with vesico-ureteral reflux are commonly present. Bladder and bowel control are often impaired.

According to Paris and Laine[1] the earliest mention of these anomalies was by Pline and Herodotus. The first modern reports were those of Hohl[2] in 1852 and Wertheim[3] in 1857, who described complete sacro-coccygeal agenesis in newborn girls. Ten single case reports were published until White and Klauber[4] in 1911 described three additional cases and noted the association with club foot. In 1924, Achard et al.[5] and then Foix and Hillemand[6] coined the term "dystrophie cruro-vesico-fessière" in cases of sacral agenesis below S1 and pointed out the associated vesical problems. They suggest the first classification. The same year, Stewart[7] described a further small series. In 1938, Pouzet[8] reported the first familial case of lumbo-sacral agenesis in a boy and his father.

Johanna Blummel[9] in 1959 extensively analyzed 50 cases collected from the United States and Hawaii with special genetic studies of their own eight cases. She suggested that diabetes in the mother might be of etiologic significance, but no evidence of a genetic pattern of inheritance can be supported. The same year, Durham-Smith[10] reported 26 cases from Australia and described the findings of six dissections in postmortem specimens.

Duhamel[11-13] in 1961 coined the term "caudal regression syndrome." Since this work, different syndromes with gut and vertebral abnormalities have been recognized as polydactyly–imperforate anus–vertebral anomalies syndrome by Say and Gerald[14]; "Vater" association (an eponym for vertebral, anal, tracheal, ectromelia, and renal abnormalities) by Quan and Smith,[15] and "OEIS complex" for omphalocele–extrophy–imperforate anus–spinal abnormalities by Carey et al.[16] Classification of sacral agenesis was suggested recently by Renshaw[17] in 1978 and by Stanley et al.[18] in 1979.

The presence of spine, limb, gut, urinary, and sometimes cardiovascular defects can be explained by one or more insults affecting the developing embryo during the third to the eighth weeks (embryonic life).

Controversies about orthopedic management in lumbo-sacral agenesis still persist between Aitken and Frantz,[19] Russel and Aitken,[20] and Frantz and Aitken[21] who recommended bilateral subtrochanteric amputation and early prosthetic fitting, and Banta,[22] who preferred preservation of the lower extremities when proprioception was present. Phillips et al.[23] prefer knee disarticulation for his patients. Spinopelvic stability must be achieved for Van Derwerker,[24] Pirkey and Purcell,[25] and Perry et al.[26] but not for Andrish et al.[27]

Classification

In 1924, Foix[6] coined the term "dystrophie cruro-vésico-fessière" in one case of partial agenesis of the sacrum. Similar conditions described by him are total absence of the coccyx, hemisacrum, and sacral agenesis with spina bifida. Then in 1959, Durham-Smith[10] described agenesis of the sacrum (total and subtotal) and hemisacrum. In 1978, Renshaw[17] included lumbo-sacral agenesis in his classification of sacral agenesis:

Type I: total or partial unilateral sacral agenesis
Type II: partial sacral agenesis, with partial but bilaterally symmetrical defects and stable articulation between the ilia and a normal or hypoplastic first sacral vertebra
Type III: Variable lumbar and total sacral agenesis, with the ilia articulating with the sides of the lowest vertebra present
Type IV: Variable lumbar and total sacral agenesis, the caudal end-plate of the lowest vertebra resting above either fused ilia or an iliac amphiarthrosis.

In 1979, Stanley[18] in the same way as Renshaw[17] included lumbo-sacral agenesis in his classification of sacral agenesis. He divided (as Foix did before) congenital sacral anomalies into groups:

Group I: Absent vertebra (agenesis). This is the true "agenetic" group which corresponds to the caudal regression syndrome of Duhamel. It is characterized by relative neurologic sparing and a relatively low incidence of visceral congenital abnormalities.
Group II: Hemivertebrae (dysgenesis). In this group the sacral defect is sometimes associated with hemivertebrae and butterfly vertebrae in the thoracolumbar spine. There is a high incidence of visceral abnormalities, but the neurologic deficit is minimal. Any limb abnormalities are usually true congenital deformities.

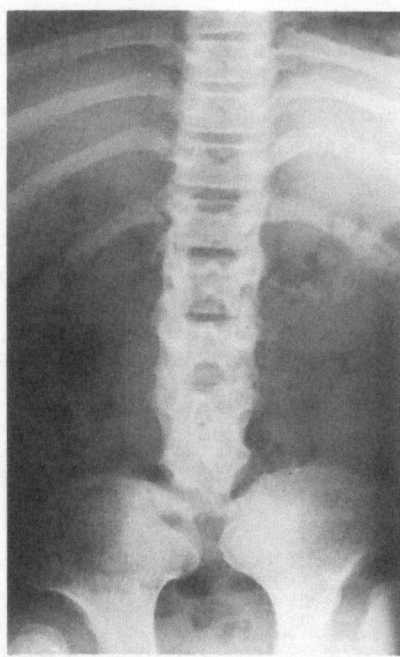

Figure 7.1. Sacral agenesis. Group I. Lumbo-sacral agenesis. Iliae amphiarthrosis. The hips are dislocated.

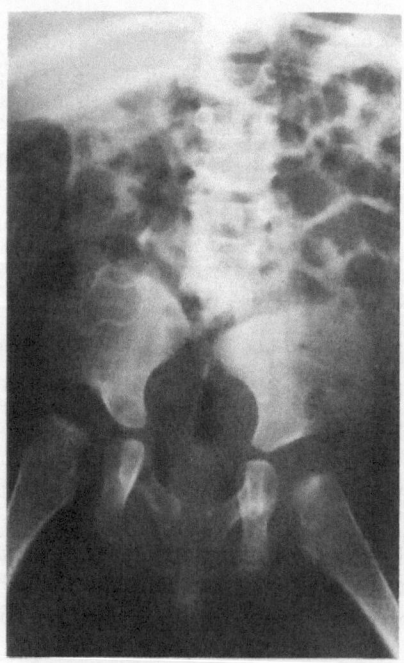

Figure 7.2. Sacral agenesis. Group I.

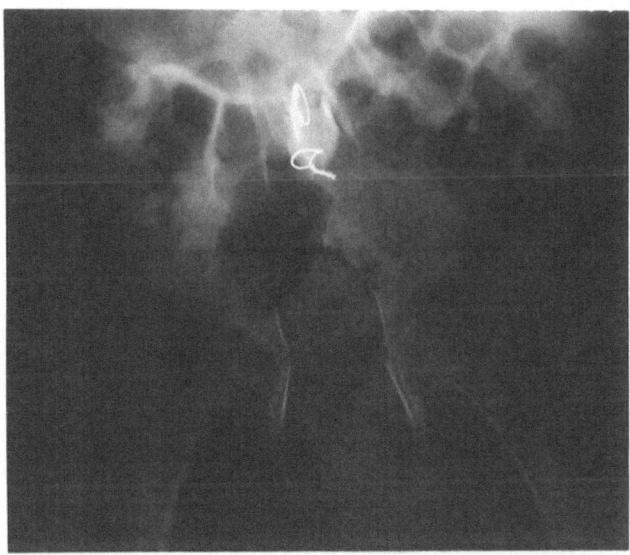

Figure 7.3. Sacral agenesis. Group I. Lumbo-sacral agenesis. The two iliac wings are fused. The hips are not dislocated.

Group III: Dysraphism. Deficiencies of the neural arch leading to spina bifida with meningocele or meningomyelocele at the sacral level.

Based on the previous classifications and our own experience with 56 thoraco-lumbo-sacral, lumbo-sacral, and sacral agenesis, we propose the following classifications:

Group I: Total sacral and variable lumbar or thoraco-lumbar agenesis. The caudal end-plate of the lowest vertebra resting above either fused ilia or an iliae amphiarthrosis. The ilia can also articulate with the sides of the lowest lumbar present vertebra (Figs. 7.1, 7.2, and 7.3).

Group II: Sacro-iliac dysgenesis (Fig. 7.4). One of the two sacro-iliac joints is agenetic or dysgenetic leading to an instability of the sacro-iliac joint. We have assessed this deformity through eighteen C.T. scans performed in sacral agenesis.

On the side of the unstable sacro-iliac joint, if the gluteus muscles work, the iliac wing rotates inward pulled by the gluteus medius (Figs. 7.5 and 7.6). At the same time, the two first sacral vertebrae move down and back inducing a congenital scoliosis.

Group III: Sacral agenesis with two stable sacro-iliac joints and partial or complete agenesis below S2 (Fig. 7.7).

We have excluded from our classification the dysraphic group with posterior meningocele or myelomeningocele.

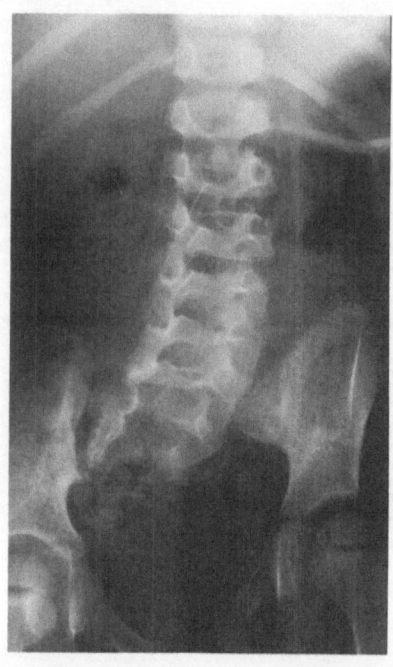

Figure 7.4. Sacral dysgenesis. Group II.

Spina bifida occulta is often associated with Group I, II, or III, but posterior meningocele or myelomeningocele is a different condition in our opinion.

Etiology

Blummel et al.'s[28] report included six children from a total of 50 cases of sacral agenesis with sacral agenesis (four complete, two partial) whose mothers were

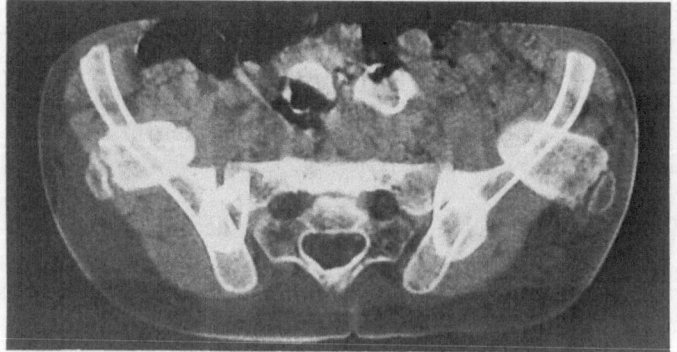

Figure 7.5. Normal relationships at C.T. scan. Reconstruction of the hips and iliac wings.

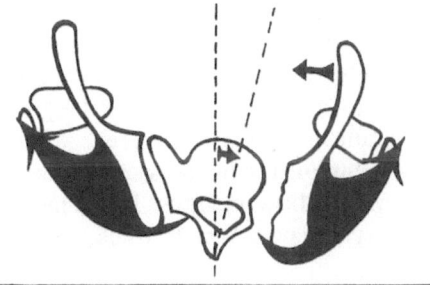

Figure 7.6. Drawing of C.T. scan reconstruction for a sacro-iliac dysgenesis Group II. The iliac wing on the side of the unstable sacro-iliac joint rotates inward pulled by the gluteus medius.

diabetic. Pedersen et al.[29] in a study of 853 infants born to diabetic mothers showed that congenital malformations were found in 6.4% of the diabetes group and in 2.1% of the control group. According to White's[4] group of pregnant diabetics, Pedersen et al.[29] found that the frequency (10.7%) and severity of the malformations were significantly higher in children of women with late diabetic vascular complications rather than in children of mothers with insulin reactions and hypoglycemia during the first trimester of pregnancy. Stern et al.[30] and Kucera[31] added cases of sacral agenesis and maternal diabetes. Three cases of

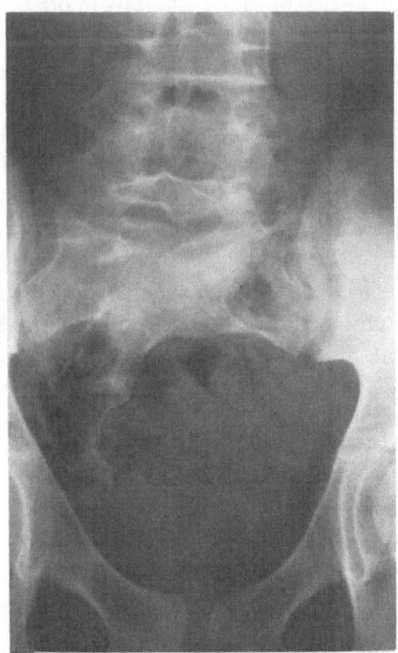

Figure 7.7. Sacral agenesis. Group III.

lumbo-sacral agenesis in infants of diabetic mothers were reported by Rusnak and Driscoll[32] who suggested a specific pathogenetic relationship to maternal diabetes mellitus in light of the rarity of these anomalies in the general population. Passarge and Lenz[84] reported that 14% of all caudal regression syndromes are associated with maternal diabetes, suggesting this could be an environmental factor. Barnetche,[33] in a review of 124 lumbo-sacral agenesis children, found an incidence of 31% of maternal diabetes mellitus. Talhammer et al.[34] described one case of caudal regression syndrome in a child whose mother, 18 years old, was prediabetic when pregnant.

Experimental studies of insulin-induced skeletal anomalies have been performed by a number of investigators. After injecting pregnant rabbits with insulin, Corda[35] noted that they either produced undersized offspring or aborted. The mechanical shaking of hens' eggs was reported by Lanauer[36] to produce "rumplessness in chickens." But the genetic background of the hen was believed to be important. He also noted that the injection of insulin into incubated hens' eggs led to an increased number of rumpless" embryos. Duraiswami[37] also reported the induction of skeletal anomalies in developing chicken embryos by injecting insulin into the yolk sac at various times during incubation. Dunn[38] described a new gene in mice producing deletion defects of the spinal column. Danforth[39] reported genetic rumplessness in fowl.

Lichtenstein et al.[40] reported anomalies in the offspring of albino rats given protamine zinc insulin during pregnancy. Runner[41] made the same investigations in mice and Sevastikoglou[42] in chicken embryos. The Collaborative Perinatal Project of Chung and Myrianthopoulos[43] concluded that insulin played no role in the production of congenital anomalies but confirmed reports of the increased incidence of sacral agenesis in offspring of diabetic mothers.

It was likely that genetic factors conditioned response of the embryo to metabolic disorders as supported by Stewart.[7] Ancel and Lallemand,[44] using colchicine on chick embryos, produced caudal regression anomalies as Cohlan[45] and Kalter and Warkany[46] did with high doses of vitamin A on mice.

Gillman et al.,[47] Beaudoin and Wilson,[48] and Kaplan and Grabowski[49] using Trypan blue, and Nogami and Ingalls[50] using 6-aminonicotinamide, showed caudal regression anomalies in rat, chicken, and mice embryos. A report of nine cases of sacral agenesis by Kucera[31] appeared to implicate exposure to fat solvents, particularly acetone, during early pregnancy, as an etiologic factor. Renshaw[17] described three mothers who had been exposed to fat solvents during the first trimester with caudal regression anomalies in children.

Several familial cases of sacral agenesis have been reported, but there is no clear-cut pattern of inheritance. Bloom et al.[51] in 1917 described two sisters with coccygeal agenesis; Pouzet[8] in 1938 reported a father and son with sacral agenesis; Rochet et al.[52] in 1966 described two sisters with sacral agenesis below S1; Finer et al.[53] in 1978 reported two brothers with total sacral agenesis and heart disease. These four publications report the only "pure" familial cases of sacral agenesis.

Stewart[7] in 1979 described siblings, brother and sister, with sacral agenesis whose mother was diabetic. Familial cases of sacral agenesis often present with

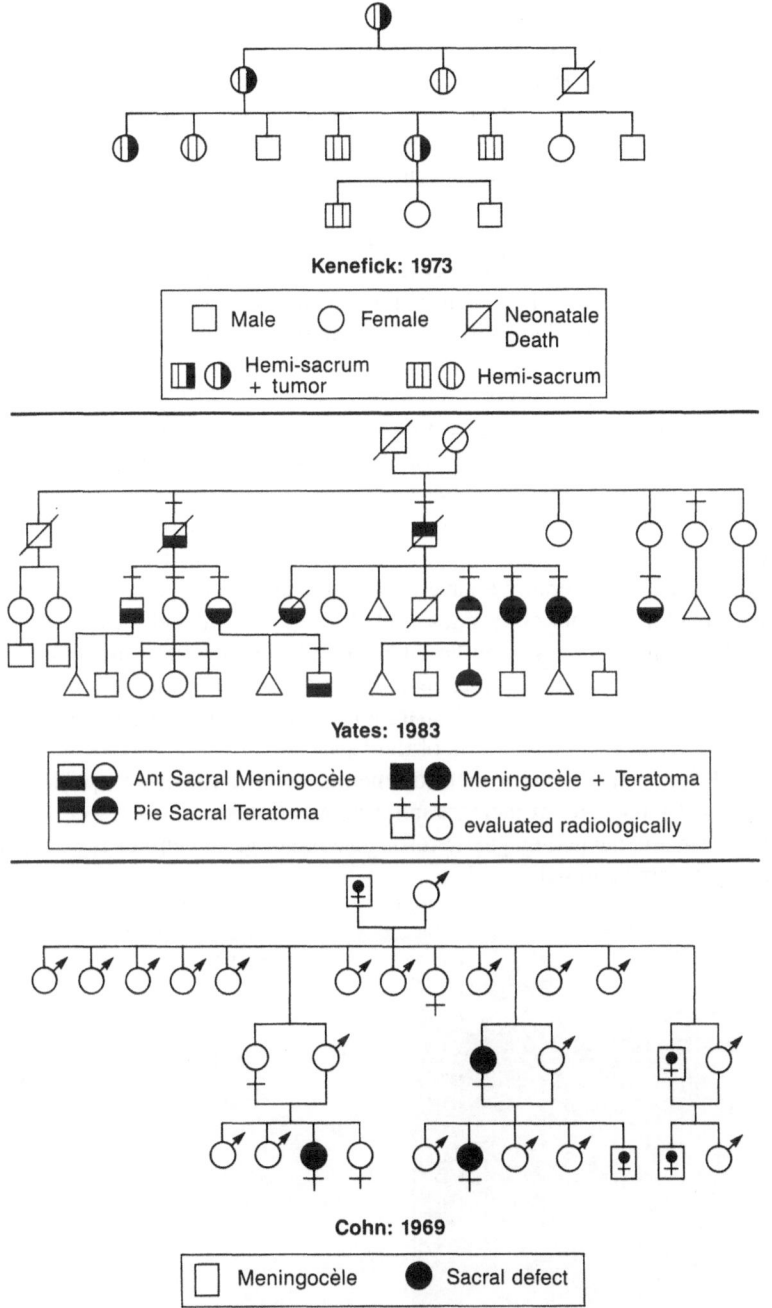

Figure 7.8. Pedigree of three families with partial agenesis and presacral tumor, meningocele, or both. Top: From: Kenefick[56] with permission.
Middle: From: Yates et al[57] with permission.
Bottom: From: Cohn et al[54] with permission.

anterior sacral meningocele or presacral tumors (Fig. 7.8). Cohn and Bay-Nielsen[54] reported that 60 of the 69 known patients with anterior sacral meningocele were women, adding six familial cases of sacral defect (in fact seven, because in case 1, he described two sisters with sacral agenesis); see Fig. 7.8. Four of the seven patients had ventral sacral meningoceles. For the author, this indicated a sex-linked dominant inheritance. Say[14] suggested that the hemizygous state in the male is lethal.

Ashcraft et al.[55] in 1965 studied presacral teratomas, describing sacral defects and presacral teratomas in 17 individuals from six different families and suggested the possibility of autosomal dominant inheritance. None of the patients studied had family members with anterior sacral meningoceles, alone or in combination with the teratomas.

Kenefick[56] in 1973 (Fig. 7.8) presented four patients of the same family with presacral tumors and sacral defect. Five more members of this family had sacral defects alone. There were six women and three men. Kenefick thought that sacral defect is transmitted as a dominant trait and presacral tumors as a sex-linked dominant trait. Paris[1] in 1973 described a mother with sacral agenesis and her daughter with sacral agenesis and anterior sacral meningocele. Anterior meningocele and presacral teratoma have been discovered in association with sacral agenesis (Cohn,[54] Kenefick,[56] Yates et al.[57]; see Figs. 7.8 and 7.9).

The following symptoms can be encountered: constipation, incontinence of urine or enuresis, residual urine, recurrent infection of the urinary tracts and localized pain, dysmenorrhea, dyspareunia, labor difficulties, disturbance of sphincter control, and paresthesia of the legs.

In addition, patients with anterior meningocele may suffer headache and nausea due to intermittent increase in intracranial pressure.

Body scan and nuclear magnetic resonance are of great help for the diagnoses of this associated anomaly.

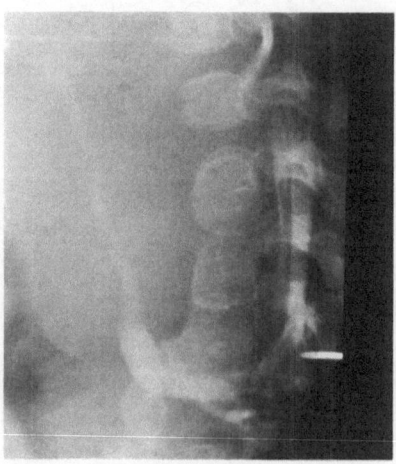

Figure 7.9. Myelography in anterior meningocele associated with sacral agenesis.

Surgical removal of the presacral teratoma is recommended because of the potential for malignancy and the increased risk of meningitis and abscess formation. The meningocele is usually diagnosed after announced by complications. This is the time for surgical removal.

Yates[57] in 1983 (Fig. 7.8) reported 11 members of the same family, four male (three with anterior sacral meningocele, one with presacral tumor) and seven female (two with anterior sacral meningocele, three with presacral teratoma, and two with both), with this defect. He proposed that anterior sacral defects associated with an anterior meningocele or teratoma, or both, be considered as an autosomal dominantly inherited condition.

Wolff[58] in 1936 destroyed, by irradiation, the axial part of the auda in chick embryos. He obtained symelie with distal spine agenesis. Roux and Martinet [59] in 1962, on the basis of the works of Kalter and Warkany,[46] gave high doses of vitamin A to the mothers of chick embryos and induced anomalies with minor and major spine defects and anal and genito-urinary malformations.

Smith et al.[60] established a relationship between monozygotic twinning and the Duhamel syndrome. Part of the excess frequency of malformation in monozygotic twins versus dizygotic twins is due to the increased likelihood of having the Duhamel syndrome. Whatever the cause of the aberration in the early morphogenesis of the embryonic center which resulted in monozygotic twinning, the same cause may give rise to a problem in the early organization within the embryonic disk and adversely affect primitive streak formation and function. This may result in an increased likelihood of the Duhamel syndrome.

Embryology

There are three distinct steps in caudal embryo development (Fig. 7.10).

1. *Formation of the primary perinea.* From the end of the third week, and during the fourth week, there is a migration of mesenchyme cells from the primitive streak surrounding the cloacal membrane and in the fifth week the mesenchyme cells join in front of the cloacal membrane giving issue to the genital bud, ischio-pubic area, and cloacal plinater.

2. *Spread of the caudal process.* At the beginning, the caudal process is the ultimate aspect of the primitive streak, then reaches its maximum in the sixth week before involuting in the seventh week after contributing to the formation of the postanal bowel and the neural canal.

3. *Constitution of the secondary perineum.* Mesenchyme cells from the caudal process induce formation of the secondary perineum with a cloacal septum.

Theoretically, there are two possibilities of inducing anomalies: abortion of the caudal process (using irradiation for example) and over-regression of the regression process. Abortion of the caudal process, if not complete, stops separation of the cloaca; if complete, it leads to disappearance of rectum and uro-genitary sinus and to syneriform monsters with sacral or lumbo-sacral agenesis. The caudal

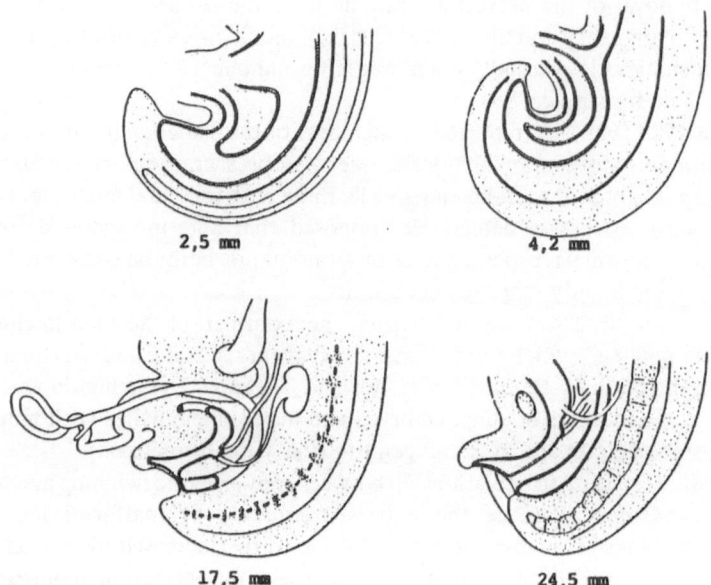

2,5 mm   4,2 mm

17,5 mm   24,5 mm

Figure 7.10. Pattern of development with involution of the caudal process. From: Duhamel[13] with permission.

regression syndrome leads to sacral or lumbo-sacral agenesis. Duhamel[11-13] thinks that if caudal abortion has a teratogenic action, the caudal regression syndrome is a specific caudal anomaly linked to some species and with a genetic pattern. In reality, caudal abortion and caudal regression syndrome may result in the same deformities. Dunn[38] crossbred short tail mice which led indifferently to caudal abortion or to caudal regression deformities.

Williams and Nixon[61] in ano-rectal malformations found an incidence of 44% of epistasis (one or more additional vertebrae between the thoracic and sacral spine). The iliac bone, instead of connecting with the 25th vertebra, connects with the 26th or 27th. Caudal regression has also been thought to reduce the spine to a constant length. In this case with an iliac bone articulating with the 27th vertebra, the sacrum ends at S3.

Abnormalities associated with sacral agenesis (heart, trachea, and esophagus; rectum; neural arches; limbs; kidneys) can be induced by anomalies in perineal mesenchymation and by dyssynchronization of the temporal relationship between the developing viscera and skeleton (Fig. 7.11).

Autopsy Case Reports

Friedel[62] in 1910 was the first to perform an autopsy on such a case. Others (Israel et al.,[63] Finer,[53] Hotston and Carty[64] reported results of postmortem dissection with special attention to visceral abnormalities but no details of the sacral region.

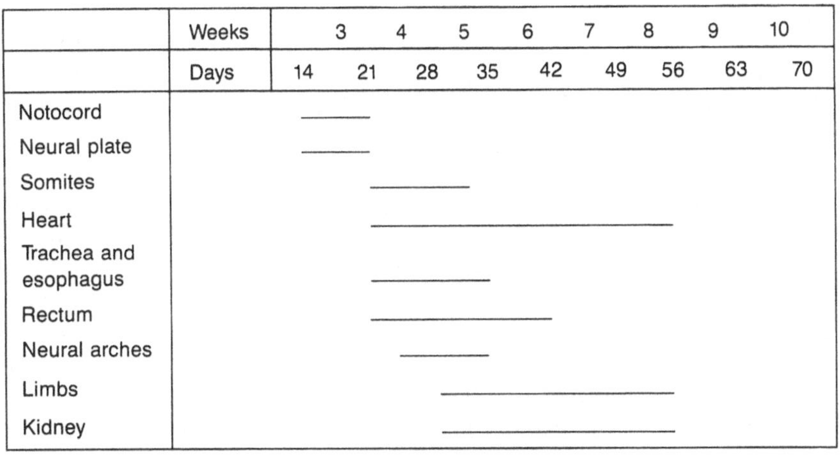

	Weeks	3	4	5	6	7	8	9	10
	Days	14	21	28	35	42	49	56	63	70
Notocord		———							
Neural plate		———							
Somites			————						
Heart				———————————					
Trachea and esophagus				————					
Rectum				—————					
Neural arches			———						
Limbs					————————				
Kidney					————————				

Figure 7.11. The temporal relationship of the developing viscera and skeleton. From: Stanley et al[18] with permission.

Frantz[21] did post-amputation lower-limb dissection in four cases. He found a normal arterial tree, no muscle tissue, and superficial subcutaneous nerve fibers along the medial aspect of the leg. Ignelzi and Lehman[65] in 1974 found ganglia cells, suggesting that the neural crest had developed normally.

Anderton and Owen[66] in 1983 dissected a lumbo-sacral agenesis specimen in which the spine ended below L1; two cartilaginous plates spanned the gap between the first lumbar vertebra and the pelvis; the spinal cord ended at the 11th thoracic vertebra and from there the cauda equina streamed distally to end in two large nodules; and histologic examination of the nodules showed well-formed ganglia with bands of nerve tissue. This specimen had no pituitary gland.

Durham-Smith[10] made careful dissections of six specimens with sacral agenesis. Two distinct patterns of spinal nerve outflow were found:

1. In four cases, the sacral roots failed to develop caudal to the lowest formed vertebra and there was a close correlation between absent sacral nerves and deficient sacral segments.

2. In two other specimens, some sacral roots were absent, some were present even where vertebrae were absent, and some of the nerves were extraordinarily persistent in reaching their destination even to the extent of crossing and recrossing the midline.

Rusnak[32] in 1965 dissected a specimen with thoraco-lumbo-sacral agenesis. The spine ended below T11 and only nerve fibers could be found below this level. Both grossly and microscopically the brain and upper segments of the cord were normal. Abraham[67,68] in 1976 reported an autopsy of a specimen with lumbo-sacral agenesis below L3. The most distal nerve root exiting beyond the lowest lumbar vertebra was the third lumbar-nerve root. Sarnat et al.[69] in 1976 dissected a specimen with lumbo-sacral agenesis below L3. He found two sacral nerve roots larger in diameter than the others.

Clinical Characteristics

There is a great difference between partial sacral agenesis and lumbo-sacral agenesis. In the first group, clinical appearance is normal leading to delay in the diagnosis. This diagnosis is usually made by the urologist when the patients complain of urinary problems, especially enuresis. On the other hand, patients with lumbo-sacral agenesis have a Buddha-like appearance, with marked narrowing of the pelvis and collapse of the ilio-lumbar articulation. This causes pelvic flexion when the patient is not supported by his upper extremities. The buttocks are uniformly flattened and have a short intergluteal cleft. Frequently, there are prominent gluteal dimples. The lower extremities are small and the hips are abducted in the coronal plane. Severe flexion contractures of the hips and knees are common, and prominent popliteal webbing is always present in severe cases (Fig. 7.12). The lower extremities are commonly cone-shaped or tapered and the feet are often in calcaneo-varus or equino varus deformity.

In the lower limb, no muscle tissue is present. Fatty infiltration and scant nerve filaments are the only identified tissue at autopsy with normal shape and distribution but a smaller than normal arterial tree.

Urologic Complications

The primary urologic deficit associated with sacral agenesis is neurogenic bladder dysfunction resulting from failure in development of one or more sacral segments (Williams[61]). But Ringertz[70] showed that even minor lumbo-sacral spine anomalies can lead to enuresis.

The innervation of the muscles of the bladder, urethra, and pelvic floor is complex and debated (Nergardh and Naglo[71]). When the bladder is distended during filling, the afferent impulses are transmitted with the parasympathetic pelvic nerve to sacral segments in the spinal cord. This spinal micturition reflex sends its efferent impulses through the pelvic nerve initiating contraction of the detrusor muscle in the bladder wall and relaxation of some of the peri-urethral muscles. The reflex is inhibited by the sympathetic hypogastric nerve via a thoraco-lumbar center and a spinal connection to the micturition and neurologic center. Koff and Derrider[72] made a careful neurologic examination of patients with sacral agenesis and neurologic bladder. Each patient displayed an individualized mixture of upper and/or lower motor neuron deficits. For a complete description of current thinking on physiologic micturition and the pathogenesis of its disturbances, see the chapter by Berlini and Vigevano in this volume.

Williams[61] and White[4] reported two series with absence of two or more sacral segments. All the patients had an abnormal bladder function. Williams[61] stressed that urinary symptoms in patients with an abnormal sacrum may not develop until later in life. Koontz and Prout[73] emphasized the catastrophic results of a late diagnosis, something that unfortunately occurs often delayed (Braren and Jones[74] and Cumes[75]).

Figure 7.12. Sacral agenesis with femoral agenesis.

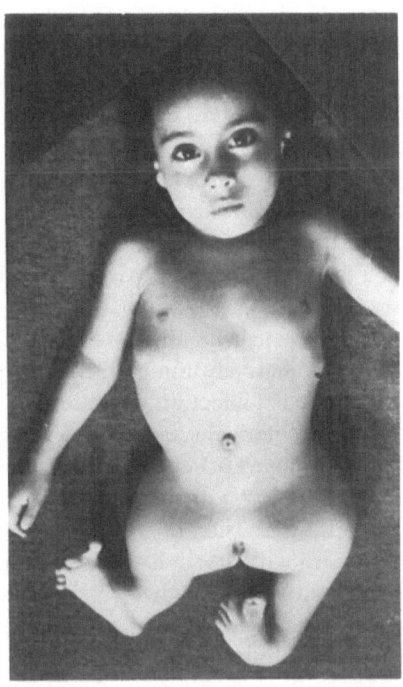

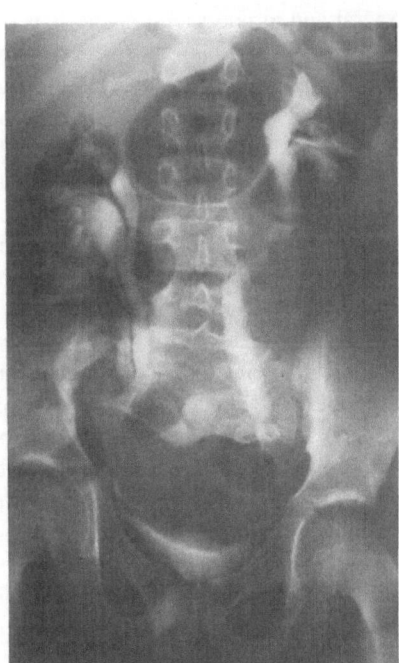

Figure 7.13. Sacral agenesis with duplication of the ureter.

The innervation of the perineal skin (S2–3–4–5) is through the same roots as the main sacral outflow to the bladder (S2–3–4). In spite of this, the presence of perineal sensation in sacral agenesis with incontinent bladder is often encountered. The main urologic problems are incontinence, whether of the spastic or overflow type; vesico-ureteral reflux, found in 91% of the patients with sacral agenesis[76]; hydronephrosis; recurrent infections of the urinary tract leading to failure in renal function; and duplication of the ureter (Fig. 7.13). Genital function has been investigated by only one author, Ruderman.[77] He reported the case of a married woman, 47 years old, with sacral agenesis, who enjoyed a normal sexual life.

In the management of a congenital neurogenic bladder secondary to sacral agenesis, there are three objectives: preservation of renal function, control or elimination of infection, and adequate urinary continence. The treatment modalities available include the Credé maneuver, which is generally unsatisfactory; bladder training, when detrusor dysfunction is mild in an older child; intermittent catheterization, rather than indwelling catheter drainage; and urinary diversion and plastic revision of the bladder neck. Actually, intermittent catheterization combined with drugs that increase urethral resistance is used to correct incontinence and upper tract deterioration. Implantation of an artificial sphincter would have to be combined with ureteral reimplantation because of the almost 100% incidence of ureteral reflux.

Neurologic Complications

Sacral and lumbo-sacral agenesis is often associated with neurologic complications other than motor neuron dysfunction in the lower limb. Posterior meningocele and meningomyelocele are the most frequent abnormalities associated with sacral agenesis. This high incidence of meningomyelocele, 16% (Table 7.1), results in the designation of a special group in the classification of sacral agenesis. Sacral agenesis has also been associated with occult spinal dysraphism. Sarnat[69] found an occult meningomyelocele in the soft tissue at the level of the sacral bony defect. Of the 73 patients reported on by Anderson[78] with occult spinal dysraphism, eight had partially absent or split sacral segments and one had complete absence of the sacrum.

Conditions such as lipoma of the cord (Andrish[27]), dermoid cyst, and tethering of the cord owing to a tight filum terminale may be encountered (Fig. 7.14). Five cases of hydrocephalus and one case of microcephalus were reported. Except for Tandon and Lall[79] and Louri,[80] myelography is not reported in literature.

In spite of pathologic mobility at the spino-pelvic junction in lumbo-sacral agenesis, no significant neurologic worsening or improvement has occurred in patients with hemisacrum or sacral agenesis with the passage of time. Little is known about the intellectual and developmental outcome of those patients. In a series of 24 patients with vertebral agenesis, Rosenfelder[81] described two patients with above normal intelligence and nine with mental retardation. Renshaw[17]

Table 7.1. Associated malformations in sacral agenesis.

	Stanley	Blummel	Durham-Smith	Renshaw	Andrish	Banta	Carlo	Total	Percent
Case number	71	50	26	23	17	7	8	202	
Male	30	27	5	8	8	3	2	83	43
Female	41	23	13	15	9	4	6	111	57
Oesophageal atresia and duodenal atresia	5	–	1	1	–	1	–	7	3.4
Rectal atresia, imperforate or ectopic anus	17	5	8	4	2	1	2	39	19
Cardio-vascular abnormalities	6	2	1	2	3	–	3	17	8
Renal agenesis	8	1	2	5	5	–	2	23	11
Renal hypoplasia or horseshoe, or double kidney	4	–	2	2	2	–	–	10	5
Dislocation of the hip	10	10	–	7	9	4	2	42	20
Club foot or lobster-claw foot	10	21	–	9	8	4	3	55	27
Arthrogryposis multiplex congenita	7	6	–	–	–	2	–	15	7
Hemivertebra and/or fused ribs	10	9	4	5	12	–	1	41	20
Short femur and/or tibia	4	–	–	–	1	–	–	5	2.4
Spina bifida occulta other than sacral	10	5	2	–	–	–	–	17	8
Absence of tibia and/or fibula	2	1	–	–	–	–	–	3	1
Meningomyelocele	6	3	13	8	3	1	–	34	16
Hypospadias, diaphragme hernia, agenesis of lung	–	–	4	–	–	–	1	5	2.4
Omphalocele	–	–	1	1	–	–	–	2	1
Cleft lip and palate	–	3	–	–	–	–	–	3	1.5
Extrophy of bladder, lipoma of cauda equina	–	–	–	–	2	–	–	2	1
Hydrocephalus	–	–	–	2	3	–	–	5	2.4
Persistent cloaca	–	–	–	3	–	–	–	3	1.5
Microcephalus	–	–	–	1	–	–	–	1	0.5
Scoliosis	–	5	–	11	4	–	1	21	10
Inguinal hernia	–	3	–	1	–	–	–	4	2
Atrophy of legs	–	4	–	–	2	–	–	6	3
Radial club hand	–	–	–	–	2	–	–	2	1

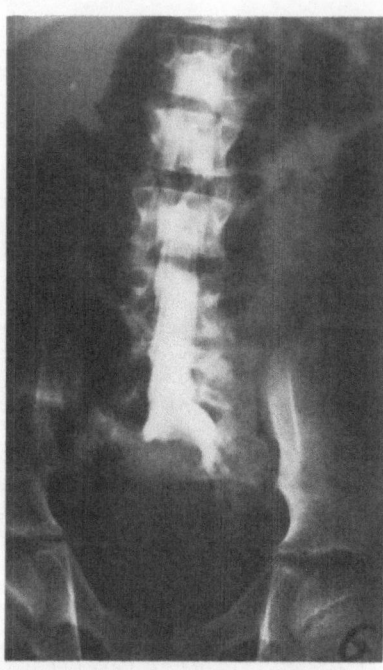

Figure 7.14. Lipoma of the cord with tight filum terminale associated with sacral agenesis.

described seven mentally retarded patients in a series of 23. Carlo[82] reported four cases with normal intelligence.

Visceral Malformation

In order to learn the frequency of associated visceral malformations, we have to analyze seven publications (Stanley,[18] Blummel,[28] Durham-Smith,[10] Renshaw,[17] Andrish,[27] Banta,[22] and Carlo[82]) that report a total of 202 well-detailed observations (Table 7.1). Sex ratio is 57% female and 43% male. Rectal atresia or imperforate anus is the most frequently associated visceral malformation (19%), followed by renal agenesis (11%) and cardiovascular abnormalities (8%). The remaining multiple visceral malformations add up to fewer than 5%. For the treatment of such multiple and different visceral malformations, one should consult the work of Carcassonne.[83]

Orthopedic Management

In his publication, Frantz[21] described orthopedic deformities of patients with lumbo-sacral agenesis:

The patient sits in a characteristic cross-legged attitude, the feet directed dorsally, the femora abducted in the coronal plan, and the knees flexed at 60 degrees. The feet usually are under the buttock in calcaneus position. There is a dorsal prominence of the twelfth thoracic vertegra. A wide popliteal web exists. When the patient sits unsupported, the pelvis seems to roll up under the thorax. When the patient supports himself on his hands, the pelvis drops forward, seeming to rest ventral to the thoracic spine. All patients reported had normal sensation down to the knees.

Aitken,[19] Frantz,[21] and Russel[20] recommend bilateral subtrochanteric amputation and early prosthetic fitting for the severe deformities of lower limbs in lumbo-sacral agenesis. The prostheses are semirigid plastic laminated pelvithoracic buckets, which ride high on the thorax and are fashioned in the nature of a funnel to allow some weight-bearing. Exterior perineal surface is made flat for stability in the sitting position.

Phillips[23] thinks that when there is inadequate quadriceps function, it is difficult to correct knee flexion contractures and to prevent them from recurring. For severe knee deformity, knee disarticulation rather than subtrochanteric amputation and prosthetic fitting is the most effective treatment. Banta[22] uses serial corrective casts, applied as early as possible, and repeated anterior supracondylar closing wedge osteotomies; the patients walk with the aid of braces and forearm crutches. Banta believes that preserved sensation and proprioception, present in most of these patients, warrant preservation of the limbs. Andrish[27] agrees with Banta that subtrochanteric amputations in the past have been overemphasized as a part of the routine management of these patients (Figs. 7.15 and 7.16).

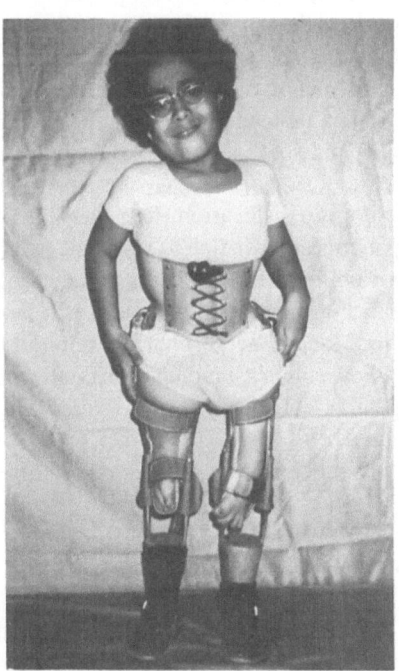

Figure 7.15. Protheses for a patient with lumbo-sacral agenesis.

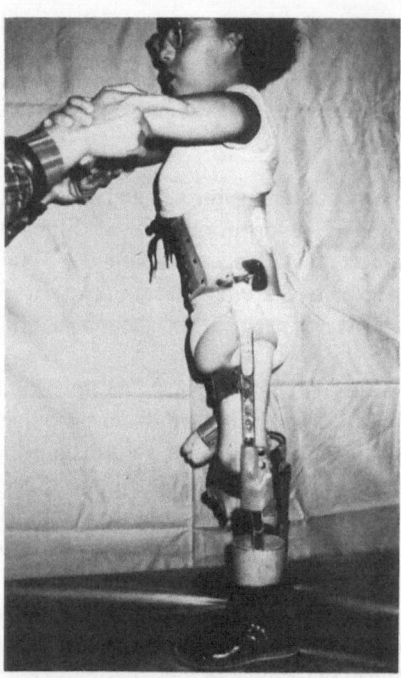

Figure 7.16. Same patient as Figure 7.15.

Perry[26] and Pirkey[25] recommend spinal-pelvic fusion because it allows patients to sit with the hands free, permits stretching of the hip-flexion contractures, and protects the viscera from unphysiologic compression. Philips[23] says "it is difficult to assess the significance of visceral compression." For Philips and Andrish[27] spinal-pelvic fusion cannot be recommended because it may cause problems with hip-flexion contractures that previously were compensated for by the hypermobile spinal pelvic junction. Seventeen of Philips' nineteen surviving patients sit without support and have no apparent problems.

For hip dislocation, Renshaw[17] thinks that many surgical procedures in some patients are justified to avoid the pain, breakdown of the skin, and increased pelvic obliquity. The benefits of reduction of dislocated hips in patients with lumbosacral agenesis may not be worth the risk of having painful stiff hips resulting from aseptic necrosis of the femoral head or infection.

For scoliosis, bracing is difficult when spinal-pelvic instability is present. Congenital scoliosis, that is progressing in an adolescent or pre-adolescent patient, is fused.

Foot deformities are treated by corrective plaster casts and/or surgical releases.

Summary

1. Patients with sacral or lumbo-sacral agenesis must be cared for by a multidisciplinary team including a neurosurgeon, an urologist, an othropedic surgeon,

and in severe cases a physiotherapist, an occupational therapist, and a prosthesist.

2. Anterior sacral defects associated with an anterior meningocele or teratoma, or both, are probably an autosomal inherited condition but no support for a familial inheritance can be found for sacral agenesis alone.

3. Sacral agenesis is associated with a high incidence of maternal diabetes mellitus.

4. The relationship between neurologic findings and skeletal defects is not always consistent.

5. A classification similar to that of Standly is proposed.

6. In minor forms of sacral agenesis, the diagnosis is often not made until patients consult an urologist for enuresis.

7. Rectal atresia or imperforate anus is the most frequently associated visceral malformation (19%), followed by renal agenesis (11%) and cardiovascular abnormalities (8%).

References

1. Paris J, Laine E: Agénésie sacro-coccygienne héréditaire avec perforation anal incomplète. Mégarectum dans l'enfance, méningocèle pelvienne à l'âge adulte. Semin Hôp Paris 49:1320–1322, 1973.
2. Hohl AF: Zur Pathologie des Beckens. I. Das schräg–ovale–Becken. Wilhelm Engelmann, Leipzig, p 61, 1852.
3. Wertheim C: Vollständiger Mangel des Kreuz-und steissbeins bei einem Neugeborenen. Monaststschr Geburtsk Frauenkr 9:127–131, 1857.
4. White RI, Klauber GT: Sacral agenesis: analysis of 22 cases. Urology 8:521–525, 1976.
5. Achard C, Foix C, Mouzon J: Syndrome de réduction numérique des vertèbres sacro-coccygiennes. Revue Neurol 1:270, 1924.
6. Foix C, Hillemand P: Dystrophie cruro-vésico-fessière par agénésie sacro-coccygienne. Rev Neurol 40:450–468, 1924.
7. Stewart TM, Stoll S: Familial caudal regression anomalad and maternal diabetes. J Med Genet 16:17, 1979.
8. Pouzet F: Les anomalies de développement du sacrum. Lyon Chirurgical, Séance du 2.2. 35:371–373, 1938.
9. Blummel J, Butler MC, Evans EB, Eggers GWN: Congenital anomaly of the sacrococcygeal spine. Arch Surg 85:982–993, 1962.
10. Durham-Smith E: Congenital sacral anomalies in children. Austr N Zeal J Surg 29:165–176, 1959.
11. Duhamel B: Malformations ano-rectales et malformations vertébrales. Arch Franç Pediatr 16:534, 1959.
12. Duhamel B: From the mermaid to anal imperforation: the syndrome of caudal regression. Arch Dis Child 36:152, 1961.
13. Duhamel B: Morphogenese pathologique, Vol. 1. Paris, 1966.
14. Say B, Gerald PS: A new polydactyly (imperforate anus) vertebral anomalies syndrome? Lancet 688, 1968.
15. Quan L, Smith DW: The Vater association, vertebral defects, anal atresia, T.E. fistula

with esophageal atresia, radial and renal dysplasia: a spectrum of associated defects. J Pediatr 82:104, 1973.

16. Carey JC, Greenbaum B, Hall BD: The O.E.I.S. complex (omphalocèle, exstrophy, imperforate anus, spinal defects). Birth Defects. Original Article Series, Vol. XIV: The National Foundation, March of Dimes, New York, 1978, p 253.

17. Renshaw TS: Sacral agenesis. J Bone Joint Surg 60 A:373–383, 1978.

18. Stanley JK, Owen R, Koff S: Congenital sacral anomalies. J Bone Joint Surg 61 B:401–409, 1979.

19. Aitken GT, Frantz CH: Management of the child amputee. In: Instructional Course Lectures, The American Academy of Orthopaedic Surgeons, Vol. 17. CV Mosby, St. Louis, 1960, pp 246–295.

20. Russel HE, Aitken GT: Congenital absence of the sacrum and lumbar vertebrae with prosthetic management. J Bone Joint Surg 45A:501–508, 1963.

21. Frantz CH, Aitken GT: Complete absence of the lumbar spine and sacrum. J Bone Joint Surg 49A:1531–1540, 1967.

22. Banta JV, Nichols O: Sacral agenesis. J Bone Joint Surg 51A:693–703, 1969.

23. Phillips WA, Cooperman DR, Lindquist TC, Sullivan RC, Millar EA: Orthopaedic management of lumbosacral agenesis. J Bone Joint Surg 64A:1282–1294, 1982.

24. Van Derwerker EE: Ilio-lumbar fusion in the management of sacral agenesis. Int Clin Inform Bull Subcommittee on Child Prosthetics. Problems and Development 5:8, 1966.

25. Pirkey EL, Purcell JH: Agenesis of lumbosacral vertebrae. A report of ten cases in living infants. Radiology 69:726–729, 1938.

26. Perry J, Bonnett CA, Hoffer M: Vertebral pelvic fusions in the rehabilitation of patients with sacral agenesis. J Bone Joint Surg 52A:288–294, 1970.

27. Andrish J, Kalamchi A, MacEwen D: Sacral agenesis. Clin Orthop 139:52–57, 1979.

28. Blummel J, Evans EB, Eggers GWN: Partial and complete agenesis of malformation of the sacrum with associated anomalies. J Bone Joint Surg 41A:497–518, 1959.

29. Pedersen LM, Tygstrup I, Pedersen J: Congenital malformations in newborn infants of diabetic women. Lancet 1:1124–1126, 1964.

30. Stern L, Ramos A, Light L: Sacral agenesis in infants of diabetic mothers. Lancet i:1393, 1965.

31. Kucera J: Exposure to fat solvents: a possible cause of sacral agenesis in man. J Pediatr 72:857–859, 1968.

32. Rusnak SL, Driscoll SG: Congenital spinal anomalies in infants of diabetic mothers. Pediatrics 35:989–995, 1965.

33. Barnetche JM: Agénésies lombo-sacrées. Thèse, Médecine, Bordeaux, 1984, no. 135.

34. Thalhammer O, Lachmann D, Scheibenreiter J: Caudale regression beim kind einer 18 jährigen Frau mit Prädiabetes. Ztsch Kinderh 102:346, 1968.

35. Corda GM: Ricerche sperimentali sulla influenza della iperglicemia e della ipoglicemia materna sul decorso della gravidanza e sullo sviluppo dei feti. Ann Obstet Gyneol 54:143, 1932.

36. Landauer W: Rumplessness of chicken embryos produced by the injection of insulin and other chemicals. J Exp Zool 98:65–75, 1945.

37. Duraiswami PK: Insulin induced skeletal abnormalities in developing children. Br Med J 2:384–390, 1950.

38. Dunn LC: The inheritance of rumplessness in the domestic fowl. J Hered 16:127, 1925.

39. Danforth CH: Artificial and hereditary suppression of sacral vertebrae in the fowl. Proc Soc Exp Biol 30:143–145, 1932.

40. Lichtenstein H, Guest GM, Warkany J: Abnormalities in offspring of white rats given protamine zinc insulin during pregnancy. Proc Soc Exp Biol Med 78:398, 1951.
41. Runner MN: Inheritance of susceptibility to congenital deformity. Pediatrics 23:245, 1959.
42. Sevastikoglou JA: Biochemical studies on the skeleton of insulin induced micromelia in chickens. Acta Paediatr 51:60, 1962.
43. Chung CS, Myrianthopoulos NC: Factors affecting risks of congenital malformations. Birth Defects. Original Article Series, Vol. XI. The National Foundation, March of Dimes, New York, 1975, p 10.
44. Ancel P, Lallemand S: Sur l'arrêt de développement du bourgeon caudal obtenu expérimentalement chez l'embryon de poulet. Arch Phys Biol 15:43(Suppl 27), 1941.
45. Cohlan SQ: Congenital anomalies in the rate produced by excessive intake of Vit A during pregnancy. Pediatrics 13:556–567, 1954.
46. Kalter H, Warkany J: Congenital malformations of the vertebral bodies. Bull John Hopkins Hosp 62:216, 1938.
47. Gillman J, Gilbert C, Gillman T: A preliminary report on hydrocephalus, spina bifida and other congenital anomalies in the rat produced by Trypan blue. S Afr J Med Sci 13:47, 1948.
48. Beaudoin AR, Wilson JG: Teratogenic effect of Trypan blue on the developing chick. Proc Soc Exp Biol Med 97:85, 1958.
49. Kaplan S, Grabowski CT: Analysis of Trypan blue-induced rumplessness in chick embryos. J Exp Zool 165:325, 1967.
50. Nogami H, Ingalls T: Pathogenesis of spinal malformations induced in the embryos of mice. J Bone Joint Surg 49A:1551, 1967.
51. Bloom CJ, Stone RE, Henriques A: Three unusual cases of congenital origin. Arch Pediatr 34:512–515, 1917.
52. Rochet E, Gacon G, Robert JM, Grunthaler C: Dystocie osseuse par agénésie sacro-coccygienne. Gynecol Obstet 65:115–124, 1966.
53. Finer NN, Bowen P, Dunbar LG: Caudal regression anomalad (sacral agenesis) in siblings. Clin Genet 13:353–358, 1978.
54. Cohn J, Bay-Nielsen E: Hereditary defect of the sacrum and coccyx with anterior sacral meningocele. Acta Paediatr Scand 58:268–274, 1969.
55. Ashcraft KW, Holder TM, Harris DJ: Familial presacral teratomas. In: Birth Defects. Original Article Series, Vol. XI. The National Foundation, March of Dimes, New York, pp 143–146.
56. Kenefick JS: Hereditary sacral agenesis associated with presacral tumours. Br J Surg 60:271–274, 1973.
57. Yates VD, Wilroy RS, Whitington GL, Simmons JCH: Anterior sacral defects: an autosomal dominantly inherited condition. J Pediatr 102:239–242, 1983.
58. Wolff E: Les bases de tératogénèse expérimentale des vertèbres amniotes d'après les résultats de méthodes directes. Arch Anat Histol Embryol (Strasb) 22:1, 1936.
59. Roux C, Martinet M: Syndrome de régression caudale chez l'animal. Arch Franc Pediatr 19:781, 1962.
60. Smith DW, Bartlett C, Harrah LM: Monozygotic twinning and the Duhamel anomalad. Birth Defects. Original Article Series, Vol. XII. The National Foundation, March of Dimes, New York, 1976, pp 53–63.
61. Williams DI, Nixon HH: Agenesis of the sacrum. Surg Gynecol Obstet 105:84, 1957.
62. Friedel G: Defekt der wirbelsaüle nom 10 Brustwirbel an abwärts bei einem Neugeborenen. Arch Klin Chir 93:944–958, 1910.

63. Israel JN, Day DW, Hirschmann A, Smith GF: Sacral agenesis and associated anomalies. Birth Defects. Original Article Series, Vol. XII. The National Foundation, March of Dimes, 1976, pp 45–51.

64. Hotston S, Carthy H: Lumbosacral agenesis: a report of three new cases and a review of the literature. Br J Radiol 55:629–633, 1982.

65. Ignelzi RJ, Lehman RAW: Lumbosacral agenesis: management and embryological implications. J Neurol Neurosurg Psychiatry 37:1273–1276, 1974.

66. Anderton JM, Owen R: Absence of the pituitary gland in a case of congenital sacral agenesis. J Bone Joint Surg 65B:182–183, 1983.

67. Abraham E: Lumbosacral coccygeal agenesis. Autopsy case report. J Bone Joint Surg 58A:1169–1171, 1976.

68. Abraham E: Sacral agenesis with associated anomalies (caudal regression syndrome): autopsy case report. Clin Orthop 145:168–171, 1979.

69. Sarnat HB, Case ME, Graviss R: Sacral agenesis. Neurology 26:1124–1129, 1976.

70. Ringertz H: Bladder capacity, urethral sensation and lumbosacral anomalies in children with enuresis. Acta Radiol Diagn 25:45–48, 1984.

71. Nergardh A, Naglo AS: Observations on the internal sphincter mechanism during the filling phase in children with hyperactive neurogenic bladder. Scand J Urol Nephrol 16:205, 1982.

72. Koff SA, Deridder PA: Pattern of neurogenic bladder dysfunction in sacral agenesis. J Urol 118:87–89, 1977.

73. Koontz W, Prout G: Agenesis of the sacrum and neurogenic bladder. JAMA 203:481–486, 1968.

74. Braren V, Jones WB: Sacral agenesis: diagnosis, treatment and follow up of urological complications. J Urol 121:543–544, 1979.

75. Cumes D: Dysraphism causing neurogenic bladder dysfunction. J Urol 117:127–128, 1976.

76. Mariani AJ, Stern J, Khan AV, Cass AS: Sacral agenesis: an analysis of 11 cases and review of the literature. J Urol 122:684–686, 1979.

77. Ruderman RJ, Keats P, Goldner JL: Congenital absence of the lumbosacral spine. A report of an unusual case. Clin Orthop 124:177–180, 1977.

78. Anderson FM: Occult spinal dysraphism. Pediatrics 55:826, 1975.

79. Tandon PN, Lall BN: Agenesis of the sacrum and coccyx. Ind Pediatr 5:274–276, 1968.

80. Louri H: Sacral agenesis. Case report. J Neurosurg 38:92–95, 1973.

81. Rosenfelder BA: Vertebral agenesis. Review of the literature and presentation of 24 new cases. I. Am Phys Ther Assoc 48:203–217, 1968.

82. Carlo WA, Kliegman RM, Dixon MS, Fletcher BD, Fanaroff AA: Vertebral agenesis. Am J Dis Child 136:533–537, 1982.

83. Carcassonne M, Bergoin M, Choux M, Montfort G, Gregoire A, Morrisson-Lacombe G, Bollini G: Les malformations de la colonne lombo-sacrée et leurs implications viscérales. Chir Pediatr 22:n=2–3, pp 69–223, 1982.

84. Passarge E, Lenz W: Syndrome of caudal regression in infants of diabetic mothers: observations of further cases. Pediatrics 37:672, 1966.

CHAPTER 8

Teratomas

J.G. Raffensperger

Teratomas are rare, puzzling neoplasms containing a diversity of tissue not ordinarily found at the tumor's site. The term *teratoma* is derived from the Greek word meaning monster and accurately suggests the dichotomy of these lesions, i.e., a combination of developmental anomaly and tumor. They are almost always found in children and frequently arise in the gonads. Extragonadal teratomas tend to occur near the midline of the body, indicating their possible origin from disorganized cells in the germinal layers of the primitive streak or notochord. The sites of origin of extragonadal teratomas are those often seen as common points of connection between conjoined twins.

Despite considerable experimental work, the exact cellular origin of teratomas remains unknown. The two oldest schools of thought suggest either germ cells or undifferentiated embryonic cells.[1] The tissue is highly variable within a single tumor. There may be derivatives from only two germ layers such as skin, skin appendages, and connective tissue. However, in most sacro-coccygeal tumors, there is tissue from all three germ layers including skin, teeth, nervous system, intestine, endocrine glands, cartilage, and bone (Fig. 8.1). There are also varying degrees of differentiation in individual tissues. The more differentiated tumors may contain well-developed extremities or a partially formed fetus (Fig. 8.2). The most immature component resembles undifferentiated embryonic cells. In general, teratomas containing well-differentiated tissue are benign; the more immature or poorly differentiated tissue is most often malignant. Unfortunately, a small nest of immature cells in an otherwise well differentiated teratoma may metastasize or lead to local recurrence.

Literature Review

Data from 405 cases of children with sacro-coccygeal teratomas were collected by the Surgical Section of the American Academy of Pediatrics in 1973.[2] Seventy-four percent of these patients were female. The diagnosis was made on the first day of life in 205 cases. Seventy-four infants (18%) had associated con-

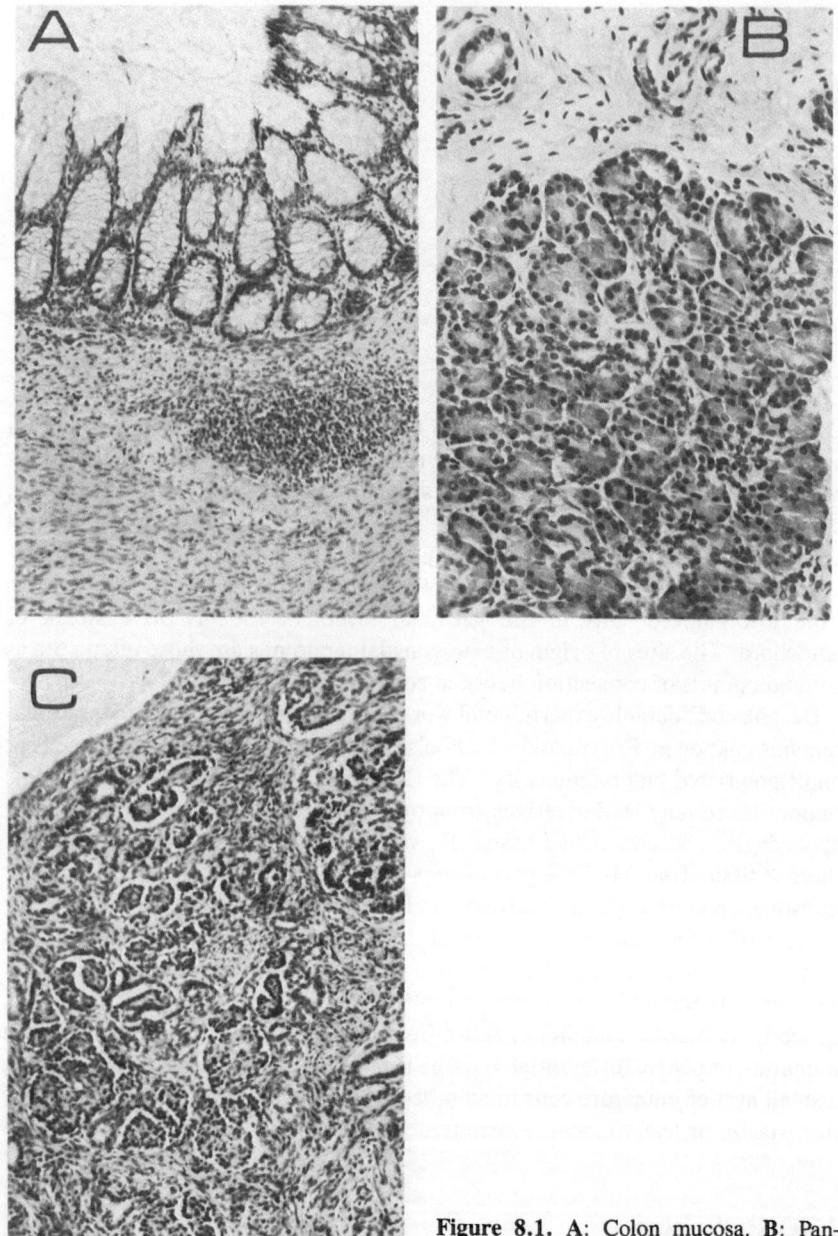

Figure 8.1. A: Colon mucosa. B: Pancreas. C: Glomeruli and renal tubules.

genital anomalies, most involving the musculoskeletal system. This large group of tumors was subdivided and classified according to the size of the intrapelvic portion of the tumor. In 186 patients, the bulk of the mass extended outside of the pelvis and was readily visible (Fig. 8.3). Only 39 patients had presacral lesions

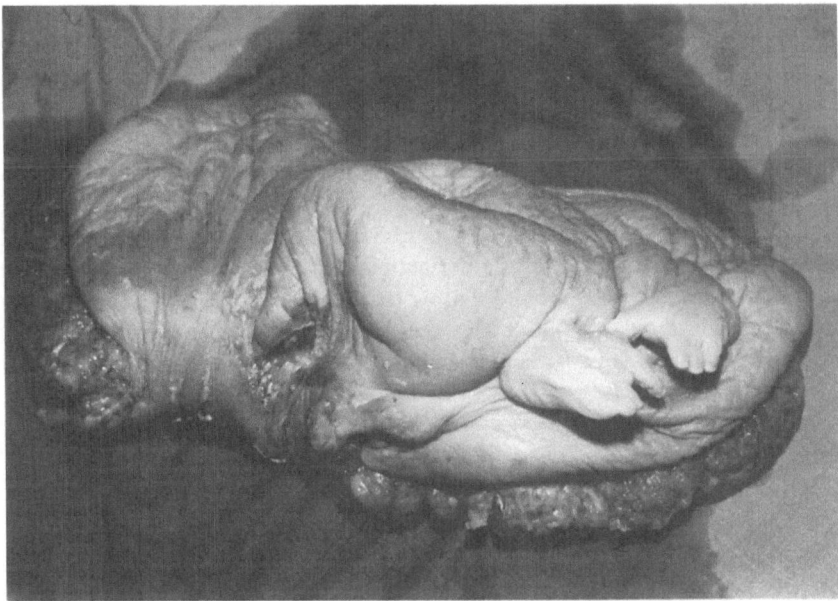

Figure 8.2. Sacro-coccygeal teratoma, lying within a sac and exhibiting extremities with formed digits.

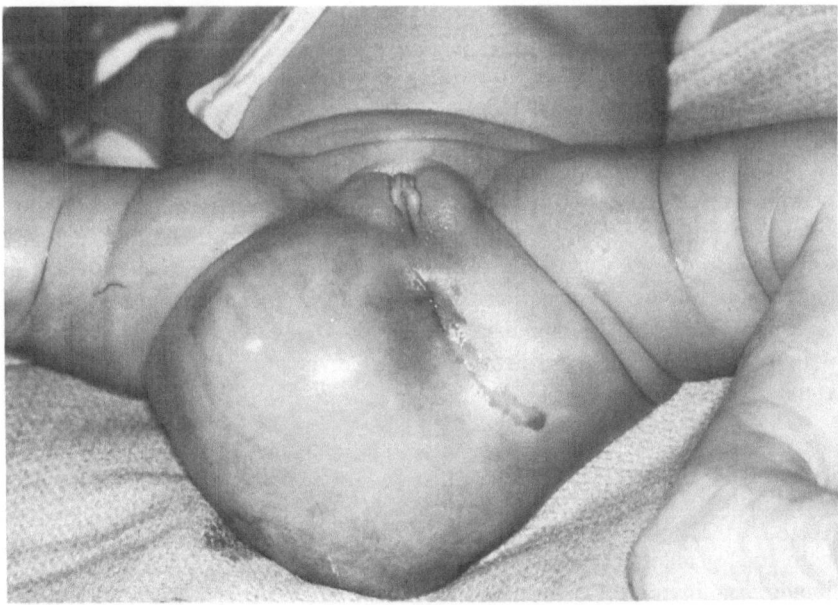

Figure 8.3. Sacro-coccygeal teratoma, lying outside the pelvic cavity in a newborn infant.

without external presentation. Intrapelvic or presacral tumors had a higher incidence of malignancy. As would be expected, there was considerable delay in the diagnosis of the presacral lesions which were invisible to exterior observation. Thus, there is considerable clinical importance in defining sacro-coccygeal teratomas as *presacral* or *postsacral*.

There may be a genetic influence in their origin, since Ashcraft and his associates have described a familial syndrome of presacral teratomas, sacral defects, and anal stenosis.[3] The familial distribution in his series suggests an autosomal dominant transmission. Several other authors have described both the familial occurrence of these lesions as well as associated birth defects.[4-6] Sacral tumors rarely present in older children and adults. Usually there has been a history of neglected draining sinuses or a long-standing mass lesion suggesting the onset at a much earlier time.[7]

Pathology

Benign teratomas are well encapsulated and contain varying degrees of solid and cystic components (Fig. 8.4). Even well-encapsulated benign lesions are often intimately adherent to the coccyx. The cystic fluid may be serous, mucoid, or bloody, and the cyst lining often consists of recognizable squamous epithelium with sebaceous material and teeth. Limb buds and male genitalia may also protrude into the cyst cavity. Predominantly cystic tumors are more likely benign, and the incidence of malignancy rises in proportion to the amount of solid tissue. The variety of tissues within a single teratoma is apparent only on careful microscopic examination which reveals varying degrees of differentiation of almost every organ system.

In spite of the heterogeneity of tissues found in these tumors, the malignant component, when present, is almost always the yolk sac or endodermal sinus tumor. This tumor is microscopically similar to the rat endodermal sinus, a yolk sac structure not found in humans but present in the early development of the fetal rat.[8] Epithelial structures predominate with a papillary and tubo-alveolar pattern of cystic spaces lined by columnar and cuboidal epithelium. Crussi and Roth have supported this origin of the endodermal sinus tumor with electron microscopic studies.[9] In our own series of seven malignant sacro-coccygeal teratomas, the malignant component was always of endodermal sinus origin.[10] Malignant sacral tumors infiltrate into the pelvic organs and metastasize to lymph nodes, liver, and lungs.

Diagnosis

Sacro-coccygeal teratomas have been diagnosed prior to birth by fetal ultrasonographic examination.[11,12] The mass contains more solid elements and is more caudal than the usual meningomyelocele. Prenatal diagnosis is important, because these tumors may be large enough to cause dystocia. Rupture of the

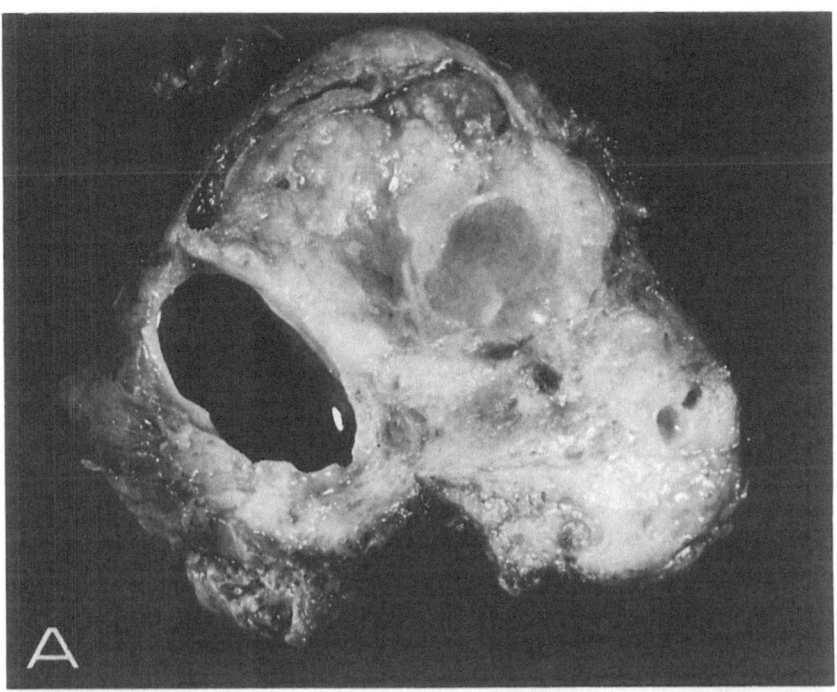

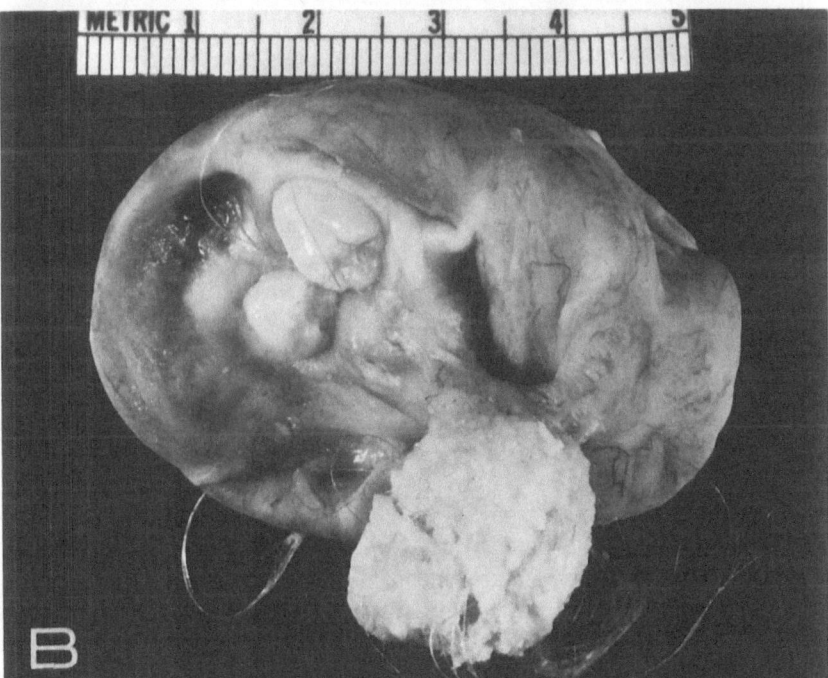

Figure 8.4. Gross section of sacro-coccygeal teratoma. **A:** Solid and cystic component. **B:** Sebaceous material and hair.

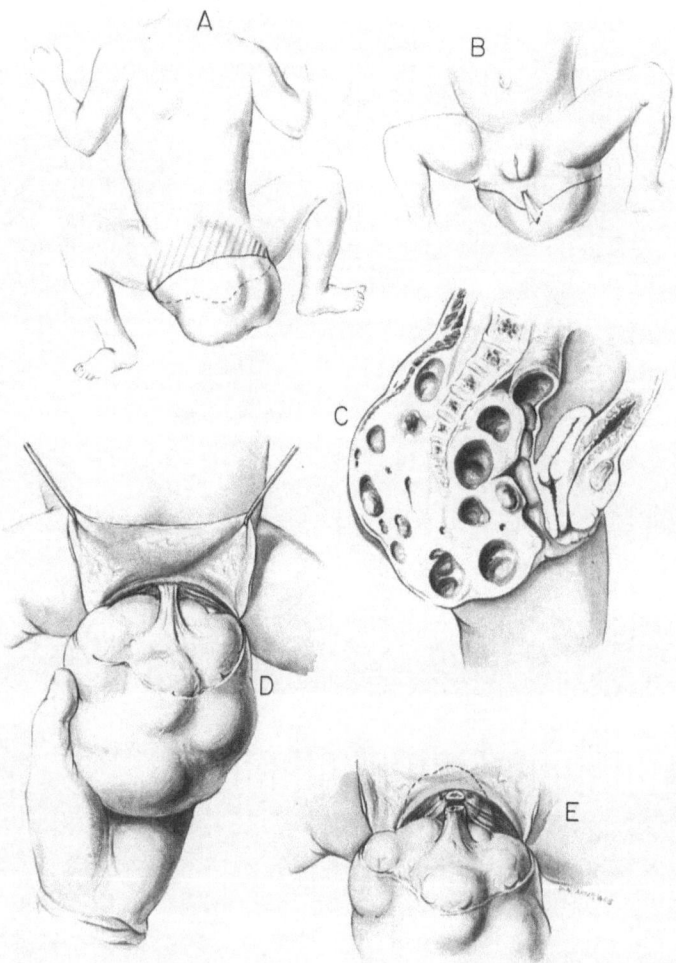

Figure 8.5. Technique for excision of a sacro-coccygeal teratoma. Elevation of skin flap (**A–D**) exposes the tumor, and the coccyx is transected (**E**), the presacral extension is removed (**F–G**), and the wound is closed with drains (**H–J**). (Reprinted with permission from: Raffensperger J: Swenson's Pediatric Surgery, fourth edition, Appleton-Century-Crofts, New York, 1980.)

tumor with massive hemorrhage may also occur during birth. Thus, it is important to have the mother delivered by cesarean section in a center where the infant can receive immediate surgical treatment.

In well over half of the reported cases, a sacro-coccygeal teratoma presents as an obvious caudal, skin covered, firm or cystic mass. The mass may weigh more than the infant or be no more than a barely noticeable lump. The larger masses often distort and push the anus anteriorly. A large presacral extension may compress pelvic veins, causing leg edema. In addition, we have observed an infant

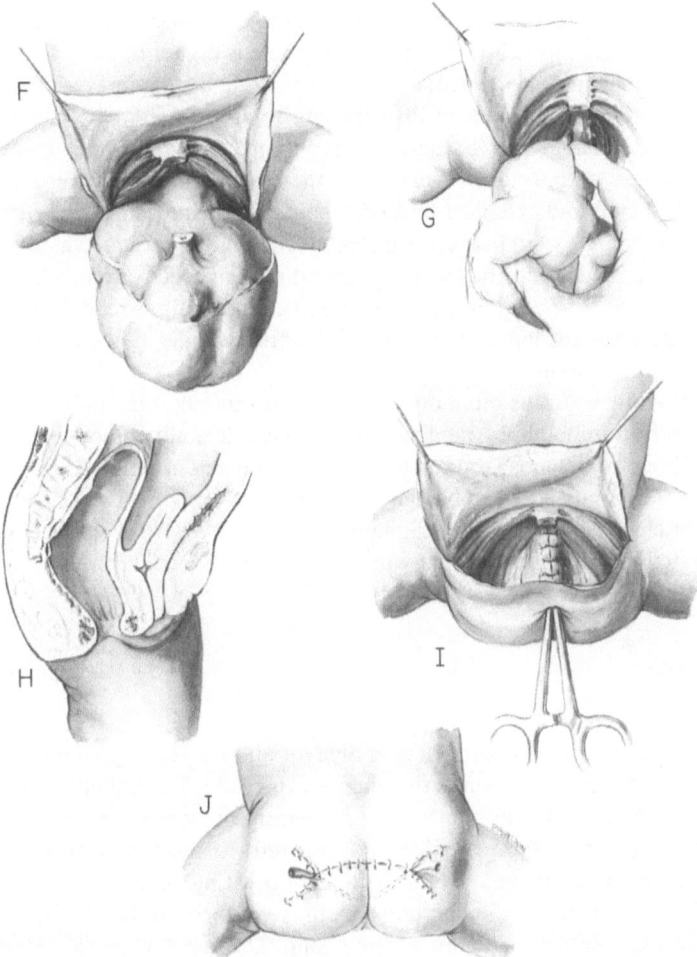

Figure 8.5. *Continued.*

whose presacral tumor obstructed the bladder, causing renal failure and vesical rupture. The skin over large tumors is thin, and may be discolored with hematoma and a network of blood vessels. Rarely a teratoma is off to one side in a buttock. In older children, presacral teratomas can present with constipation or nonspecific pelvic pain. There may be no obvious external mass but rectal examination will reveal a firm tumor, often fixed to the sacrum. Draining sinus tracts or repeated episodes of abscess formation posterior to the anus also suggest an undiagnosed teratoma.

Other tumors such as neuroblastoma, hemangioma, hamartoma, and chordoma could be confused with a teratoma. However, all of these require excision for diagnosis and therapy. A cystic duplication of the rectum is palpable as a smooth, rounded lesion in the presacral space; imaging studies would clearly indicate its cystic nature. It is most important to differentiate a lipomeningocele from a teratoma. Clinically, the lipomeningocele is higher up the back and overlies the spinal canal. Roentgenograms demonstrate a spina bifida. Naidich and associates found it difficult to differentiate teratomas from lipomeningoceles with B-mode sonography because the teratoma was homogeneous and echogenic.[13] These authors did observe that the lipomeningoceles were above the intergluteal cleft and extended through a spina bifida into the canal. Teratomas, on the other hand, were below the intergluteal cleft and extended anterior to the sacrum rather than into the canal. Presacral meningoceles are much softer and more fluctuant than a teratoma. Any imaging study (ultrasound, computerized tomography, or myelogram) should easily differentiate the presacral meningocele from a teratoma.

Plain roentgenograms often demonstrate teeth or calcification in a teratoma. Computerized tomography demonstrates septae and solid components in otherwise difficult to diagnose teratomas. The serum α-fetoprotein (AFP) is a useful test to differentiate between benign and malignant teratomas. In one series, the AFP was elevated in 31 of 32 malignant teratomas.[14] AFP has also been found to be elevated in the amniotic fluid when the infant has a teratoma.[15]

Treatment

Surgical excision is the treatment of choice for all sacro-coccygeal teratomas and should be carried out as soon as the diagnosis is made. The infant is prepared for a major operation. In the newborn, preoperative management consists of the administration of antibiotics, vitamin K, and intravenous fluids. Blood is always typed, cross-matched, and available in the operating room. To prevent intraoperative hypothermia, the operating room is warmed, and the infant is placed on a warming mattress under an infrared lamp. The baby's upper extremities and head should be wrapped in clear plastic sheeting to conserve body heat. Vital signs are monitored with an esophageal temperature probe, a precordial stethoscope, electrocardiogram, and blood pressure cuff. A radial artery catheter is extremely useful for constant recording of the blood pressure and for intraoperative arterial blood gas determinations. When the infant has been anesthetized, he is placed on his abdomen over a roll to elevate his hips. The rectum is irrigated and the skin is cleansed with a solution of povidone iodine and the entire lower back, sacrum, perineum, thighs, and abdomen are draped into the sterile field. The infant can be turned easily onto his back for an abdominal incision if there is extensive intrapelvic tumor. A curved transverse or inverted "V" incision is made over the mass with the apex of the V overlying the coccyx (Fig. 8.5A–J). When the skin is thinned out over a large mass, some is left adherent to the tumor and excised with the specimen. The blood supply of a sacrococcygeal teratoma comes almost entirely from the middle sacral vessels; consequently, the dissection is extended superior to the mass into the subcutaneous tissues overlying the sacrum.

After the upper margins of the tumor and the sacrum have been exposed, the coccyx and lowest sacral segment are transected. The exposure provided allows for ligation of the sacral vessels. In any case, the coccyx must always be removed to prevent tumor recurrence. The fascia over the gluteus muscle is next divided, and the tumor dissected away from the muscle with electrocautery. There may be no clear demarcation of normal tissue from malignant tissue. Consequently, normal muscle should be transected with the electrocautery to obtain a tumor-free margin. As the dissection proceeds about the mass, the surgeon should insert his finger into the rectum in order to identify a safe plane of dissection which will not injure the bowel. Finally, the mass is removed with any excess skin and the wound is irrigated with an antibiotic solution. The levator ani muscles, often thinned and distorted by the mass, should be identified and sutured together in the midline behind the rectum. The wound is drained and separated from the anus with an adherent plastic dressing.

Extensive malignant presacral tumors often require a combined abdominal and presacral excision to separate the tumor from the ureters, bladder, rectum, and pelvic nerves. These children must be prepared and draped to allow a combined abdominal and perineal incision. It is sometimes necessary to remove a portion of the rectum. However, with the advent of effective chemotherapy, tumor may be left behind if necessary to spare vital structures.

Tumor recurrence is almost inevitable unless the coccyx is removed along with the mass.[16] In one personally operated case the mass did not involve the coccyx which was left behind. Five years later, malignant endodermal sinus tumor developed even though the original teratoma was well differentiated. In an extended review of 254 teratomas of all types, Tapper found that the most important single prognostic sign of malignant recurrence was the complete removal of the tumor at the first operation.[17] There is a definitely higher incidence of malignancy when the diagnosis is made after 3 months of age. This observation is also correlated with the increased incidence of "hidden" or presacral tumors. In our own hospital, there have been eight children with malignant sacro-coccygeal teratomas diagnosed over the past 10 years. All were endodermal sinus tumors, diagnosed from 4 months to 7 years of age. Two of these children had "benign" tumors resected in the newborn period. Radiation combined with multiple drug chemotherapy has allowed surgical resection of residual tumor and cure in four of these patients.

Summary

Sacro-coccygeal teratomas are tumors that contain a variety of tissues from two or three germ layers. They most commonly present in newborn infants and must be differentiated from sacral lipomas and low meningoceles. The diagnosis may be made by physical examination, supplemented when necessary by ultrasound, plain x-ray, or computerized tomography. Treatment consists of surgical removal of the tumor and coccyx. Delayed diagnosis beyond 2 months of age or incomplete removal is associated with malignancy.

References

1. Crussi FG (ed): Extragonadal Teratomas. Series 2, Fascicle 18 Atlas of Tumor Pathology. Armed Forces Institute of Pathology, Washington, DC, 1982.
2. Altman RP, Randolph JG, Lilly JR: Sacrococcygeal teratoma: American Academy of Pediatrics Surgical Section Survey – 1973. J Pediatr Surg 9:389–398, 1973.
3. Ashcraft KW, Holder TM, Harris DJ: Familial presacral teratomas. Birth Defects 11:143–146, 1975.
4. Kenefick JS: Hereditary sacral agenesis associated with presacral tumors. Br J Surg 60:271–274, 1973.
5. Smith J, Wixon D, Watson RC: Giant cell tumor of the sacrum: clinical and radiologic features in 13 patients. J Can Assoc Radiol 30:34–39, 1979.
6. Izant RJ, Filston HC: Sacrococcygeal teratomas. Am J Surg 130:617–621, 1975.
7. Miles RM, Stewart GS: Sacrococcygeal teratomas in adults. Ann Surg 179:676–683, 1974.
8. Teilum G: Endodermal sinus tumors of the ovary and testis: comparative morphogenesis of the so-called mesonephroma ovarii (Schiller) and extraembryonic (yolk sac-allantoic) structures of rat's placenta. Cancer 12:1092–1105, 1959.
9. Crussi FG, Roth LM: The yolk sac and yolk sac carcinoma; an ultrastructural study. Human Pathol 7:675–691, 1976.
10. Olsen MM, Raffensperger JG, Crussi FG, Luck SR, Kaplan WE, Morgan E: Endodermal sinus tumor: a clinical and pathological correlation. J Pediatr Surg 17:832–840, 1982.
11. Sherowsky RC, Williams CH, Nichols VB, et al: Prenatal ultrasonographic diagnosis of a sacrococcygeal teratoma in twin pregnancy. J Ultrasound Med 4:159–161, 1985.
12. Seeds JW, Mittelstaedt CA, Cefalo RC: et al: Prenatal diagnosis of sacrococcygeal teratoma: an anechoic caudal mass. JCU 10:193–195, 1982.
13. Naidich TP, Fernbach SK, McLone DG, Shkolnik A: Sonography of the caudal spine and back: congenital anomalies in children. AJR 142:1229–1242, 1984.
14. Tsuchida Y, Hasegawa H: The diagnostic value of alpha fetoprotein in infants and children with teratomas: a questionnaire survey in Japan. J Pediatr Surg 18:152–155, 1983.
15. Hecht F, Hecht BK, OKeefe D: Sacrococcygeal teratoma: prenatal diagnosis with elevated alphafetoprotein and acetylcholinesterase in amniotic fluid. Prenat Diag 2:229–231, 1982.
16. Donnellan WA, Swenson O: Benign and malignant sacrococcygeal teratomas. Surg 64:834–846, 1968.
17. Tapper D, Lack EE: Teratomas in infancy and childhood: a 54 year experience at the Children's Hospital Medical Center. Ann Surg 198:398–410, 1983.

CHAPTER 9

The Tethered Spinal Cord

Harold J. Hoffman

The tethered spinal cord includes a group of dysraphic conditions in which the conus medullaris is located in an abnormally low position and is fixed there in a relatively immobile state. During fetal life, the spinal cord grows much more slowly than the vertebral column. This leads to a progressive disparity between the termination of the spinal cord and the termination of the spine, in effect to a progressive ascent of the conus medullaris. Barson's studies showed that in the 20-week embryo, the conus medullaris terminated at the L4–5 level.[1] By term, the conus had ascended to L3 and by two months of postnatal age, the conus reached the adult L1–2 level (Fig. 9.1). Tethering of the conus prevents this normal ascent. Yamada's studies have conclusively shown that if stretch is placed on the conus medullaris, progressive ischemia occurs, leading inevitably to neurologic sequelae.[2]

The anatomic studies carried out by Breig have shown that as the normal spine flexes, the spinal cord moves toward the fourth cervical spinal level.[3] This upward movement during flexion is prevented in a conus medullaris that is tethered. A sudden flexion movement of the spine in a patient with a tethered conus can produce further traction on the conus and lead to symptomatic onset even after cessation of growth in adult life.

Conditions Associated with Tethered Spinal Cord

A wide variety of dysraphic conditions can be associated with tethering. In such patients, the spinal canal is always abnormal, displaying some form of spina bifida below the L3 level. The dural sac may be normal or may show some developmental defect. In patients with a normal dural sac, the spinal cord is tethered by a thick filum (Fig. 9.2), by a filum infiltrated with lipoma (Fig. 9.3), or by an elongated conus medullaris which reaches the end of the dural sac (Fig. 9.4).

The spinal cord can be tethered by a lipomeningomyelocele.[4] In this condition, a lipomatous stalk emerges from the spinal cord to pass through a dural defect and to continue as a subcutaneous lipoma below the surface of the skin. The spinal cord is therefore tethered to overlying skin by this lipomatous stalk, and it may

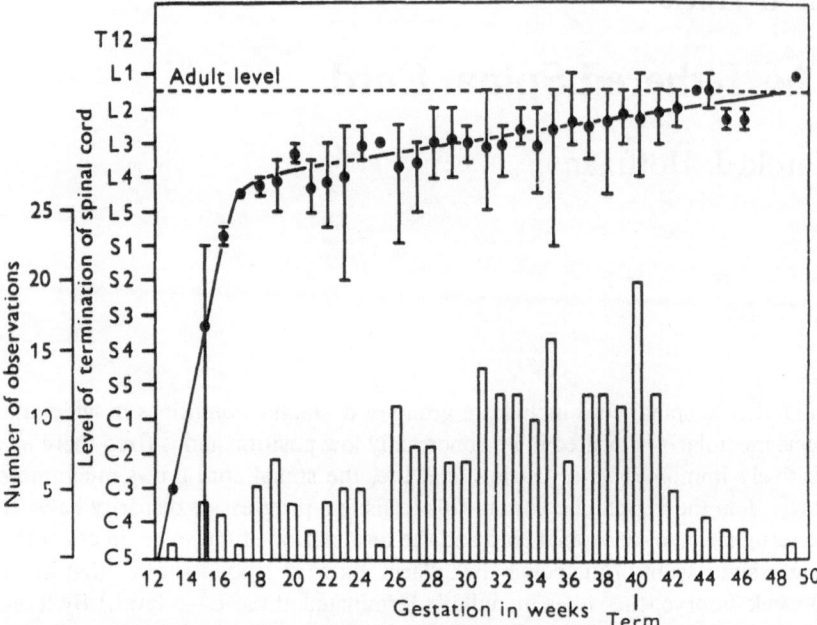

Figure 9.1. Graphic depiction of vertebral level termination of spinal cord at different gestational ages. From: Barson[1] with permission.

also be tethered by a thick filum which may go down to the bottom of the dural sac (Fig. 9.5). In patients with diastematomyelia, a bony spike emerges from the dorsal aspect of the vertebral body and passes through a split in the dural sac and an associated split in the spinal cord. The spinal cord is tethered by the dural tube which surrounds the bony spike. Furthermore, in diastematomyelia there is usually a thick filum which tethers the end of the spinal cord to the end of the dural sac (Fig. 9.6).

In addition to diastematomyelia, it is not uncommon to see patients who have a split spinal cord within a single dural sac (Fig. 9.7). In such patients, symptomatology is due to the associated tethering of the spinal cord by a thick filum which terminates at the end of the dural sac. In some of these patients, the conus itself is split and there may be two separate fila that extend to the end of the dural sac (Fig. 9.1). More often, however, the split spinal cord reunites above the level of the conus and there is a single thick filum that terminates at the end of the dural sac.

The patient with a repaired meningomyelocele can present years later with evidence of progressive deficit due to tethering. In such cases, the dural repair has typically been inadequate, allowing mesodermal tissue to grow in through the inadequate dural repair and attach itself to the dorsal aspect of the neural placode, preventing normal ascent and movement of the spinal cord. The patient with a

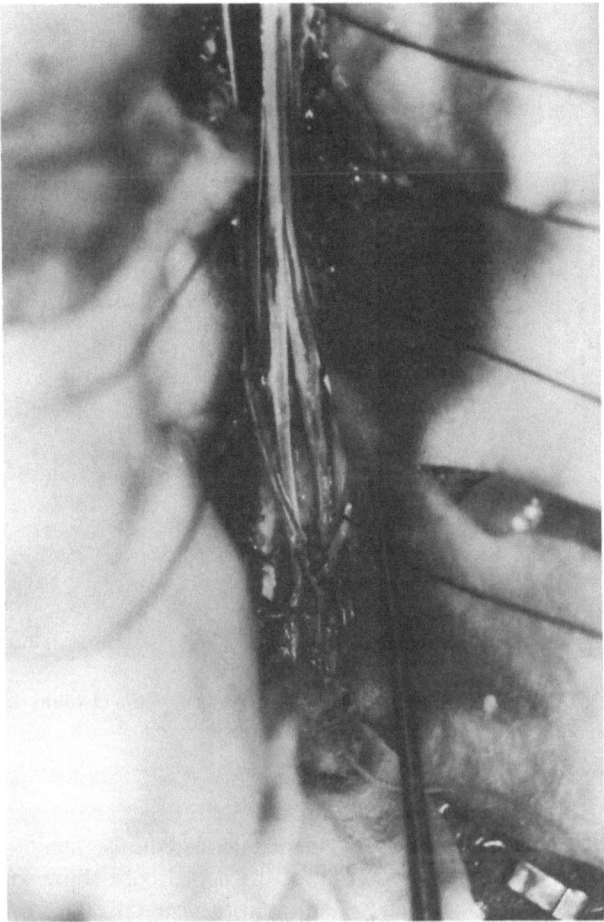

Figure 9.2. Thickened and bifid filum terminale seen at operation.

repaired meningomyelocele who shows late deterioration of leg function may do so for a variety of reasons including a missed diastematomyelia, hydromyelia, a Chiari malformation, and shunt malfunction. Investigation of such patients includes ruling out the above conditions since all patients with a meningomyelocele will have an abnormally low-lying conus medullaris.

Clinical Manifestations

Cutaneous manifestations in patients with a tethered spinal cord are common. Patients with a lipomeningomyelocele usually have a fatty lump frequently associated with some other cutaneous manifestation. Patients with diastemato-

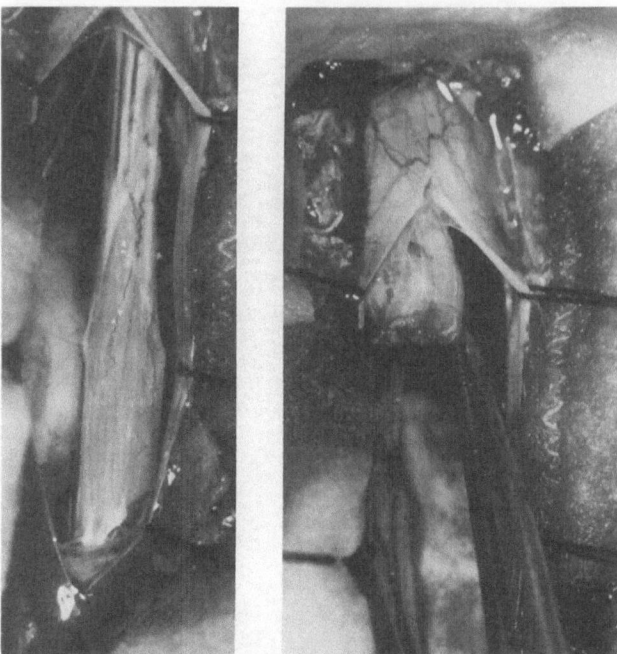

Figure 9.3. *Left*: Filum infiltrated with fat. *Right*: After division of filum the cord shows remarkable ascent.

myelia usually have a large hairy patch in the region of the dysraphic spine. About 30% of patients with simple tethering of the spinal cord show some form of cutaneous lesion. These cutaneous manifestations can take the form of a hairy patch, hemangioma, dimple, an area of thin atrophic skin, or a subcutaneous lipoma.

The child with a tethered spinal cord frequently presents with progressive motor or sensory deficit in his lower limbs. Many are seen in the orthopedic surgeon's office because of a gait disturbance. They may display foot deformities, such as pes cavus or equinus deformity of a foot. They can present to a plastic surgeon because of trophic ulceration in a foot due to sensory loss. Scoliosis alone or in combination with other problems is common in patients with a tethered spinal cord. If a spine straightening procedure (spinal instrumentation) is carried out without the tethered cord having been dealt with, sudden and precipitous deterioration in neurologic function may occur. Untethering the spinal cord in a patient with mild scoliosis can frequently prevent progression of the scoliosis or even improve the scoliosis and thus avoid the need for spinal instrumentation. Patients with a tethered spinal cord frequently develop a neurogenic bladder. Many present with signs of neurogenic bladder as the major manifestation. In inves-

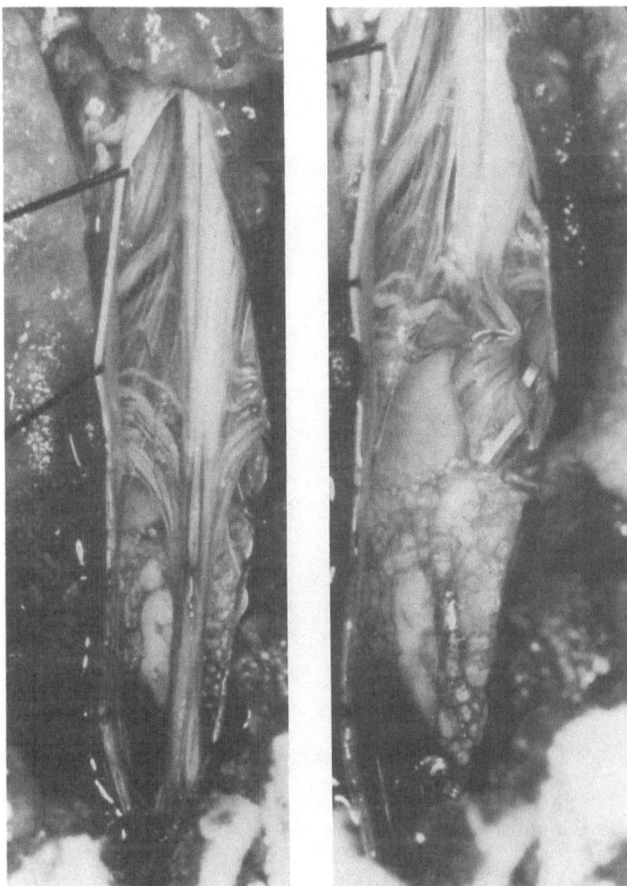

Figure 9.4. *Right*: Tethered conus medullaris which reaches bottom of dural sac. Lower spinal nerve roots ascend in cephalad direction to reach their exit foramina. *Left*: After release of conus, the lowermost spinal nerve roots take a more natural course.

tigating such patients, the urologist frequently sees evidence of the dysraphic spine on the intravenous pyelogram.

Back pain and sciatic pain occur in patients with a thickened filum or low-lying conus. The pain is typically intractable and aggravated by movement. Pain, however, is rarely a presenting feature in patients with diastematomyelia or lipomeningomyelocele.

Although some patients with a tethered spinal cord present early in infancy, many develop their symptoms during spurts of growth. Moreover, patients with a tethered spinal cord can show deterioration following sudden flexion movements of the spine when normal upward movement of the conus is prevented by

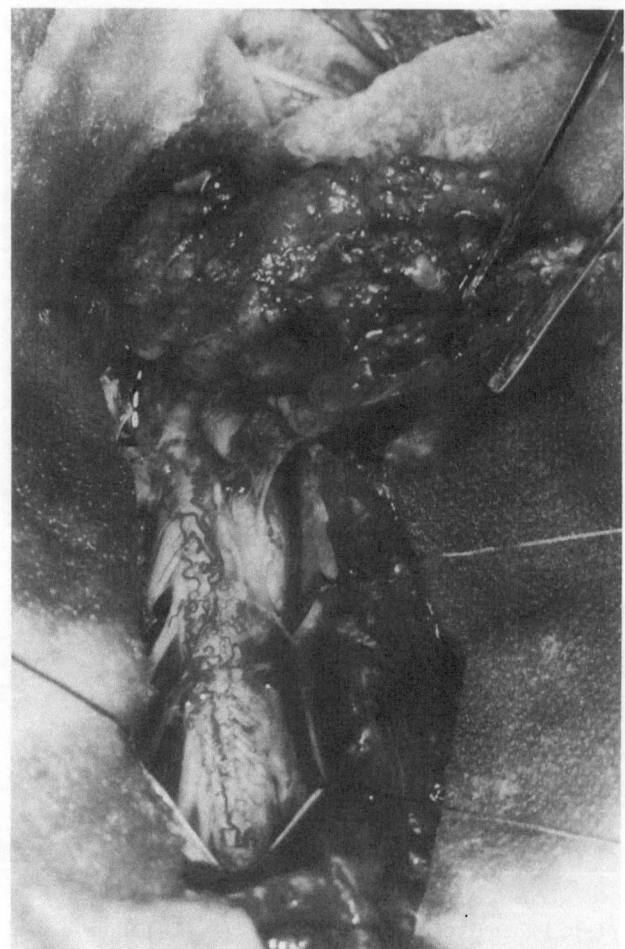

Figure 9.5a. Dorsal lipomeningomyelocele arising from dorsal aspect of spinal cord.

the tethering. This can lead to a sudden onset of symptoms, and no doubt accounts for those tethered spinal cord patients who do not present until adult life. The patient with a lipomeningomyelocele, in addition to tethering, is prone to local injury to the fatty lesion which can transmit trauma to the underlying attached spinal cord.

Investigation

Plain radiographs of the lumbosacral spine always show evidence of dysraphism. The bifid spine is usually below the L3 level, and it may involve several segments. Ultrasound can be used in the infant to delineate the low-lying conus. Computed

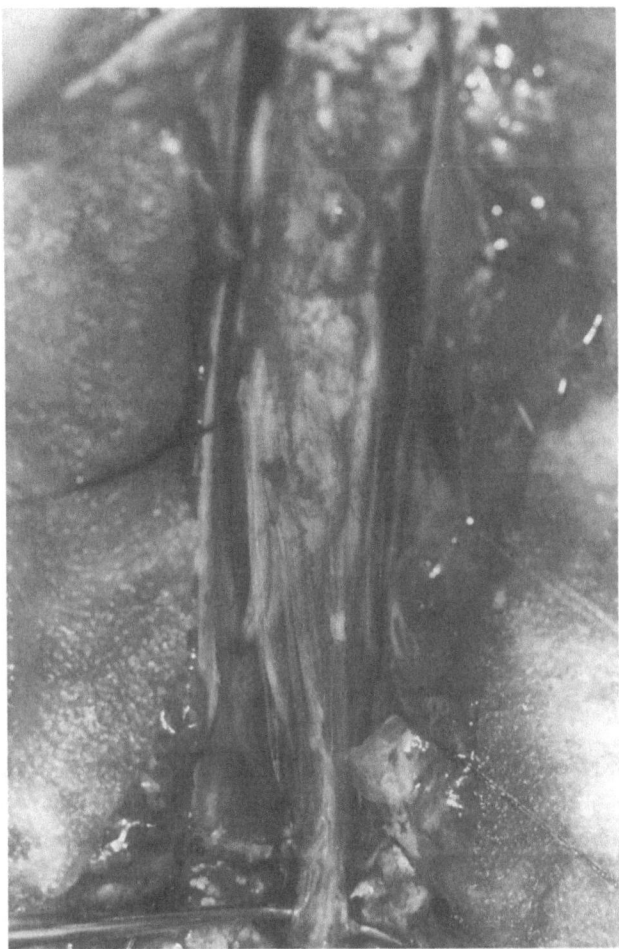

Figure 9.5b. Thickened filum in same patient as Fig. 5a.

tomographic metrizamide myelography (CTMM) reveals the abnormally low conus and the thickened film. A normal filum is 1 to 2 mm thick, whereas patients with a tethered cord have a filum that is greater than 2 mm in diameter. Furthermore, the thickened filum is situated dorsally right up against the dural sac. In patients with lipomeningomyeloceles, one can see the fat on plain CT scan. With CTMM the dural defect and tethered spinal cord become apparent. The few patients with tethering at the site of meningomyelocele repair show on CTMM a low conus, dorsally situated, with nerve roots emanating from the anterior aspect of placode and showing evidence of stretch. The CTMM clearly shows the split spinal cord as well as the split dural sac and the bony spike of diastematomyelia. Magnetic resonance imaging has added a marvelous new

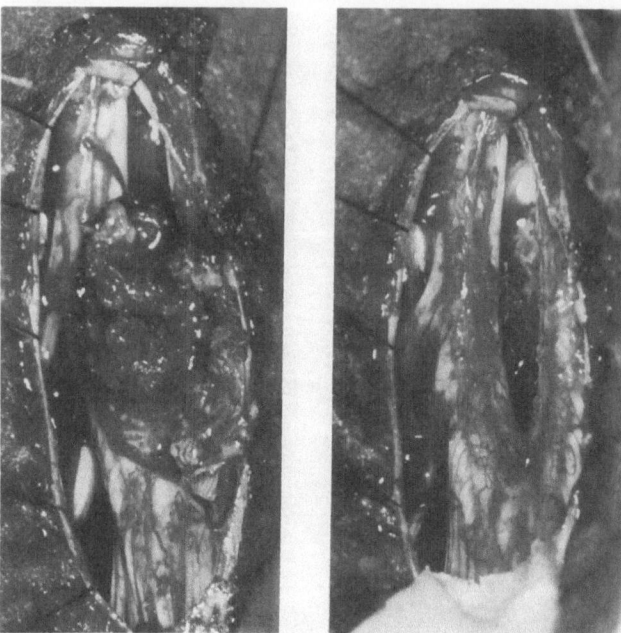

Figure 9.6a. Diastematomyelia spike (*left*) and split cord (*right*) at surgery.

investigative tool to the study of the patient with a tethered spinal cord. Without injection of agents or the need of anesthesia in the child, one can vividly see the disordered anatomy.

Treatment

Patients with a tethered spinal cord can show deterioration of function not only during childhood growth spurts, but also throughout adult life as a result of trauma and flexion movements of the spine. Even under close observation, these patients are prone to sudden and irreversible deterioration in neurologic function. I, therefore, feel that patients with a tethered spinal cord should be treated when first diagnosed. In a patient with an obvious lipomeningomyelocele, treatment can be carried out early in infancy when the vast majority of these children are neurologically intact. In patients with a tethered spinal cord and some cutaneous manifestation of dysraphism, investigation, including CT metrizamide myelography or MRI scanning, should be done to demonstrate whether a tethered spinal cord is present, and thus allow for early and prompt treatment of the condition. In those patients who present with signs and symptoms of their tethered cord, treatment must be carried out expeditiously. Although the main

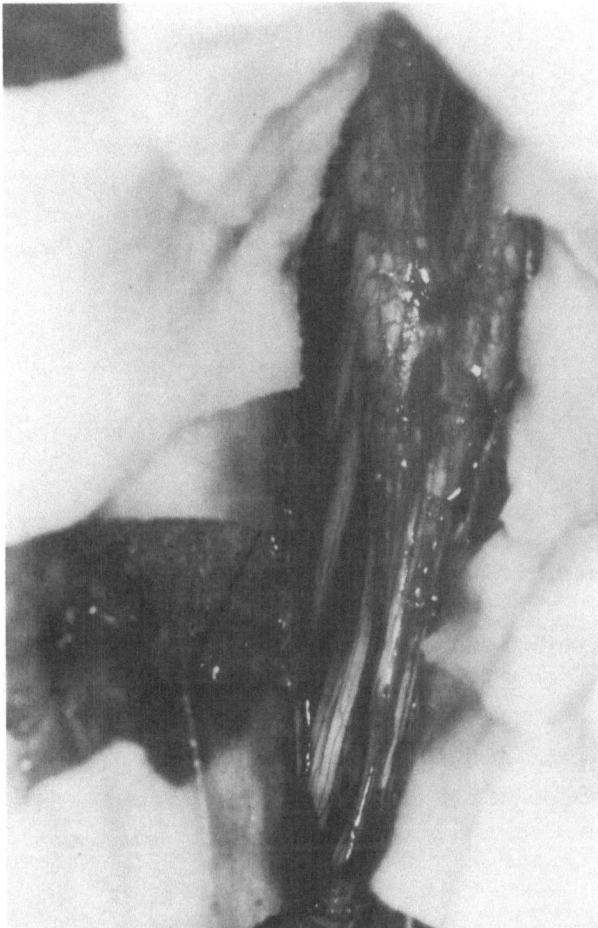

Figure 9.6b. Thickened filum in same patient as Fig. 6a.

aim of such treatment is the prevention of further deterioration, many of these patients show improvement of function following untethering. In patients with a single intact dural sac, the tethered cord is simply released. There may be adhesive bands that have to be severed. In those patients with a thickened filum, the filum is cut and one can see the severed ends literally spring apart. In patients with a conus attached to the end of the dural sac, one can safely cut through the attachment and allow the conus to ascend. Frequently, in such patients, the lowermost spinal nerves ascend to their exit foramina.

In the case of patients with lipomeningomyeloceles, there has always been fear that an attempt to untether the lipomeningomyelocele at the same time as it is

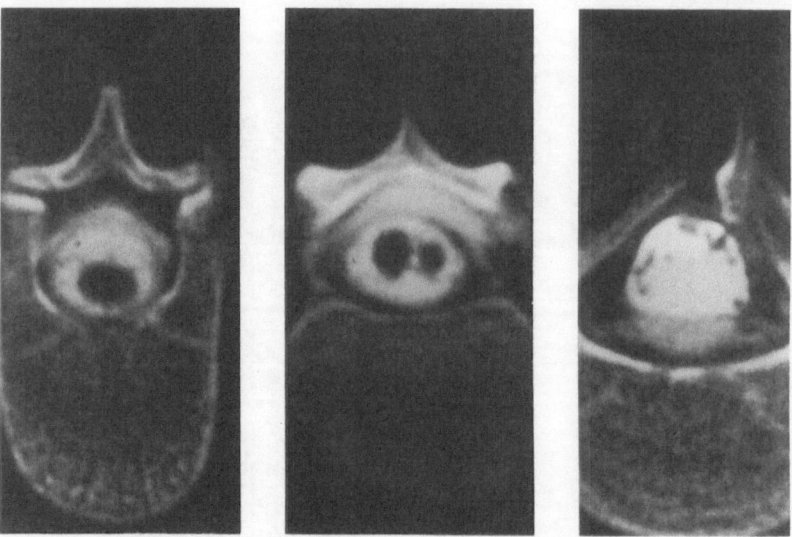

Figure 9.7a. Split spinal cord in single dural sac as seen on CTMM.

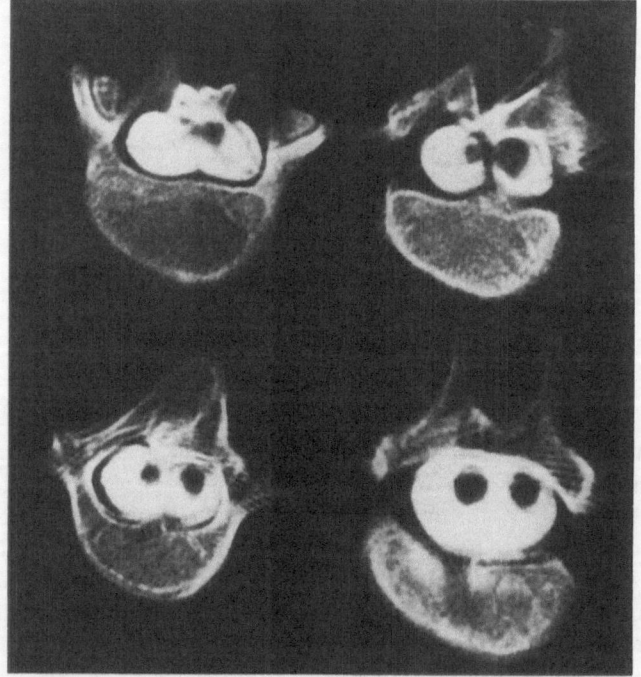

Figure 9.7b. Split spinal cord (*lower right*) eventually being encased in separate dural tubes (*upper right*) and then uniting into a thickened filum in a single dural tube (*upper left*).

repaired would produce neurologic disturbance, and cause the surgeon rather than the natural course of the disease to be blamed for the development of any deficit. Thus, in the past, patients with lipomeningomyeloceles usually had a cosmetic repair of their lesion, with no attempt at untethering the cord. It has now been clearly shown that patients with lipomeningomyeloceles are at risk for progressive neurologic deterioration. Most of these patients are neurologically intact before the age of 6 months, and with early and appropriate repair of their lesion, this state can be preserved. I never cease to be amazed at how patients with such a terribly disordered anatomic configuration of their spinal cord can maintain normal neurologic function as long as they are appropriately untethered (Fig. 9.5).

In addition to removing the bony spike in patients with diastematomyelia, one must remove the dural tube that surrounds the bony spike and reconstitute a single dural sac for the split spinal cord. These patients frequently have an associated thick filum or low-lying conus, with tethering of the spinal cord at the end of the dural sac. Again, the tethering at the end of the dural sac must be treated to ensure alleviation of the tethered cord syndrome.

In patients with tethering secondary to repair of a meningomyelocele, one invariably finds deficient dura with mesodermal tissues invading through this deficient dura into the neural placode. Repair involves freeing up the neural placode from this mesodermal tissue, finding the edges of the deficient dura, and repairing the dural defect with cadaver freeze-dried graft.

During untethering one can monitor neurologic function by stimulating nerve roots and recording bladder pressure, anal sphincter pressures, EMG activity in legs and anal sphincter, as well as somatosensory evoked responses. However, in most cases of tethering, the anatomy is patently obvious, and only rarely is such monitoring of value.

Conclusion

The patient with a tethered spinal cord is at risk for neurologic deterioration. This deterioration can be slow and insidious, or can come on quite suddenly following a flexion injury of the spine or a spurt of growth. Ideally, patients with a tethered spinal cord should be treated prophylactically while they are still normal and when appropriate therapy can preserve normal neurologic function. However, many patients with a tethered spinal cord have no clinical stigmata to point to the fact that they have a tethered cord. These patients may present with a gait disturbance to the orthopedic surgeon, or with a sphincter disturbance to the urologist. If such patients are promptly investigated and referred for appropriate therapy at an early stage, they frequently improve and sometimes regain normal function. On the other hand, if they are allowed to continue with their tethered cord, they will eventually suffer irreversible damage to the conus, presumably on an ischemic basis, and will be left with a permanent deficit despite successful untethering.

References

1. Barson AJ: Vertebral level termination of spinal cord during normal and abnormal development. J Anat 106:489, 1969.
2. Yamada S, Zinke DE, Sanders D: Pathophysiology of tethered cord syndrome. Neurosurgery 54:494–503, 1981.
3. Breig A: Overstretching of and circumscribed pathological tension in the spinal cord — a basic cause of symptoms in cord disorders. J Biomech 3:7–9, 1970.
4. Hoffman HJ, Hendrick EB, Humphreys RP: The tethered spinal cord: its protean manifestations, diagnosis and surgical correction. Childs Brain 2:145–155, 1976.
5. Hoffman HJ, Taecholarn C, Hendrick EB, Humphreys RP: Management of lipomeningomyeloceles. Experience at the Hospital for Sick Children, Toronto. J Neurosurg 62:1–8, 1985.

CHAPTER 10

Neuromuscular Scoliosis

Lawrence A. Rinsky and Eugene E. Bleck

Scoliosis and other spinal deformities have long been recognized to occur associated with any of the diverse neuromuscular diseases. In fact, patients with scoliosis secondary to poliomyelitis were the source of experience for many of the world's first scoliosis surgeons and centers.[1-5] As early as 1957, Moe wrote of his experience with "paralytic scoliosis"... all patients with poliomyelitis.[6] Since then, there has been a quantum leap in our ability to understand the natural history and operatively to control or correct spinal deformity.[11] With the advent of polio immunization, the attention of most spinal surgeons turned more toward idiopathic scoliosis (IS).[12] However, as the number of patients with polio deformity decreased, attention also began to be paid to the many other types of neuromuscular scoliosis (NMS). Simultaneously, other improvements in general medical care and especially adaptive devices have improved the quality and length of life in these patients.[13,14]

The pathogenesis, natural history, goals, and treatment often vary widely in NMS and differ considerably from those for IS.[14] In general, the treatment of spinal deformity in neuromuscular patients is more difficult than in IS patients because of the special problems related to the underlying diseases. Pseudoarthroses are more common following fusion in paralytic curves.[15] Because of the wide variation in the level and laterality of paralysis, the progressive or stable nature of the deficit, the mental status, the respiratory ability, etc., the rules and lessons learned in treating polio and IS do not always apply in the other types of NMS.

Classification and Incidence

The causes of NMS are generally divided into neuropathic and myopathic.[7,14] Neuropathic etiologies are divided according to the level of involvement: upper motor neuron lesions, including brain and spinal cord; and lower motor neuron lesions, including anterior horn cell disease, polio, and traumatic lesions. The causes of scoliosis in spinal dysraphism include, in most cases, both upper and lower motor neuron factors as well as mechanically displaced muscle and

Table 10.1. Known causes of NMS

I. Neuropathic
  A. Upper motor neuron
    1. Cerebral palsy
    2. Acquired static encephalopathy, e.g., hypoxia, post-traumatic
    3. Spino-cerebellar degeneration and other progressive neurologic degenerative diseases
       (Friedreich's ataxia, Charcot–Marie–Tooth (CMT), etc.)
    4. Syringomyelia
    5. Spinal cord injury and tumor

  B. Lower motor neuron and peripheral neuropathies
    1. Anterior horn cell disease (Werdnig–Hoffman, Kukelberg–Welander, some variants of
       Charcot–Marie–Tooth, etc.)
    2. Polio
    3. Viral myelitis
    4. Traumatic
    5. Familial dysautonomia

  C. Meningomyelocele (often considered separately, because it commonly has upper and lower
       motor neuron causes as well as congenital vertebral anomalies)

II. Myopathic
  A. Muscular dystrophies
  B. Arthrogryposis
  C. Congenital myopathies
  D. Myotonias

frequently congenital vertebral anomalies. A summary of the various known causes of NMS is shown in Table 10.1.

Neuropathic, Upper Motor Neuron

Lesions of the brain may produce any type of focal or diffuse neurologic damage. Cerebral palsy is probably the archetype and most common cause here, but acquired cerebro-spastic conditions such as due to head injury or hypoxia may also produce any type of spinal deformity. In general, the incidence of NMS in a population varies directly with the severity of the brain damage. Depending on the stringency of criteria used for diagnosis, the incidence in cerebral palsy varies between 15 and 38%.[14,16-19]

In institutionalized patients, the incidence is closer to 25% with large numbers of severe curves. Most of these severe curves tend to be in the ("total body involved") spastic quadriplegic patient.

Spinal cord injury is a frequent cause of scoliosis, depending on the age at onset and whether it is purely traumatic, or associated with spinal cord tumor, radiation, or other form of injury.[20-23] Complete paraplegia in infants produces a spinal deformity in nearly 100%. In one group of 64 children suffering from traumatic quadriplegia, those with complete lesions before the age of 13 had a 100% incidence of scoliosis,[24] those with an age at onset > 16 had a 50% incidence. The chance of deformity decreases as the age at onset increases, but the combination of spinal tumor, partial paralysis, and laminectomy with x-ray therapy is particularly likely to produce a severe deformity even in patients near skeletal maturity.

Spino-cerebellar degenerative diseases include Friedreich's ataxia; peroneal muscular atrophy, and other familial, chronic, often slowly progressive, degenerative states. These are usually compatible with fairly long life span and vary widely in degree of severity. The incidence of spine deformity varies between a low of 10% in Charcot–Marie–Tooth (CMT) and 50% in other diseases, although some series report scoliosis in up to 75 to 80%.[14,25-29] This incidence is dependent on the genetic subtype (there are many even within individual disease categories), the length of follow-up, and the criteria for diagnosis.

Syringomyelia is also very commonly associated with scoliosis.[14,30] The important point in syringomyelia is that the curve patterns produced often look idiopathic with typical right thoracic curves. In the early stages, the neurologic findings are often quite subtle. As a result, the underlying neurologic diagnosis is often missed in the cases considered to be simply idiopathic.

Neuropathic, Lower Motor Neuron

The anterior horn cell can be damaged diffusely, as in spinal muscular atrophy, or segmentally, as in poliomyelitis. Since the onset of weakness in spinal muscular atrophy is early, the percentage of scoliosis is probably higher than in polio. Both Hensinger[26] and Pekak[27] found an incidence >60%, with significant scoliosis, in spinal muscular atrophy.

Poliomyelitis is still common in underdeveloped areas, so new cases are seen by spine surgeons everywhere because of the general mobility of the world's immigrant population (in the US typically Southeast Asians or Latin Americans). Since polio can affect the cord at any level and at any age, with varying degrees of recovery, wide variations in the pattern of deficit occur. The precise incidence of patients developing scoliosis is not really well known.[6,7] However, in patients with profound paralysis at a very young age the incidence approaches 100%. The reported incidences in the literature including all cases have varied between 5 and 35%.[14]

Familial dysautonomia is a very rare genetic defect found in children of Ashkenazi Jewish origin. There is very little experience, but scoliosis is reported to occur in the majority of patients followed to adulthood.[14,31]

Meningomyelocele

Spinal deformity secondary to spinal dysraphism merits special consideration because many simultaneous etiologic factors are operative. Nearly all patients with meningomyelocele suffer some degree of lower motor neuron deficit. However, many, if not most, also have some upper motor neuron dysfunction secondary to either hydrocephalus, syringomyelia, or autonomously functioning areas of the cord. Furthermore, besides the failure of posterior midline fusion, congenital vertebral anomalies are common (e.g., hemivertebrae, failure of segmentation, etc.). Lastly, the paraspinous muscles are mechanically displaced, most notably in those patients with congenital kyphosis. In a large series of 250 patients with myelodysplasia, Piggott found that the incidence of spinal deformity sufficiently severe to require fusion was almost 50%.[32] However, because of the referral nature of his practice, his series was probably skewed toward the more severe cases. In our own spina bifida clinic, the incidence of scoliosis is probably 50% overall but only 10 to 20% of patients are severe enough to require fusion.

Myopathy

Duchenne's muscular dystrophy is the most common of the muscular dystrophies and is usually associated with some degree of spinal deformity.[14,33-35] In the young (still ambulatory) patient, scoliosis is rare, but in teenagers spinal deformity is the rule, with an incidence ranging from 60 to nearly 100%. In the other dystrophies (limb girdle, fascio-humeral scapular) the degree of impairment is less as is the degree of trunkal weakness during growth.[33,36] Correspondingly, the incidences of curvature would seem to be less. Pecak reports an incidence of 54% with some degree of scoliosis in limb girdle dystrophy.[27]

Arthrogryposis multiplex congenita is a group of syndrome complexes of multiple contractures present at birth.[29] It is not necessarily myopathic in origin, but probably represents a final common outcome of a neurologically nonprogressive disorder of muscle, anterior horn cell, or both. Although often originally described as involving primarily the extremities and sparing the trunk, it has become increasingly evident that the spine is often severely involved.[37] Drummond found that the incidence of scoliosis was 28%, with 16% of patients having severe curves.[38]

The congenital myopathies represent a recently described group of genetically determined disorders of muscles which have only recently been differentiated on the basis of electron microscopy and histochemical staining.[36] These include such conditions as nemaline myopathy, central core disease, congenital fiber type disproportion, central nuclear myopathy, etc. Experience with these individual diagnoses is limited; however, in general these conditions are either stable or only slowly progressive. The natural history regarding the spinal deformities is not known, but the overall incidence seems lower in our cases.

Etiology and Pathogenesis

In all the above neuromuscular conditions, there is always dysfunction of the skeletal muscle in one sense or another. It is tempting to think that asymmetric muscle weakness is the common etiology that produces the spinal deformity.[7]

This supposition derives from our knowledge of polio and is easy to conceptualize. However, on closer review, it becomes apparent that many other factors, known and unknown, contribute toward development of scoliosis in neuromuscular disease. Known factors include age at onset of the deficit, degree and type of paralysis, life span, effect of gravity, progressive nature of the neurologic deficit, hip contracture and dislocation, etc. However, how these factors relate to an individual scoliosis patient is not always predictable.

In general, a congenital onset with profound weakness results eventually in severe curvature. Examples include infantile traumatic paraplegia, Werdnig–Hoffman's disease, and severe cases of arthrogryposis. Because the neurologic deficit is persistent or progressive, it is not surprising that the curves often continue to increase after skeletal maturity more so than do idiopathic curves.[12]

The many unknown factors with regards to etiology of NMS are emphasized when one considers that many young patients with profound weakness still do not develop spinal deformity. In one study of 110 patients with muscular dystrophies and atrophies, overall 56% had scoliosis.[27] However, 44% did not. Why not? Many patients develop scoliosis early in the course of their disease, when there is little or no weakness, while they are still walking. The incidence of scoliosis also does not relate directly to the degree of weakness or its duration: many profoundly weak patients do not suffer spinal deformity. Furthermore, neither the site nor the side of the scoliosis was related to the distribution of muscle weakness as determined by manual testing. It is difficult to explain the marked tendency for lumbar curves to be predominantly to the left and for thoracic curves to be predominantly to the right in the face of symmetric muscle weakness. Weakness of the paravertebral muscles is often thought to be the predominant mechanism but this can hardly apply to scoliotic patients with Charcot–Marie–Tooth disease, who have predominantly distal limb involvement.

Many believe that sensory or proprioceptive defects are also contributory as this has been shown to exist in some studies of IS.[39] However, this too is controversial. In our own study we were unable to find any proprioceptive or coordination deficits in IS.[40] Gregoric reported similar conclusions after looking for sensory deficits and comparing patients with early mild Duchenne's dystrophy and IS.[41] On the other hand, the obvious proprioceptive and stereognostic deficits in brain injury, syringomyelia, etc., may well contribute to the development of spinal deformity. The best evidence for this is the production of scoliosis in experimental animals by controlled sensory lesions.[42]

It, therefore, seems that the abnormality of spinal muscle function is an important factor in the etiology of NMS, but muscle weakness itself is not the cause. Once a small curvature develops, for whatever reason, gravitational forces on the vertebral end-plate become asymmetric. This paves the way for a progressive curve, especially during adolescence. Alterations of vertebral body shape, disc, and facet joint occur secondarily. The effects of defective proprioception (spinal cord injury), equilibrium deficits (CP), and hip contracture (polio) all may contribute.

Natural History

The natural history of scoliosis in neuromuscular disease differs from that of IS. In IS, it is rare for scoliotic curves <30° to increase after skeletal maturity.[14,21] Spinal deformity in neuromuscular disease is capable of increasing a fair amount even after skeletal maturity. This increased tendency is especially true in spastic patients.

Although any curve pattern may exist in NMS, the long single "collapsing" C-curve is characteristic of extensive paralysis.[12,21] Single thoracic curves are uncommon except in syringomyelia, and sometimes in Friedreich's ataxia.[25] Most neuromuscular curves are primarily lumbar or thoraco-lumbar. It is rare for IS to involve the pelvis, whereas this is common in paralytic curves. The unhappy tendency for pelvic obliquity gives rise to many functional complications in NMS. Sitting patients without sensation in the buttock have abnormally high pressure under the low ischium and a tendency to develop pressure sores. Sensate sitting patients, such as in cerebral palsy, who have pelvic obliquity have pain under the low buttock and thus decreased sitting tolerance, or the need to use their hands for support.

Patients with NMS nearly always have decreased vital capacity and pulmonary function, mainly due to the underlying neuromuscular disease. Even with small paralytic curves, alteration of the lung's volume may be profound, but it is not necessarily related to the chest deformity. Most neuromuscular curves are lumbar or thoraco-lumbar and, as in IS, *lumbar* curves have little effect on pulmonary function tests (PFTs). Thoracic curves by themselves are not associated with a significant decrease of vital capacity until the curves are over 60°. Thus, the scoliosis may contribute to decreased pulmonary function, but is rarely primarily responsible in NMS.

The onset of the curvature generally relates to the onset of the neurologic deficit. For example, the onset following polio usually begins 1 to 2 years after the clinical disease.[12] For the many heritable neurologic conditions, age at onset of the curvature varies widely, depending on the appearance of the weakness. However, in most conditions, there is a greater likelihood of the curve being seen before age 10, the more common age of appearance of IS. There is no female preponderance in NMS.

Spinal deformities that do not affect functional independence of patients with IS affect adversely the independence of the neuromuscular patient because of the many commonly associated abnormalities. For example, sphincter dysfunction secondary to spinal cord injury often requires catheterization, either intermittent or continuous. A severe curve may decrease the ability of a patient for self-catheterization by tying up the upper extremities for support. The TLSO brace used for nonoperative treatment may also diminish the ability for self-catheterization. Decreased mental function, hyperactivity, or seizures in a brain-injured patient makes cooperation with brace wearing difficult. Similarly, the tendency for loosening of implanted hardware will be increased in an athetotic or spastic patient. Cardiac problems are seen in the cardiomyopathy of Duchenne's muscular dystrophy and in the arrhythmias of Friedreich's ataxia.[29,36]

Hip dislocation is common in many neuromuscular diseases, especially cerebral palsy, spina bifida, and polio. The commonly found adduction contracture associated with the dislocated hip usually accentuates the lumbar scoliosis and pelvic obliquity, although it is sometimes difficult to distinguish cause from effect.[6,15] The pelvic obliquity greatly increases the difficulty in obtaining solid fusion, since fixation across the lumbo-sacral joint is necessary. This is the most difficult level at which to obtain fusion.

Finally, in all of the flaccid conditions and in many of the spastic conditions, osteopenia is much more common. This also has the effect of making it more likely that implanted hardware will loosen. Furthermore, there is less available autologous bone available for grafting.

Literature Review of Treatment

As early as 1957, Moe, writing about his experiences with polio, emphasized many of the most basic principles true today.[6] (At that time, he was operating without the advantage of internal fixation.) He stressed the importance of releasing hip contractures (ilio-tibial band) and of maintaining or gaining spinal flexibility (with casts). He noted that bracing can deform ribs, and that fusion should not be delayed if the curve was increasing even in patients as young as 8 years. Finally, he stated the undesirability of fusing to the sacrum in the ambulatory patient, but the necessity of doing so in the wheelchair-bound patient with pelvic obliquity. The fusion results were best when facet fusions were supplemented with iliac autologous graft.

In 1962, Harrington introduced the modern era of internal fixation of the spine in his report of a system of rods and hooks affixed to the lamina.[4] This greatly improved the maintenance of correction, but experience showed that prolonged external fixation and fusion were still necessary to avoid hardware failure and loss of correction. In 1975, Bonnett et al. summarized the evolution of treatment of paralytic scoliosis at Rancho de los Amigos Hospital.[15] During the period 1954 to 1970, the technique of correction and stabilization evolved from cast correction and fusion in situ to that of preliminary halo-femoral traction with posterior fusion and Harrington instrumentation. All surgery was posterior, and two-thirds of the patients had polio. Tracheostomy was used extensively. The percentage correction improved from 20 to 57% even though the period of recumbency was reduced from 1 year to as little as 3 weeks in the last group of patients. However, in truth, nearly all of the correction was that obtainable due to intrinsic flexibility in the curves (e.g., the younger flexible patients had the best average correction). Complications were many. They included failure of Harrington fixation across the lumbo-sacral joint in almost one-half of the patients. A developmental lordosis occurred in some, years after long posterior

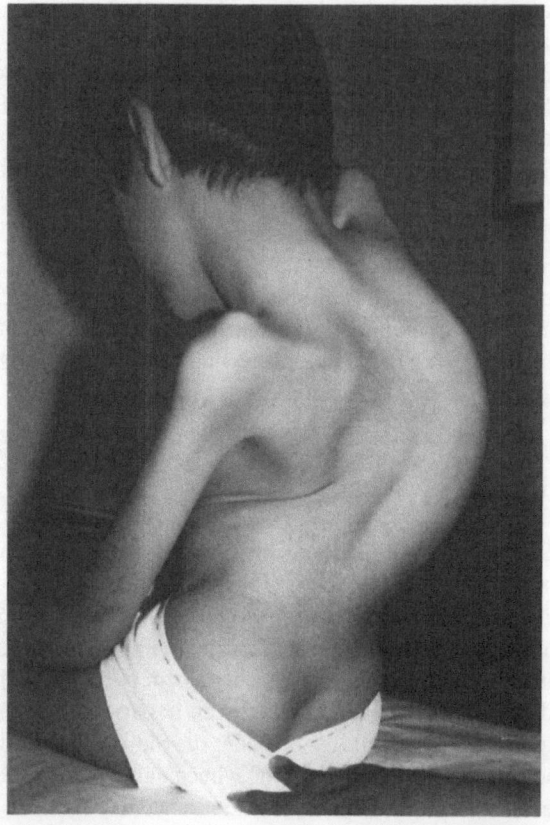

A

Figure 10.1. *A*: Eleven-year-old boy with severe thoracic curve secondary to polio. *B*: Same patient in halo-wheelchair traction. This was used for 2 weeks pre-operatively.

fusions from the cervical spine to the pelvis. Stiff hips were seen after some halo-femoral traction and pseudarthroses were seen in almost 30% of the group, including those with Harrington rods.

Although the halo became popular in the 1960s and 1970s, its popularity has waned recently in view of the occasional complications seen such as avascular necrosis of the odontoid, cranial nerve palsies, pin tract infections, and especially a lack of clear cause and effect with improvement in the degree of correction.[15,43-45] A survey of spinal surgeons revealed the controversy in the use of pre-operative traction to gain correction.[46] Although some reported excellent correction with the use of prolonged skeletal ambulatory traction using the pelvic halo fixator, reports of disastrous complications (perforation of the abdominal viscera, pelvic osteomyelitis) were responsible for decreasing use of this technique. The most reasonable traction technique, in our opinion, with the least complications is the so-called halo wheelchair or halo gravity traction originally

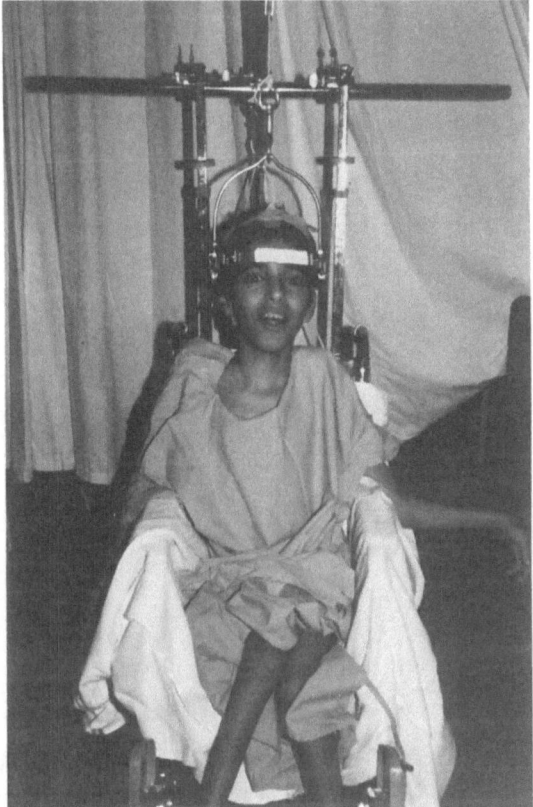

B

Figure 10.1. *Continued.*

popularized by Stagnara.[14,45] This has the advantage of maintenance of upright posture during the period of traction and minimum interference with either the hip or the area of the pelvis from which bone graft is taken (Fig. 10.1).

In 1969, Dwyer introduced the first true system of anterior instrumentation.[47-50] This technique uses anterior staples and a cable across the convexity of the curve. It allows a much improved percentage of correction, especially in rigid thoraco-lumbar and lumbar curves associated with pelvic obliquity. However, loss of correction and hardware failure were common to many early investigators unless a posterior fusion was added. Furthermore, there was an unhappy tendency to reduce the normal lumbar lordosis.

In an effort to improve the defects of the Dwyer system, Zielke changed the cable to a slightly more rigid threaded rod.[11] This allowed better maintenance of lordosis and better de-rotation and overall correction. However, most authors still prefer to add a secondary posterior fusion or a circumferential fusion, especially in spastic patients or those with severe rigid deformity.[7,8]

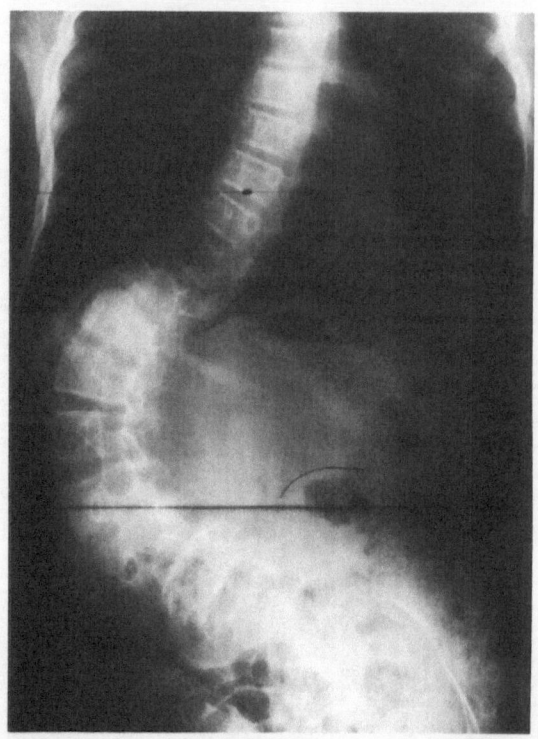

A

Figure 10.2. A: Fifteen-year-old Vietnamese boy with 100° thoraco-lumbar curve secondary to polio. B: Postoperative radiograph at 4 months status-post anterior fusion followed by posterior fusion with Luque instrumentation. Anterior view. C: Lateral radiograph of same patient showing contouring of rods for the normal sagittal plane contours of lumbar lordosis. Note fixation of lower end of rods into ilium. Patient was allowed up walking immediately after the Luque instrumentation.

Probably the most useful recent addition to the surgical armatarium is segmental spinal instrumentation (SSI), using sublaminar wires, introduced by Dr. Eduardo Luque of Mexico.[51-53] The greatly improved security of fixation has allowed avoidance of any postoperative immobilization in most patients, and much earlier return to normal activities. When combined with posterior or circumferential fusion, results have been excellent. (Fig. 10.2).

Luque also described the technique of using SSI in growing children without fusion until spinal growth was achieved.[54] The biologic basis for the continued growth of the spine despite instrumentation has been proven in dog experiments.[55] However, despite early promising results, delayed complications such as hardware failure and especially significant recurrence of the curvature are universal. The procedure is not often indicated (Fig. 10.3).[56] For those unfortunate patients with severe curves who are too young for fusion, Moe recommends

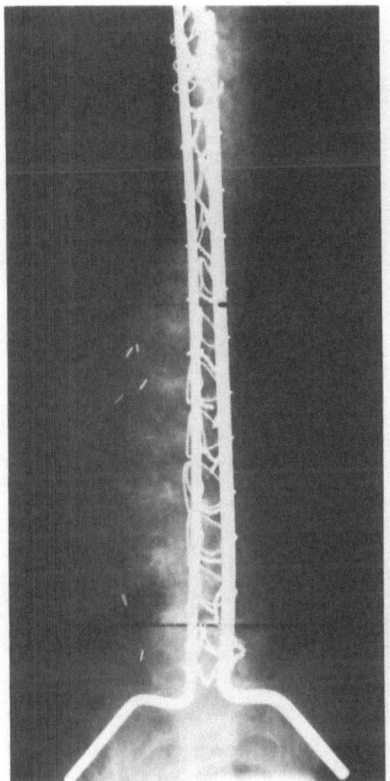
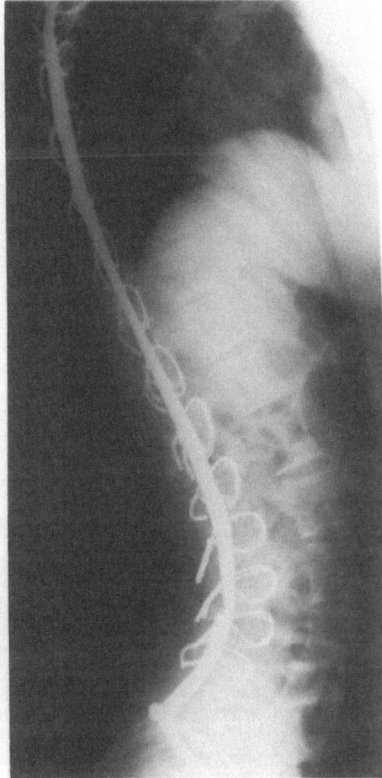

B

C

Figure 10.2. *Continued.*

modified Harrington instrumentation without fusion.[57] This technique requires periodic rod adjustments or replacements. Patients may need four or five operations before they finally have a fusion. Many "manageable" problems arise during the period of years while the patient's growth is being "guided" by the rod.

Many articles have been written summarizing the evolution of the surgical treatment for spine deformity associated with a specific neuromuscular disease such as spinal muscular atrophy (SMA),[58,59] muscular dystrophy,[34,60] cerebral palsy (CP),[16,23,61–65] Friedreich's ataxia,[25,26] spinal cord injury,[20–23] etc. Some of the most important principles have been summarized by Allen and Ferguson, who used the technique of anterior spinal release without instrumentation, followed by posterior SSI.[61,66,67] They have stated that the first task is to attain correctability. This is either inherent in the curve (a flexible curve) or accomplished by anterior removal of discs and vertebrae: basically a restatement of the original principles of Moe. Maintenance of the attained correctability is usually best accomplished by posterior SSI.

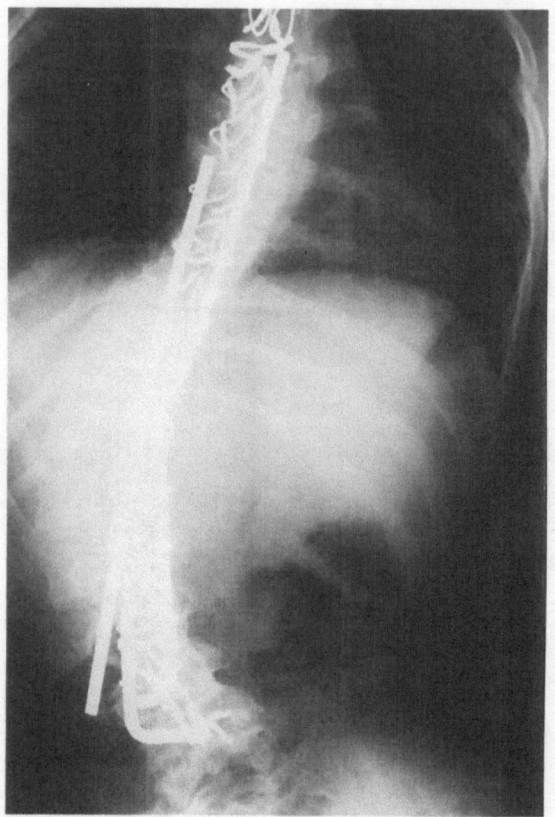

Figure 10.3. Typical postoperative result after segmental spinal instrumentation *without* fusion performed 4 years previously. Although initial correction had been good, the hardware is now broken, there are many loose wires, and the correction has been lost. SSI should not be performed without fusion.

Current Treatment

There are three modalities to consider in treatment, each with its place: observation, orthotic treatment, surgery.[12]

Observation is important for recognition of the many patients with NMS for whom no intervention is appropriate. It allows the surgeon to get to know the patient and at least the early natural history of the curvature. Not all curves progress and, clearly, not all paralyzed patients develop curves. Furthermore, intervention can be a double-edged sword. A total contact orthosis may improve spinal alignment but may also decrease chest expansion and compliance, thereby predisposing a weak patient to pneumonia (Fig. 10.4). Most children with struc-

Figure 10.4. This 11-year-old patient with severe congenital muscular dystrophy is literally too weak to tolerate any type of TLSO. Vital capacity is under 200 cc and episodes of pneumonia frequent. With surgery and bracing impossible, rehabilitative devices and observation are the only treatment alternatives.

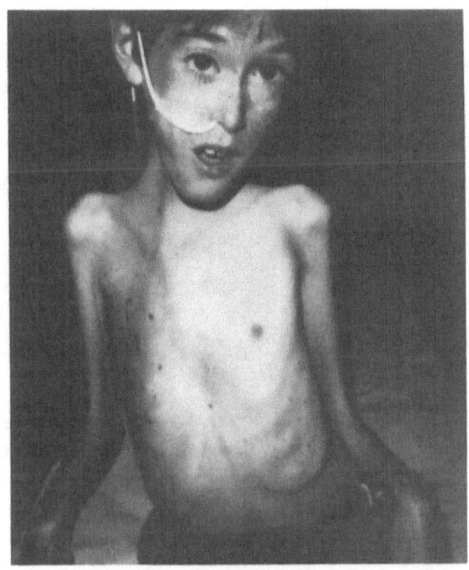

tural curves under 20° may simply be followed, seated in ordinary wheelchairs, cushions, and seatbelts if they are nonambulatory.

Those patients who are just barely able to walk (such as a 9-year-old boy with a 30° scoliosis and Duchenne's muscular dystrophy) would have greater difficulty walking either braced or fused. Because such a patient may soon be in a wheelchair, it is probably best simply to observe his scoliosis and wait to fuse him when he no longer walks. A final example of the use of observation would be the severely retarded, cortically blind, institutionalized, quadriplegic, cerebral palsy patient. Some of these unfortunate patients are totally out of contact with their environment. Although we try to make it possible for all patients to be seated, it is sometimes inappropriate to embark on heroic surgery because of the complication rate and the difficulty assessing any functional benefit. This, of course, becomes a rather philosophical issue and has to be dealt with on an individual basis. We use an informal test of responsiveness to assess whether a patient is too retarded to consider a candidate for surgery. Although we operate on many retarded patients, any child who will not respond to food (e.g., a cookie) in some way either visually, verbally, or by some directed movement, should be treated by adaptive devices without surgery.

Orthotics

Orthotics have a definite role in treatment of *some* patients with NMS.[13,68-71] We include here both bracing and special seating systems. A Milwaukee brace can occasionally be used in a mild, ambulatory (almost idiopathic) type patient.

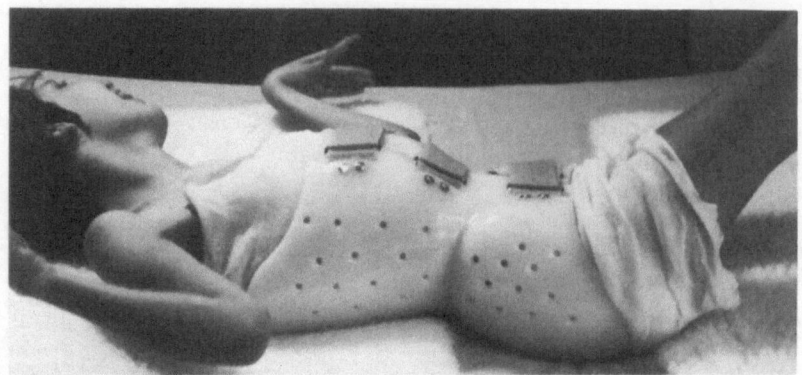

Figure 10.5. Use of a molded plastic TLSO in patient with cerebral palsy. Note perforations and simplified Velcro anterior opening straps.

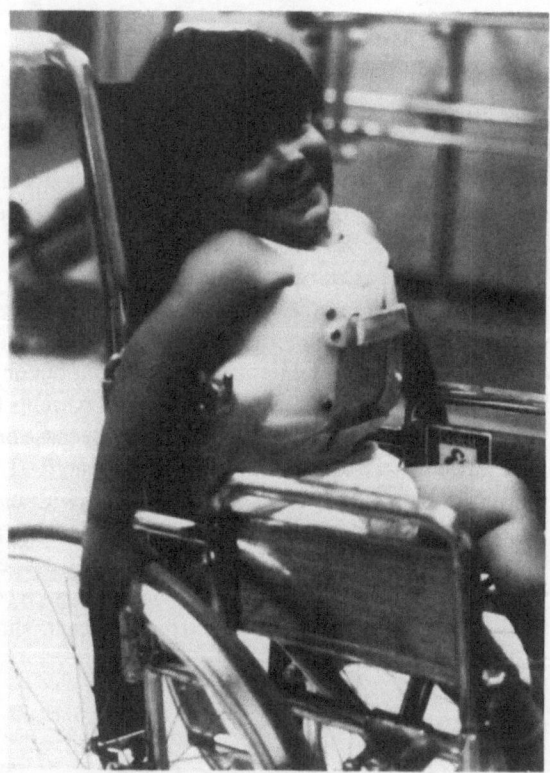

Figure 10.6. Seven-year-old girl with paraplegia secondary to meningomyelocele. In a thoracic suspension orthosis she is suspended by the lower rib cage.

However, cosmetically it has poor acceptance and furthermore depends more on the dynamic ability of the patient to pull away from the pads and throat mold. This is an ability usually lacking in the paralytic patient. Much more commonly used in NMS are a variety of underarm body jackets (TLSOs). The TLSO is usually fabricated of a stiff plastic (e.g., polypropylene, Kydex). It is formed from a plaster mold of the body. The brace is often lined with plasteazote or other foam type lining (Fig. 10.5). The brace can be front-, back-, or side-opening, depending on who is to apply it. It is usually perforated to allow sweat evaporation, and has a variably large anterior window to permit free respiration. The brace functions as a passive container and can retard the progression of some curves, especially in nonspastic patients. The greatest usefulness of bracing is in flaccid "collapsing" type patients with flexible curves who are still too young to fuse. Many of these patients cannot sit up without their orthoses. The brace helps free up the upper extremities.

Underarm bracing can be used over anesthetic skin when it is made by a skilled orthotist and when the parent or caretaker is cooperative and intelligent. Most neuromuscular patients do not need to wear their orthoses during sleep. An occasionally useful modification is the so-called thoracic suspension orthosis for wheelchair-bound patients. In this situation, the torso is suspended by the lower rib cage (Fig. 10.6). The weight of the pelvis and lower limbs serves as a kind of traction to tend to hang the spine "straight." The greatest usefulness of this technique is with lumbar curves in non-obese, wheelchair-bound patients with anesthetic skin under the ischiae.

There are a number of situations where bracing cannot be used. As curves increase >50 to 60°, bracing becomes increasingly ineffective biomechanically. Furthermore, it is usually uncomfortable due to the necessary forces of corrections. Severely spastic or drooling patients often cannot comfortably adjust to bracing. Adult supervision is usually required for donning and doffing the braces. Even a large chest window in the TLSO may restrict chest expansion unacceptably in a very weak, flaccid patient. The more obese a patient becomes, the more futile bracing is. Bracing ambulatory patients with mild curves (<20°) is rarely justified.

Specialized seating systems come in two forms.[13] Prefabricated multi-adjustable component systems, such as the Mulholland chair, allow upright sitting for many patients with a variety of deformities (Fig. 10.7). Lateral trunk and head supports, adduction posts, and various arm and leg supports are individually adjusted. The author usually prefers a custom system of molded foam inserts. These can accommodate pelvic obliquity and allow upright sitting, gently maintaining the spine in the most optimal alignment possible. An advantage is that these inserts may be transferred between wheelchairs, for example, manual to electric, and can be used as car seats or even feeding seats in the home (Fig. 10.8).

The indication for using an orthosis or seating system is usually the need to maintain upright, hands-free, sitting posture in a patient for whom fusion is not appropriate. Although this is usually the patient under 10, some children who

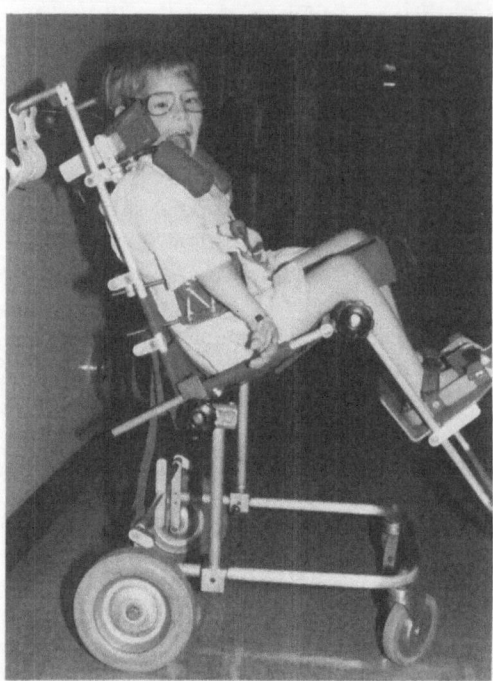

Figure 10.7. Young cerebral palsy boy in component system chair.

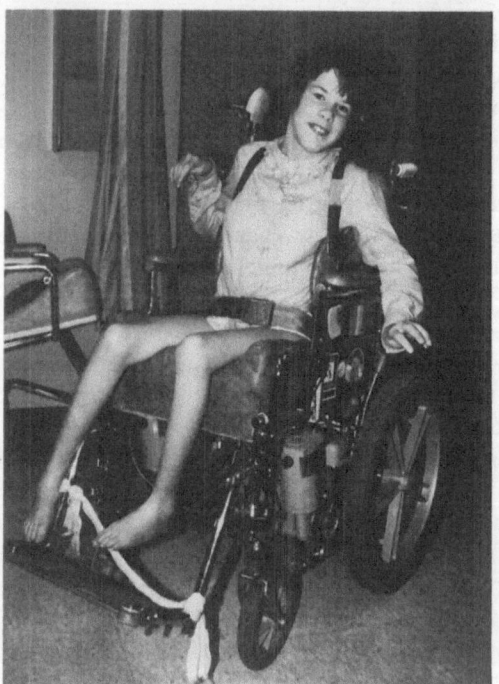

Figure 10.8. Patient with cerebral palsy and scoliosis in custom seating insert. This is adapted for use with electric wheelchair. Hands are freed from support functions.

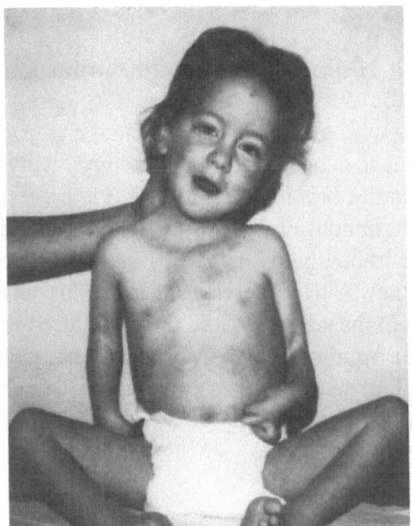

A

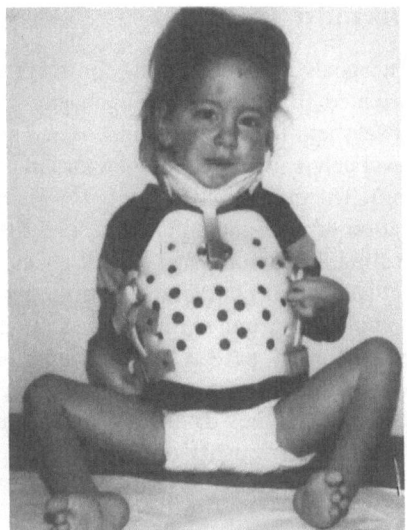

B

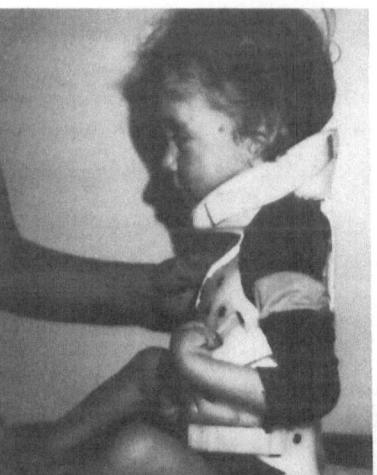

C

Figure 10.9. *A*: Three-year-old boy with severe arthrogryposis. He is not able to support his head. *B*: Frontal view of patient in custom TLSO with head support. *C*: Lateral view of same patient as in Fig. 10.9B.

will never be operative candidates can be maintained in braces. As long as the spine remains flexible bracing can be continued. In general, bracing delays progression, but as in IS, bracing does not really correct developing deformity (Fig. 10.9).

Operative Treatment

The goals and indications for surgery in NMS are much more functionally oriented than dependent upon any specific degree of curvature. One should always aim to obtain a compensated spine with a vertical torso centered over a level pelvis.[7,14] An equally important goal is to avoid loss of function (e.g., walking). The indications relate to the maintenance of hands-free sitting, the preservation of respiratory function, and the attainment of a level pelvis to facilitate seating. Maximum correction is always desirable, but is secondary to safety. The actual degree of curvature is not so important. A healthy respect for the possible complications and realistic goal setting help the surgeon avoid the temptation to correct every patient. By the same token, our currently available techniques allow us to consider safely correcting patients with diseases previously shunned (e.g., Duchenne's dystrophy, severe quadriplegic cerebral palsy, etc.) and thus improve their quality of life.

The main decision-making steps include:

1. General pre-op evaluations
2. Determination of flexibility
3. The use of traction pre-operatively or between procedures
4. Selection of levels to be fused
5. Techniques of internal fixation, anterior, posterior, or both.

Pre-operative evaluation should focus on general medical status and respiratory function. A cooperative patient with fairly significant clinical weakness should probably have formal pulmonary function testing (PFTs). A vital capacity below 30% predicted (based on arm span) is cause for considering pre-operative tracheostomy.[15,62] However, this can usually be avoided with use of intensive respiratory care.[14] If the vital capacity is below 25%, the probability of severe respiratory complication becomes prohibitive. Routine PFTs are not necessary in all patients with NMS. First, most do not have primary thoracic curves, and there is little evidence that their lumbar curves affect lung function. Second, many patients are not cooperative (such as the retarded cerebral palsy patient) which negates the accuracy of PFTs. Despite severe spasticity, the arterial blood gases are usually normal in most quadriplegic cerebral palsy patients. More important than PFTs is the history of respiratory problems or lack of them and the ability of the patient to cough, gag, and clear secretions. The most risky patients from a respiratory standpoint are those with severe peripheral myopathic or lower motor neuron weakness (e.g., Duchenne's dystrophy, severe polio, Werdnig–Hoffman disease).

Many patients need attention to specific problems resulting from the primary disease itself. Those with meningomyelocele need pre-operative evaluation, especially with regard to their genito-urinary function and whether their ventricular shunts are working well; patients with seizure disorders will need re-evaluation of their antiseizure medication. Postoperative seizures are always undesirable and may dislodge Harrington hooks or anterior fixation. Friedreich's ataxia and muscular dystrophy patients should be evaluated pre-operatively by a cardiologist.

Patients with NMS undergoing spinal surgery should be evaluated by an anesthesiologist accustomed to the frequent massive blood loss and prolonged surgery. Usually two large intravenous lines and/or a central venous pressure line, an arterial line, and urinary catheter are recommended. Use of controlled hypotension and a blood scavenging system (e.g., Cell Saver®) are becoming more common. We use it routinely.

Pre-operative determination of spinal flexibility is critical in all cases of surgery aimed at correcting spinal deformity. This can be obtained by bending films, or those taken on a Risser frame or other similar traction device.[7,61] The doctor should supervise directly the bending films to be sure they are accurate (Fig. 10.10). In general, flaccid deformities in younger patients are more flexible; spastic deformities are more rigid. However, some of the most rigid curves occur in nonspastic conditions such as arthrogryposis.[37] The important fact is that the surgical correction by posterior instrumentation alone cannot be much better than the intrinsic flexibility of the curve. If a 12-year-old patient with polio has a collapsing 90° curve that corrects to 20° on simple supine stretch, a posterior fusion alone with some form of SSI will be able to "capture" an acceptable position. The same patient, at age 24, will not only have a curve of greater degree but will also be much more rigid.

A rigid curve can be loosened by either prolonged traction, or, better yet, an anterior discectomy or even corpsectomy. Simply removing discs over the entire length of the curve from an anterior procedure is the simplest and safest method to obtain correctability. Removing discs alone gives 2 to 6° correctability per disc (a greater percentage in younger patients where the disc and cartilaginous endplate occupy a greater percent of the anterior column) (Fig. 10.11). Furthermore, all the segmental vessels to the cord can be saved if no hardware is implanted. Removing one or two vertebrae attains greater flexibility, but greatly increases the blood loss and potential for injury to the cord (Fig. 10.12). Luque has introduced the concept of decancelization of the anterior column of bone through anterior semiclosed curettage (the "sausage" procedure). Although this gains flexibility and preserves the segmental vessels, few have the expertise to perform it, and the risk of blind curettage near the cord seems obvious.

Certain patients, older children with muscular dystrophy, may not be able to stand the rigors of prolonged traction or two procedures. They should be operated earlier, when their curves are smaller and supple, such as to be controlled by posterior surgery alone. Thus, today, an 11-year-old with Duchenne's muscular dystrophy and a 30° curve will be recommended to undergo posterior fusion and SSI.[60]

The use of traction, as mentioned earlier, remains controversial.[46] We use it less and less, though we still find it useful on occasion (halo gravity only, never halo femoral), mainly in the cooperative patient with severe deformity, 7 to 14 days between anterior and posterior fusion procedures. Traction has disadvantages. It requires excellent nursing care and constant monitoring to avoid complications, is usually applied quite distal to the deformity (e.g., traction is to the head while the curve is in the thoraco-lumbar spine). This means most of the traction force is dissipated in the cervical spine ligaments. Traction also exerts a psychologic toll on the patient and family. After an anterior six- or seven-level discectomy, most patients are better off out of bed, in therapy, or walking, if possible, rather than in a circle-o-bed or femoral traction, while awaiting their second surgery. Finally, despite the theoretical feeling that it should help with correction, there is little proof to document the efficacy of traction. Certainly, the use of pre-operative traction in most IS has been abandoned as a method of increasing correction.

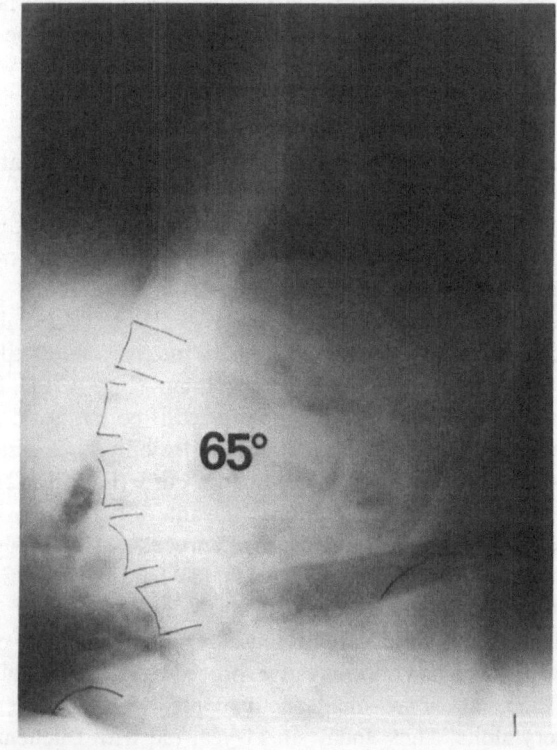

Figure 10.10. A: Sixty-five-degree curve in twelve-year-old boy with Duchenne's muscular dystrophy. B: Supine stretch and push film. Notice lead-gloved surgeon's hand straightening the spine directly. This degree of flexibility suggests that only a posterior fusion alone would be successful. C: Results 1 year after Luque instrumentation. No anterior surgery was necessary since spine was sufficiently flexible.

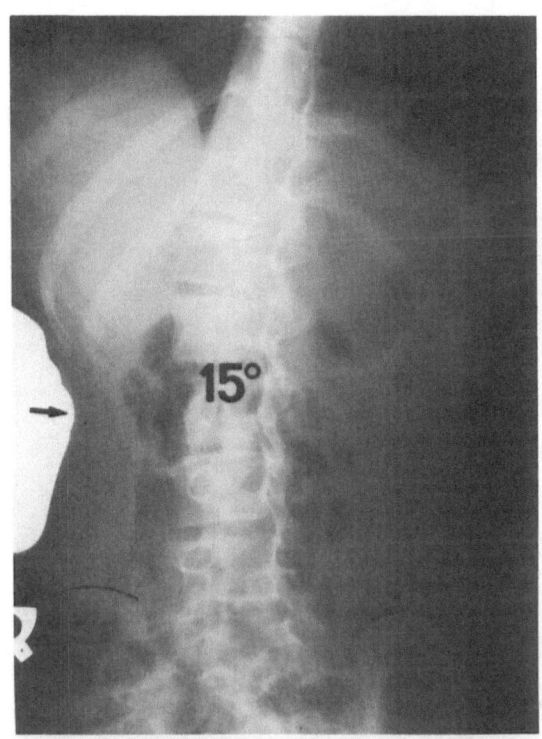

15°

B

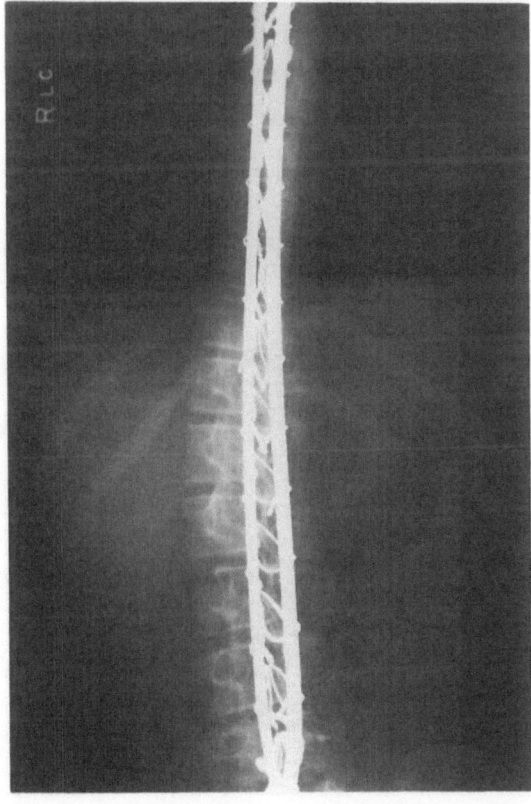

R L C

C

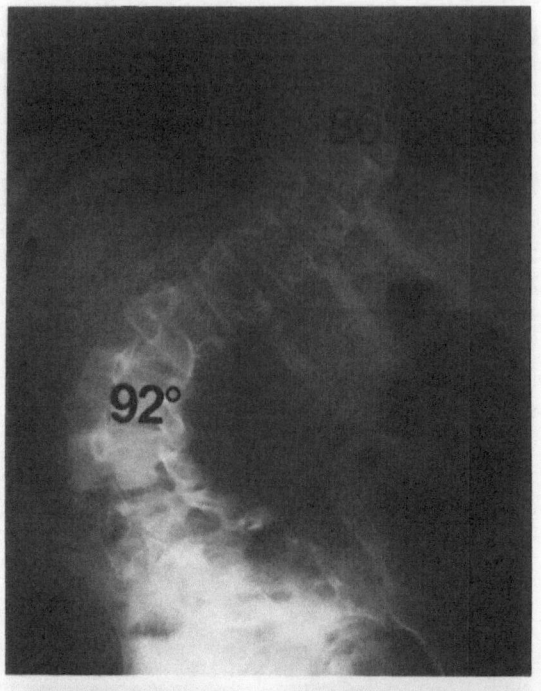

A

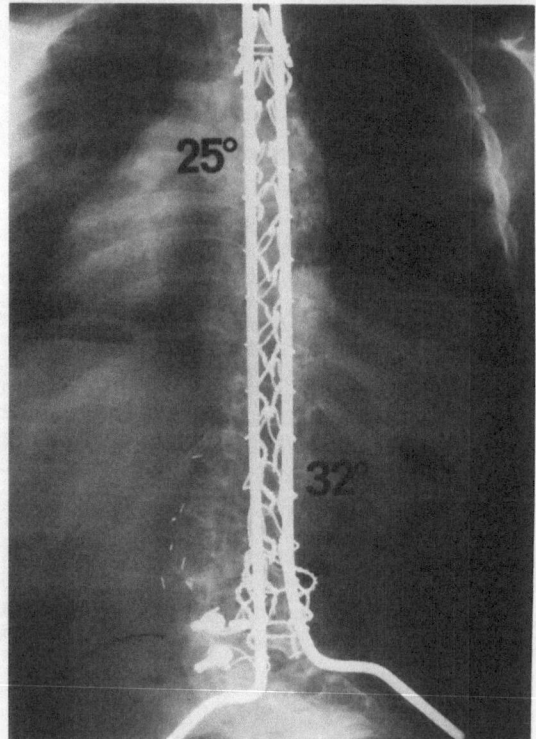

B

Selection of fusion levels is a critical step requiring evaluation of x-ray films and knowledge of the natural history, the level of function, and the type of instrumentation planned. In general, long fusions are necessary: it is rarely possible to place the lower end of the fusion at L1 or 2 unless the curve is purely thoracic (idiopathic in appearance). In most cases of syringomyelia or Friedreich's ataxia, it is possible to end the fusion at L3 or L4 since there is rarely pelvic obliquity.[25] The essential question, however, in most of the other patients is whether or not to include the sacrum. In most sitters with NMS requiring fusion, instrumentation must extend to the sacrum.[7,9,15,66,73] Exceptions, of course, are those with little or no true pelvic obliquity and little tendency for the curve to increase or lengthen. It is always desirable to maintain mobility of the lower lumbar levels (L4 to the sacrum) in children who are still ambulatory and with some expectation to continue to walk.[6] This is true even if a mild degree of obliquity will still be left postop. In these patients, fusion needs to extend from T2 or 3 to L4. In some cases where significant fixed pelvic obliquity exists, the first stage, anterior Dwyer or Zielke instrumentation, may produce enough correction to permit posterior fusion to be extended only to L4.[10]

In general, we advise against fusing to the fifth lumbar vertebra in any patient with sensation. Although others have done this successfully, we maintain that if it appears that a fusion needs to extend to L5, it should be brought down to the sacrum. A long fusion, to L5, concentrates stress across the L5–S1 joint, leading to possible back pain.

The final important decision is whether surgical correction should be anterior, posterior, or both, and which type of fixation system should be used. It is beyond the scope of this chapter to describe the technical details of each procedure, but the theoretic generalizations will be given. First, if a curve is not intrinsically flexible, flexibility must be obtained by anterior surgery.[7,8,51,62,64,67] Very occasionally, a severe curve causes spontaneous fusion posteriorly. In this case, flexibility cannot be obtained without posterior spinal osteotomy and anterior release. Since the curve always rotates into the convexity, the anterior column of bone is longer than the spinal cord and posterior elements. A rigid thoracolumbar curve needs "loosening": at least removal of the discs within the curve, or even discs and apical vertebrae. Since lumbar discs are larger, more correction is obtained by removal of lumbar discs than of thoracic discs. Furthermore, the rib cage adds an element of rigidity, not found in the lumbar spine, to the entire thoracic spine.

◀

Figure 10.11. A: Pre-operative radiograph of 11-year-old boy with spina bifida and double curve of 86° and 92°. There is significant pelvic obliquity and spinal imbalance. B: Postoperative antero-posterior radiograph following multiple level discectomy anteriorly and posterior spinal fusion with SSI. The pelvis is now level. No postoperative immobilization was used.

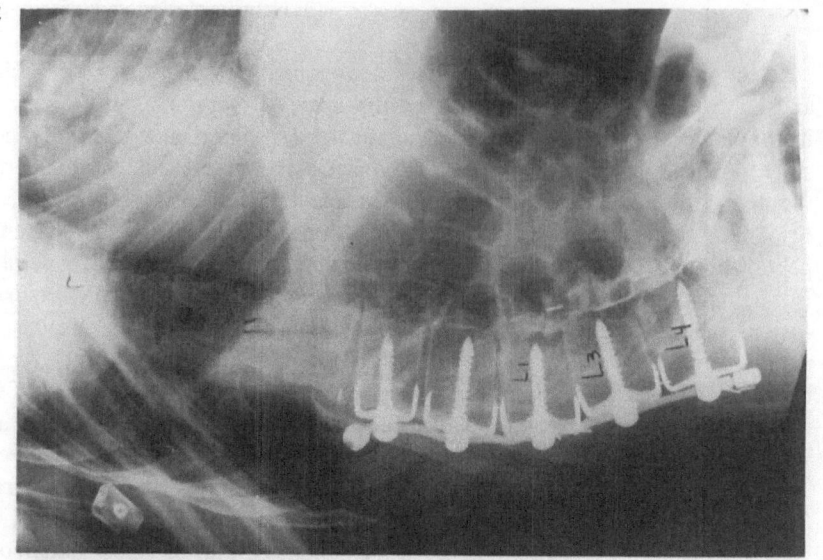

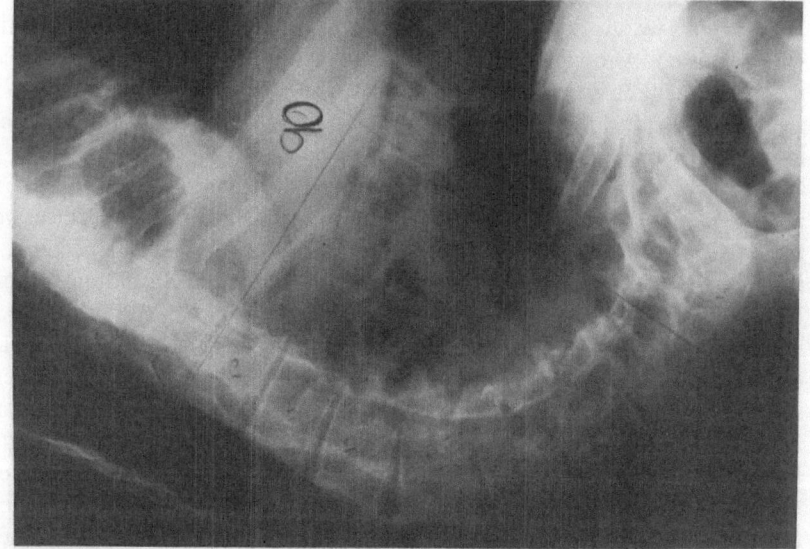

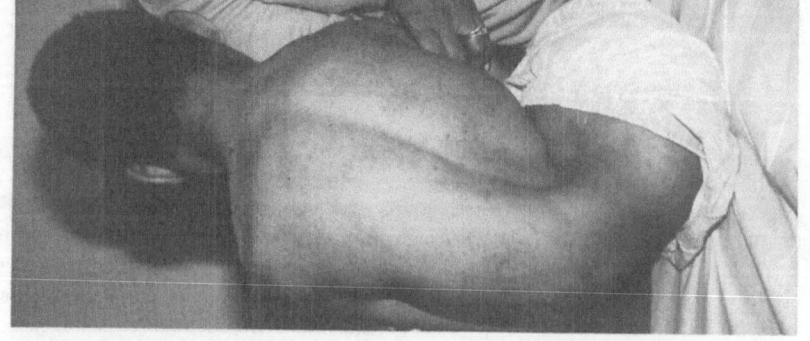

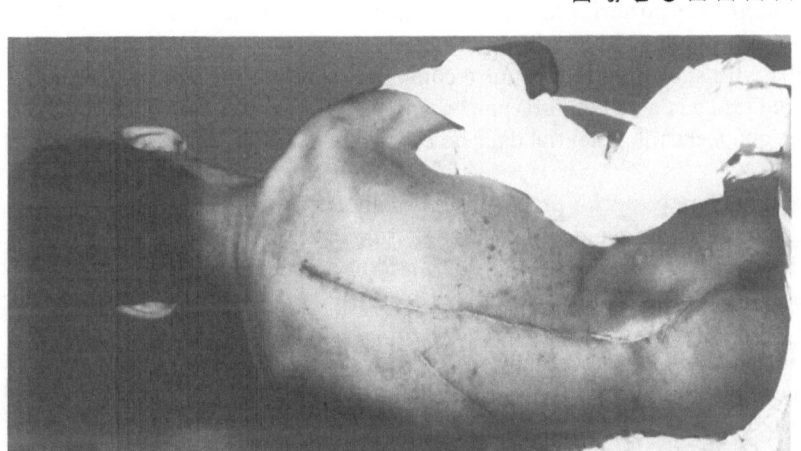

D

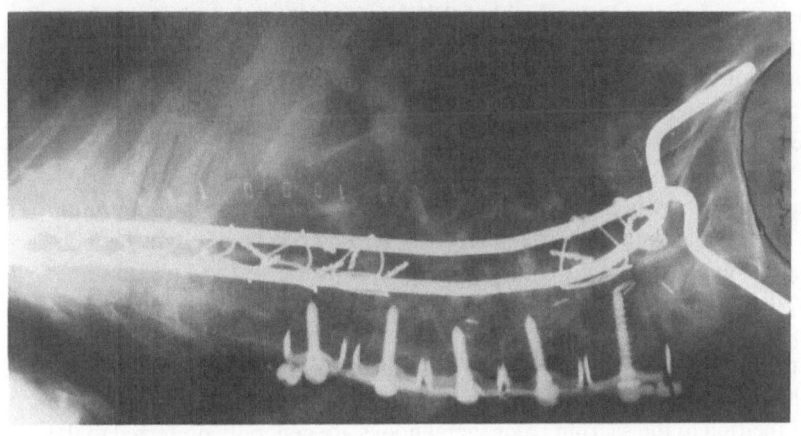

E

Figure 10.12. A: Pre-operative photograph of 20-year-old with severe cerebral palsy, severe pelvic obliquity, and normal mental function. Patient cannot sit. B: Pre-operative radiograph. Curve is extremely rigid. C: Following complete removal of the L2 vertebrae by simultaneous front and back procedure with Dwyer instrumentation anteriorly. D: Radiograph following Luque instrumentation. E: Postoperative clinical appearance. Pelvis is now essentially level.

Second, a circumferential (front and back) fusion is a stronger fusion than a posterior-only fusion. Following posterior-only fusion in a 10-year-old, the anterior elements still grow somewhat despite the posterior tether. This results in either an increasing lordosis, partial loss of correction or, usually, both.[15] In some cerebral palsy patients, severe spasticity will be "fighting" the posterior fusion in trying to bend it. Therefore, the severely spastic patient represents a relatively strong indication for front and back surgery.

Additionally, early return to function requires secure fixation if external immobilization is to be avoided. Anterior instrumentation, whether with Dwyer or Zielke apparatus, allows tremendous correction by directly opposing the vertebral endplates along the convexity. However, neither form of fixation is really very secure even though both devices are loaded in tension. The Dwyer cable may fray and break; screws may pull out of cancellous bone with either technique.[7] The semirigid Zielke rod is certainly not strong enough to withstand motion, especially abnormal athetoid or other movement disorders if the spine does not fuse solidly.

For the above reasons, almost any time anterior instrumentation is performed in NMS, a secondary posterior fusion with some form of SSI should be used. This can be either a standard SSI with smooth L-rods and sublaminar wires, a Harrington rod with sublaminar wires, or a combination of both. Recently, Drummond introduced a concept of intraspinal segmental wiring over small buttons.[74] This technique lacks the potential dangers of sublaminar wires and is almost as strong.

Since a secondary posterior procedure is usually necessary, in most cases our preferred technique is to avoid any anterior instrumentation at the time of discectomy and anterior fusion. This shortens the anterior procedure and decreases the blood loss. Avoiding anterior hardware also decreases the risks of late damage to the great vessels, the ureter, and cisterna chyli, all having been reported following anterior instrumentation.[75] Additionally, with any form of anterior hardware there is the tendency to decrease the normal lumbar lordosis. This kyphosing tendency can be combatted by placing screws posteriorly in the bodies and by inserting anterior grafting as well as by using the Zielke rod with its de-rotation apparatus instead of the Dwyer cable.[7,11,34] Nonetheless, we prefer simply to remove the discs and bone anteriorly to obtain all the *correctability* at that time. Using posterior Luque instrumentation subsequently permits one to "contour-in" as much lordosis as desired.

For the same goal of maintaining normal lumbar lordosis, we recommend using standard Luque rods posteriorly rather than wired-in Harrington rods. Harrington distraction rods, by being posterior to the axis of flexion, have an antilordotic effect on the lumbar spine. This tendency can also be combatted by using contoured square-ended rods and adding a compression rod to the lumbar spine. However, distraction rods tend to flatten the lumbar lordosis, even if contoured. It has been suggested that this decrease in lordosis secondarily decreases the effectiveness of the diaphragm muscle action, decreasing vital capacity.[51]

A further disadvantage of Harrington instrumentation is the lack of a secure system of fixation to the sacrum. Alar sacral hooks are generally preferred to the transacral bar, but both have a tendency to loosen or disengage. Our preferred technique of instrumentation across the lumbo-sacral joint is to contour the Luque rods into the "Galveston" fashion, extending for at least 6 cm between the two tables of the ilium.[66] Using this technique and generous bone grafting, the pseudarthrosis rate across the lumbo-sacral joint should decrease to <5%.

With all of the attention paid to the instrumentation, the spinal surgeon should not forget that all hardware will eventually fail unless a solid arthrodesis is obtained. To accomplish this, the posterior exposure must be wide, from tip to tip of transverse process. Supplemental bone graft, either bank bone or iliac bone, is always needed for posterior fusion. We have used commercially available lyophilized bank bone in most neuromuscular patients without having encountered any particular problems. There is often a lack of sufficient iliac bone, especially when fixation of the pelvis is used.

Postoperative immobilization is not always necessary now that there is widespread use of segmental spinal instrumentation.[52,76] However, in patients with severe spasticity, athetosis, or other movement disorders, a postoperative TLSO is probably prudent while the patient is upright for the first 3 to 6 months. This allows easy access to the skin for bathing, is lighter in weight, and more comfortable than a cast. When only Harrington instrumentation is used, without supplemental segmental fixation, it is best to use full-time bracing initially because of the risk of hook loosening. Whatever system is used, however, every effort should be made to get the patient upright immediately postop. It would be disastrous for a 14-year-old patient with Duchenne's dystrophy to be kept at bedrest for 3 months postoperatively.

Results

Before 1980, we used the Harrington system for posterior internal fixation of spinal deformity. Dwyer instrumentation was used anteriorly on extremely rigid curves. Since 1981, we have changed almost entirely to SSI. We often perform a preliminary anterior spinal release of discs (usually without instrumentation) on any curve that is rigid. Of the over 150 patients on whom we have performed SSI, approximately 60 have had NMS. We do not emphasize the degree of correction per se, but rather achieving the goal of a vertical torso over a level pelvis. Nonetheless, our correction has usually averaged 60 to 70% by the Cobb method. No postoperative casts are used; there is a rapid return to the pre-operative functional level. In 10 patients a postoperative TLSO was used arbitrarily during the daytime.

Complications

There have been no infections; one patient died postoperatively from a delayed perforation of the right atrium from a central venous catheter. Blood loss has been high (usually 2,000 to 4,000 cc), especially in meningomyelocoel patients.

In order to prevent neurologic injury from excessive correction, we monitor patients with somatosensory evoked cortical potentials (SSEP) and, if possible, an intraoperative wake-up test. We had one permanent neurologic injury. This (partial cord) injury occurred in a patient with severe cerebral palsy who had no control pre-operatively of her sphincter or lower limbs and had a very rigid, 150° curve. There was some loss in sensation below L3 postoperatively, but no real functional change. Inexplicably, the SSEPs monitored during the procedure were entirely normal. None of our idiopathic scoliotic patients had any neurologic deficit postoperatively although a few had complained of transient thoracic hyperesthesias.

Of the over 3,000 sublaminar wires passed, there has been no neurologic injury or dural tear secondary to wire passage. We have removed segmental spinal instrumentation on three occasions (in the so-called "growing Luque" procedure where no fusion was performed). Although there were no ill effects from removing the wires, it is impossible to control the path of the wire at the time of wire removal and one must recognize the danger of dural laceration. If rod removal is necessary, it is suggested that the wires simply be tightened down against the lamina after cutting out the rod.

Of the 60 patients, three pseudarthroses have occurred. In two patients these were repaired and re-instrumented. In one patient the pseudarthrosis was asymptomatic, associated only with a small loss of correction. The instrumentation was removed.

Conclusions

NMS is associated with almost all of the congenital or acquired neuromuscular diseases. The pathogenesis of the scoliosis is related at least in part to trunkal muscle weakness, but many other factors play a role. The treatment is usually more difficult than the treatment of IS because of many associated abnormalities. These problems relate to the underlying neuromuscular deficit as well as the associated problems of the heart, genito-urinary system, respiratory system, etc.

Although the multifactorial pathogenesis remains obscure, the methods of treatment are better defined. Recent advances and surgical instrumentation have increased the surgeon's options. In correcting formerly ignored deformities, the indications for intervention remain functionally oriented rather than related just to the degree of the curve. The patient's quality of life can often be dramatically improved by straightening and stabilizing his spine. The surgical goal is always that of obtaining a balanced torso centered over a level pelvis. One should not operate on every patient with a curve since the risk/benefit ratio is poor in certain severely brain-injured patients. Our usual preferred surgical technique is Luque instrumentation with sublaminar wires. If the curve is not inherently flexible, a pre-operative anterior excision of discs and occasionally vertebrae is used. If instrumentation to the pelvis is necessary, we use the Galveston technique as the most secure fixation.

References

1. Garrett AL, Perry J, Nickel VL: Paralytic scoliosis. Clin Orthop 21–117, 1961.
2. Garrett AL, Perry J, Nickel VL: Stabilization of the collapsing spine. J Bone Joint Surg 43A:474, 1961.
3. Gucker T: Experience in poliomyelitic scoliosis after correction and fusion. J Bone Joint Surg 38A:1281, 1956.
4. Harrington PR: Treatment of scoliosis: correction and internal fixation by spine instrumentation. J Bone Joint Surg 44A:591–610, 1962.
5. Leong JCY, Wilding K, Mok CK, Ma A, Chow SP, Yau CMC: Surgical treatment of scoliosis following poliomyelitis. A review of one hundred cases. J Bone Joint Surg 63A:726–740, 1981.
6. Moe JH: The management of paralytic scoliosis. South Med J 50–67, 1957.
7. Brown JC, Swank S: Paralytic spine deformity. In: Bradford D, Hensinger RM (eds): The Pediatric Spine. Thieme, New York, 1985.
8. DeWald RL, Faut MM: Anterior and posterior spinal fusion for paralytic scoliosis. Spine 4:401–409, 1979.
9. O'Brien JP, Yau AC: Anterior and posterior correction and fusion for paralytic scoliosis. Clin Orthop 86:151–153, 1972.
10. Swank SM, Brown JC, Williams L, Stark E: Anterior fusion with Zielke instrumentation. Orthopaedics 5:1172–1182, 1982.
11. Zielke K, Stunkat R, Beaujean F: Ventral Derotations-Spondylodese. Arch Orthop Unfallchir 85:257–277, 1976.
12. Fisk JF, Bunch WH: Scoliosis in neuromuscular disease. Orthop Clin N Am 10:863–875, 1979.
13. Bleck EE: Severe orthopedic disability in childhood: solutions provided by rehabilitation engineering. Orthop Clin N Am 9:509–523, 1978.
14. Moe JH, Winter RB, Bradford DS, Lonstein JF: Scoliosis and Other Spinal Deformities. WB Saunders, Philadelphia, 1978, pp 20B–287.
15. Bonnett C, Brown J, Perry J, Nickel V, Walinski T, Brooks HL, Hoffer M, Stiles C, Brooks R: The evolution of treatment of paralytic scoliosis at Rancho Los Amigos Hospital. J Bone Joint Surg 57A:206–215, 1975.
16. Balmer GA, MacEwen GD: The incidence and treatment of scoliosis in cerebral palsy. J Bone Joint Surg 52B:134–137, 1970.
17. Robson P: The prevalence of scoliosis in adolescents and young adults with cerebral palsy. Dev Med Child Neurol 10:447–452, 1968.
18. Rosenthal RK, Levine DB, McCarver CL: The occurrence of scoliosis in cerebral palsy. Dev Med Child Neurol 16:664–667, 1974.
19. Samilson R, Bechard R: Scoliosis in cerebral palsy: incidence, distribution of curve patterns, natural history, and thoughts on etiology. Curr Pract Orthop Surg 5:183–205, 1973.
20. Kilfoyle RM, Foley JJ, Norton PL: Spine and pelvic deformity in childhood and adolescent paraplegia—a study of 104 cases. J Bone Joint Surg 47A:659–682, 1965.
21. Lancourt JE, Dickson JH, Carter RE: Paralytic spinal deformity following traumatic spinal cord injury in children and adolescents. J Bone Joint Surg 63A:47–53, 1981.
22. Makin M: Spinal problems of childhood paraplegia. Isr J Med Sci 9:732, 1973.
23. Mayfield JK, Erkkila JC, Winter RB: Spine deformity subsequent to acquire childhood spinal cord injury. J Bone Joint Surg 53A:1401–1413, 1981.

24. Brown JC, Swank SM, Matta J, Barras D: Late spinal deformity in quadraplegic children and adolescents. J Pediatr Orthop 4:456–461, 1984.
25. Daher Y, Lonstein J, Winter R, Bradford D: Spinal deformities in patients with Friedreich's ataxia. J Pediatr Orthop 5:553–557, 1985.
26. Hensinger RN, MacEwen GD: Spinal deformity associated with heritable neurological conditions: spinal muscle atrophy, Friedreich's ataxia, familial dysautonomia, and Charcot–Marie–Tooth disease. J Bone Joint Surg 58A:13–24, 1976.
27. Pecak F, Trontelj J, Dimitrijevie M: Scoliosis in neuromuscular disorders. Int Orthop 3:323–328, 1980.
28. Shapiro F, Bresnan MJ: Current concepts review. Management of childhood neuromuscular disease. Part 1: Spinal muscular atrophy. J Bone Joint Surg 64A:785–798, 1982.
29. Shapiro F, Bresnan MJ: Current concepts review. Orthopaedic management of childhood neuromuscular disease. Part 2: Peripheral neuropathies, Friedreich's ataxia and arthrogryposis multiplex congenita. J Bone Joint Surg 64A:949–953, 1982.
30. Simmons E, Weber FA: The association of syringomyelia and scoliosis. J Bone Joint Surg 58B:589, 1974.
31. Yoslow W, Beeker MH, Bartels J, Thompson W: Orthopaedic defects in familial dysautonomia: a review of 65 cases. J Bone Joint Surg 53A:1541–1550, 1971.
32. Piggott H: The natural history of scoliosis in myelodysplasia. J Bone Joint Surg 62-B:54–58.
33. Siegel IM: Scoliosis in muscular dystrophy. Clin Orthop 93:235–238, 1973.
34. Swank SM, Brown JC, Perry RE: Spinal fusion in Duchenne's muscular dystrophy. Spine 7:484–49, 1982.
35. Wilkins KE, Gibson DA: The patterns of spinal deformity in Duchenne muscular dystrophy. J Bone Joint Surg 58A:24–32, 1976.
36. Shapiro F, Bresnan MJ: Current concepts review. Orthopaedic management of childhood neuromuscular disease. Part 3. Diseases of muscle. J Bone Joint Surg 64A: 1102–1107, 1982.
37. Daher Y, Lonstein J, Winter R, Moe J: Spinal deformity in patients with arthrogryposis. Spine 90:609–613, 1984.
38. Drummond DS, Mackenzie DA: Scoliosis in arthrogryposis multiplex congenita. Spine 3:146–181, 1978.
39. Sahlstrand T, Ortengren R, Nachemson A: Postural equilibrium in adolescent idiopathic scoliosis. Acta Orthop Scand 49:354–365, 1978.
40. Adler NA, Bleck EE, Rinsky LA, Young W: Balance reactions and eye–hand coordination in idiopathic scoliosis. J Orthop Res 4:1, 1986.
41. Gregoric M, Pecak F, Trontelj J, Dimitrijevic M: Postural control in scoliosis. Acta Orthop Scand 52:59–63, 1981.
42. McEwen GD: Experimental scoliosis. Clin Orthop 93:69–74, 1973.
43. Brinckmann P, Horst M, Polster J: Preoperative halo gravity traction in scoliosis. Internal Report SFB88/C1#19, Munster, 1979.
44. Kalamchi A, Yau AC, O'Brien JP, Hodgson AR: Halopelvic distraction apparatus. J Bone Joint Surg 58A:1119–1125, 1976.
45. Wilkins C, MacEwen GD: Cranial nerve injury from halo traction. Clin Orthop 126:106–109, 1977.
46. Lawhon SM, Crawford AH: Traction in the treatment of spinal deformity. Orthopedics 6:447–451, 1983.

47. Dwyer AF, Newton NC, Sherwood AA: An anterior approach to scoliosis. A preliminary report. Clin Orthop 62:192–202, 1969.
48. Dwyer AF: Experience of anterior correction of scoliosis. Clin Orthop 93:191–206, 1973.
49. Dwyer AF, Schaler MF: Anterior approach to scoliosis. Results of treatment in fifty-one cases. J Bone Joint Surg 56B:218–224, 1974.
50. Hall J: Current concepts review. Dwyer instrumentation in anterior fusion of the spine. J Bone Joint Surg 53A:1188–1190, 1981.
51. Cardoso: Paralytic Scoliosis. In: Luque ER (ed): Segmental Spinal Instrumentation. Slack, Thorofare, NJ, 1984.
52. Luque ER: Segmental spinal instrumentation for correction of scoliosis. Clin Orthop 163:192–198, 1982.
53. Wenger D: Biomechanics of segmental spinal instrumentation. In: Luque ER (ed): Segmental Spinal Instrumentation. Slack, Thorofare, NJ, 1984.
54. Luque ER: Paralytic scoliosis in growing children. Clin Orthop 163:202–209, 1982.
55. McAfee PC, Lubick JP, Werner FW: The use of segmental spinal instrumentation to preserve longitudinal spinal growth. J Bone Joint Surg 65A:935–942, 1983.
56. Rinsky LA, Gamble JG, Bleck E: Segmental instrumentation without fusion in children with progressive scoliosis. J Pediatr Orthop 5:687–690, 1985.
57. Moe J, Kharrat K, Winter R, Cummine J: Harrington instrumentation without fusion plus external orthotic support for the treatment of difficult curvature problems in young children. Clin Orthop 195:35–45.
58. Riddick M, Winter RB, Lutter L: Spinal deformities in patients with spinal muscle atrophy. Spine 8:476–483, 1982.
59. Schwentker EP, Gibson DA: The orthopaedic aspects of spinal muscular atrophy. J Bone Joint Surg 58A:32–38, 1976.
60. Sussman MD: Advantages of early spine stabilization and fusion in patients with Duchenne muscular dystrophy. J Pediatr Orthop 4:532–537, 1984.
61. Allen BL Jr, Ferguson RL: L-rod instrumentation for scoliosis in cerebral palsy. J Pediatr Orthop 2:87–96, 1982.
62. Bonnett C, Brown J, Brooks HL: Anterior spine fusion with Dwyer instrumentation for lumbar scoliosis in cerebral palsy. J Bone Joint Surg 55A:425, 1973.
63. Bonnett CA, Brown JC, Grow T: Thoracolumbar scoliosis in cerebral palsy. Results of surgical treatment. J Bone Joint Surg 58A:328–336, 1976.
64. Brown JC, Swank SM, Sprecht L: Combined anterior and posterior spine fusion in cerebral palsy. Spine 7:570–573, 1982.
65. Stanitski CL, Mitchell LJ, Hall JD, Rosenthal RK: Surgical correction of spinal deformity in cerebral palsy. Spine 7:563–569, 1982.
66. Allen BL, Ferguson RL: The Galveston technique for L rod instrumentation of the scoliotic spine. Spine 7:276–284, 1982.
67. Ferguson RL, Allen B: Staged correction of neuromuscular scoliosis. J Pediatr Orthop 3:555–562, 1983.
68. Bunch WH: The Milwaukee brace in paralytic scoliosis. Clin Orthop 110:63–68, 1975.
69. Bunnell WP, MacEwen GD: Non-operative treatment of scoliosis in cerebral palsy. Preliminary report on the use of a plastic jacket. Dev Med Child Neurol 19:45–49, 1977.

70. Duval-Beaupere G, Polifaut A, Bovier CL, Garibol JC, Assicot J: Plexidur jackets for correction of paralytic scoliosis. Results after seven years. Acta Orthop Belg 41:652, 1975.

71. Winter RB, Carlson JM: Modern orthotics for spinal deformities. Clin Orthop 26:74–86, 1977.

72. Luque ER: Vertebral column transposition. Orthop Trans (by J Bone Joint Surg) 7(1):29, 1983.

73. O'Brien JP, Dwyer AP, Hodgson AR: Paralytic pelvic obliquity—its prognosis and management and the development of a technique for full correction of the deformity. J Bone Joint Surg 57A:626–631, 1975.

74. Drummond D, Guadagni J, Keene JS, Breed A, Narenchania R: Interspinous process segmental spinal instrumentation. J Pediatr Orthop 4:397–404, 1984.

75. Probst-Proctor SC, Rinsky L, Bleck E: The cisterna chyli in orthopedic surgery. Spine 8:787–792, 1983.

76. Sullivan JA, Conner SB: Comparison of Harrington instrumentation and segmental spinal instrumentation in the management of neuromuscular spinal deformity. Spine 7:299–204, 1982.

77. Aprin H, Bowen JR, MacEwen GD, Hall JE: Spine fusion in patients with spinal muscular atrophy. J Bone Joint Surg 64A:1179–1187, 1982.

78. Campbell J, Bonnett C: Spinal cord injury in children. Clin Orthop 112:112–114, 1975.

79. Dwyer AP: A fatal complication of paravertebral infection and traumatic aneurysm following Dwyer instrumentation. J Bone Joint Surg 61:239, 1979.

80. Lonstein JE, Akbarnia BA: Operative treatment of spinal deformities in patients with cerebral palsy or mental retardation. An analysis of one hundred and seven cases. J Bone Joint Surg 65A:43–55, 1983.

CHAPTER 11

Current Concepts in Long-Term Care of the Deformed Spine

William J. Kane

Introduction

The term *orthopaedics* was derived by Nicolas Andry[1] in 1741 by combining *orthos* and *paes*, *straight* and *child*, respectively. He also conceived the symbolism of the bent sapling being straightened by being tied to a sturdy stake as being emblematic of orthopaedics. In no part of orthopaedics is that symbolism more appropriate than in the management of the deformed spine.

To understand what is involved in the care of the deformed spine, it is imperative that a few essential fundamentals be understood about the normal pediatric spinal column.

Normal Curves

The spinal column of a growing child is an excellent example of the observation that phylogenetic changes are recapitulated during ontogeny.[2] During the evolutionary transition from a four-legged to a two-legged state the spine changed from what was a single concave-anterior curve to a complex curved structure with four concave-convex curves in the sacral-lumbar-thoracic-cervical regions. In a like manner, as the child passes from fetal to infant to juvenile to adolescent to adult posture, the spinal column manifests different characteristic shapes and has different potentials for mobility and growth. It is clear that the "norms" and their degree of acceptable variability in each stage must be recognized before the diagnosis of "deformity" can be made justifiably. Unfortunately, it also must be stressed that these "norms" have wide ranges and depend not only on sex but also on age and genetic make-up.

Motion Segment

The mention of mobility requires definition of a "motion segment," which is "the smallest segment of the spine that exhibits biomechanical characteristics similar to those of the entire spine." It consists of two adjacent vertebrae and the connecting ligamentous tissues."[3] The behavior of a motion segment is dependent on, among other things, the physical properties of its components, such as the inter-vertebral disc, ligaments, and articulating surfaces. Because the spine may be considered as a structure composed of multiple motion segments connected in series, its total behavior is a composite of the individual motion segments.

Coupling

An additional aspect of spinal mobility is the phenomenon of "coupling."[3] This is the concept that, because of the geometry of the individual vertebrae, the con-necting ligaments, and the spinal curves, it is not possible to cause one motion without producing another "coupled" motion at the same time. For example, in the lumbar spine the frontal rotation seen in lateral bending is "coupled" to lateral translation as well as both axial and sagittal rotation. In the thoracic spine the sagittal rotation of a flexion or extension movement will be "coupled" to antero-posterior translation. From this phenomenon flows the fact that in scoliosis the lateral curve is also associated with a rotational component and a cephalo-caudal deformity. It becomes obvious then that spinal deformity cannot be considered as though it were in just one plane: it must be considered from a three-dimensional viewpoint.

Four Dimensions

Before the inexactitude of the previous sentence makes too much of an impres-sion on the reader, let it be corrected to recognize the impact of the fourth dimension—time—or more precisely the phenomenon of spinal growth over time. Because progressive spinal deformities deteriorate most rapidly during the periods of growth acceleration it is important to relate spinal growth and the potential for progressive spinal deformity. The vertebral column forms at the 23rd fetal day with the formation of somites and the sclerotomes which in turn become first the mesenchymal vertebral column, then the cartilaginous and finally the osseous spine. Ossification begins at the 33 mm crown–rump stage in the arches in a cranio-caudal direction from the cervical spine, and it starts simul-taneously in the vertebral bodies at the thoraco-lumbar junction and extends cranially and caudally.[4]

Tanner has shown that growth is not linear but is subject to two spurts, the first from birth to age 3 and the second during adolescence; the intervening period is essentially uniform and linear.[5-7] Duval-Beaupere identified, after an analysis of 560 scoliotic patients, that their curves increased at a steady rate until puberty, and then accelerated during the adolescent growth spurt until growth ceased.[8] This is the clearest correlation of growth with deformity progression.

Another important aspect of spinal growth is the relationship between the premature cessation of growth caused by a spinal fusion and the ultimate effect on the patient's total height. Winter has demonstrated that on the average 0.07 cm will be lost per spinal segment fused for each year of growth remaining.[9] This assumes that the growth in the deformed spine was normal which is a contrary-to-fact premise; consequently, because of the improvement in curve angulation occasioned by a spinal fusion and instrumentation it can be stated that ordinarily the loss of height caused by the fusion is less than the loss of height that would be caused by unattended progressive curves. Nordwall has shown that between 10 and 13 years of age the effect of fusion on final total height is only mildly negative, whereas the correction of a scoliotic deformity after 13 years results in greater final total height despite the mild stunting effect of the fusion.[10] It may sound trite but there is much truth in the aphorism "A short, straight spine is better than a short, crooked spine."

Spinal Deformities

Having described a few basic concepts important in understanding the normal spine, let us turn to the concept of "spinal deformity." A deformity is the result of the failure to develop according to anatomic norms. Because of the spine's previously described unique biomechanical characteristics, all planes are affected by a deformity predominantly seen in one, but for didactic purposes they are herein covered in the following order: (1) coronal: scoliosis; (2) sagittal: kyphosis and lordosis; (3) horizontal: spondylolysis and spondylolisthesis, diastematomyelia, spina bifida, and sacral agenesis.

In the broadest sense, it is clear that other causes of spinal deformity would fit within the dimensions of this chapter (osseous tumors, tuberculous and pyogenic abscesses, herniated nucleus pulposus, etc.) but they will more appropriately be described in other sections.

Coronal Deformities

Scoliosis

Scoliosis is a deformity of the spinal column that can be the consequence of any of a number of different causes and diseases.[11] Not only is there an abnormal lateral curvature of the spine in the frontal plane, there is also an antero-posterior deformity due either to an increase or a decrease in the normal kyphotic and lordotic curves in the sagittal plane. Because any bending or angular motion is associated with rotation, there are also alterations in the horizontal plane. An additional consequence of these three-plane deformities is the shortening of the individual spine when measured in a cephalo-caudal direction.

Since scoliosis can develop as a result of a variety of different causes and diseases, it is important for prognosis to know what has initiated a specific individual's scoliosis. Although scoliosis is classified according to its specific etiology, it is more fundamentally characterized as either structural or nonstructural.[12]

Structural Versus Nonstructural Scoliosis

A nonstructural scoliosis is mild, flexible, and totally correctable on side bending toward the convex side. It is commonly associated with various conditions that usually can be corrected, and once the problem has been eliminated the scoliosis disappears. Two examples of nonstructural scoliosis are scoliosis secondary to a leg-length discrepancy and scoliosis secondary to a vertebral osteoid osteoma. Treatment of the underlying cause usually leads to resolution of the scoliosis, unless it has developed in an immature individual to such an extent that it has taken on an independent and progressive existence. After a certain point, even elimination of the primary etiologic factor does not lead to resolution of the curve that had once been nonstructural – it has now become structural.

A structural curve is more severely angulated, less flexible, and not totally correctable on side bending to the convex side. In a sense, all scoliotic curves during their early stages are nonstructural; then, at some point in time, they lose their correctability and take on a nature independent of whatever their original etiology. They now sustain further progression.

Nonstructural scoliosis includes those postural curves that are seen in the latter part of the first decade. The noticeable thing about them is that they disappear in the recumbent position. Hysterical curves are seen mainly in females in the latter half of the second decade; rotation is not a prominent feature nor is there any wedging of the vertebrae; usually there is an emotional basis to the curvature; and psychiatric treatment is indicated. Sciatic scoliosis can be secondary to the irritation and pressure on nerve roots due to a herniated disc or a tumor.

Classification of Structural Scoliosis

The largest category of structural scoliosis is the so-called idiopathic scoliosis which has strongly hereditary and familial characteristics. Idiopathic scoliosis usually accounts for more than 80% of the population requiring treatment in most scoliosis clinics. Other large categories of structural scoliosis include neuromuscular, which is divided into either neuropathic or myopathic, and congenital scoliosis which, in turn, is divided into either failure of formation or failure of segmentation. Other causes of structural scoliosis are included in Table 11.1.

Measurement of Scoliosis

Scoliosis is measured by the Cobb method on an x-ray film parallel to the coronal plane of the body;[13] rotation is measured on the same film by the method of Moe and Nash;[14] a kyphotic or lordotic component is measured by the Cobb measurement of an x-ray film parallel to the sagittal plane of the body. Other methods are used to measure the progression of deformity such as Moire fringe topography, the scoliometer to measure the angle of trunk rotation, and other devices to measure the inclination of the rib hump (the angle of thoracic inclination).

Table 11.1. Classification of structural scoliosis

I. Idiopathic
  A. Infantile (0–3 years)
    1. Resolving
    2. Progressive
  B. Juvenile (3–10 years)
  C. Adolescent (> 10 years)
II. Neuromuscular
  A. Neuropathic
    1. Upper motor neuron
      a. Cerebral palsy
      b. Spino-cerebellar degeneration
        i. Friedrich's disease
        ii. Charcot-Marie-Tooth disease
        iii. Roussey-Lévy disease
      c. Syringomyelia
      d. Spinal cord tumor
      e. Spinal cord trauma
      f. Other
    2. Lower motor neuron
      a. Poliomyelitis
      b. Other viral myelitides
      c. Traumatic
      d. Spinal muscular atrophy
        i. Werdnig-Hoffmann
        ii. Kugelberg-Welander
      e. Meningomyelocoele (paralytic)
    3. Dysautonomia (Riley–Day)
    4. Other
  B. Myopathic
    1. Arthrogryposis
    2. Muscular dystrophy
      a. Duchenne (pseudohypertrophic)
      b. Limb-girdle
      c. Facioscapulohumeral
    3. Fiber type disproportion
    4. Congenital hypotonia
    5. Myotonia dystrophica
    6. Other
III. Congenital
  A. Failure of formation
    1. Wedge vertebra
    2. Hemivertebra
  B. Failure of segmentation
    1. Unilateral (unsegmented bar)
    2. Bilateral
  C. Mixed

IV. Neurofibromatosis
V. Mesenchymal disorders
  A. Marfan's
  B. Ehlers–Danlos
  C. Others
VI. Rheumatoid disease
VII. Trauma
  A. Fracture
  B. Surgical
    1. Post-laminectomy
    2. Post-thoracoplasty
  C. Irradiation
VIII. Extraspinal contractures
  A. Post-empyema
  B. Post-burns
IX. Osteochondrodystrophies
  A. Diastrophic dwarfism
  B. Mucopolysaccharidoses (e.g., Morquio's syndrome)
  C. Spondylo-epiphyseal dysplasia
  D. Multiple epiphyseal dysplasia
  E. Other
X. Infection of bone
  A. Acute
  B. Chronic
XI. Metabolic disorders
  A. Rickets
  B. Osteogenesis imperfecta
  C. Homocystinuria
  D. Others
XII. Related to lumbo-sacral joint
  A. Spondylolysis and spondylolisthesis
  B. Congenital anomalies of lumbo-sacral region
XIII. Tumors
  A. Vertebral column
    1. Osteoid osteoma
    2. Histiocytosis X
    3. Other
  B. Spinal cord

From: Bradford DS, Lonstein JE, Moe JH, Ogilvie JW, Winter RB. In: Moe's Textbook of Scoliosis and Other Spinal Deformities, 2nd edit. WB Saunders, Philadelphia, 1987, with permission.

The Cobb method identifies the two "end" vertebrae, which are the maximally tilted vertebrae at the top and the bottom of the curvature. A line is drawn along the superior surface of the cephalad end vertebra and a perpendicular erected on that line. Similarly, a line is drawn on the inferior surface of the caudad end vertebra, a perpendicular is erected, and the intersecting angle of the two perpendiculars is measured as the degrees of vertebral angulation.

Each scoliotic curve has rotation that is maximal at the "apical vertebra" (vertebra most removed laterally from the vertical axis of the patient, and which commonly is the middle vertebra between the two extreme "end" vertebrae). The rotation of a scoliotic curve is measured by evaluating the relationship of the vertebral pedicles to the lateral margin of the vertebral body, according to the method of Nash and Moe. When the vertebral pedicles are symmetrically situated within the lateral margins of the vertebral body, the vertebra is not rotated and is considered to be "neutral."

Progression of Scoliosis

The progression of scoliosis is related to the etiology of the curve, and the age and level of skeletal maturation of the individual because the maximum amount of vertebral deformation takes place during growth. Further skeletal deformity can occur after maturation, as a result of stretching of the soft tissues of the spinal column (the ligaments, periarticular soft tissues, and the intervertebral discs); and, finally, in the end stages of adult scoliosis, by microfractures at the concavity of the curve and a result of lateral spondylolisthesis due to facet joint degeneration and destruction. However, it is in the growing spine that the asymmetric forces of compression and distraction will cause the greatest amount of angular deformation, due to the Heuter–Volkman Law which states that increased compression on one part of a growth plate will lead to retardation of growth, whereas decreased compression on the other part of a growth plate will lead to acceleration of growth. Naturally, this leads to aggravation of the process since the convex side of a curve is under greater compression, grows less, and becomes more severely angulated. It's a positive feedback loop—tending to worsen itself—rather than to correct itself.

Management of Scoliosis

The management of scoliosis requires that it be viewed from two perspectives. In the first instance scoliosis as a community problem can, and should, be diagnosed early through school screening which is in time for nonsurgical treatment of the mild, but potentially progressive, curves. Considerable emphasis should be given to this aspect of the evaluation and management of scoliosis.[15-17]

The second part of the answer will form the major part of this chapter and will provide a framework upon which additional information and experience can be positioned.

Evaluation of Scoliosis

The orthopaedic work-up of a scoliotic patient is essentially identical to the management of any patient — history, physical, lab, and x-ray studies, followed by treatment.

It is essential that a complete history of the patient be taken, including a background history of siblings, parents, and other known family members. The examining physician should determine when and how the curvature was first noted, how much time has elapsed, whether there has been a recognized progression of the curvature since detection, and whether any prior treatment has been given to the patient.

Attention should be given to determining the consequences of the spinal deformity in terms of physical endurance, fatigability, susceptibility to respiratory infections, discomfort, or pain, and the patient's own psychologic response to the presence of the curvature.

In addition to a detailed history of the scoliosis and its effect on the individual, there should also be a careful history of the patient's general health going back to birth history, developmental and growth milestones, as well as the occurrence of any childhood and adolescent illnesses. A family history should also be taken particularly with regard to the presence of spinal deformity, orthopaedic conditions in general, as well as the more common hereditable orthopaedic diseases.

Documentation of the patient's physical maturation, including the appearance of secondary sex characteristics and, in the case of females, the onset of menstrual cycles is also essential in order to determine what treatment options are available in each instance.

The physical examination should be performed with the patient completely undressed, except for underpants, although a gown can be utilized to accommodate the natural shyness and modesty of most teenagers. The patient's height and weight should be recorded and the general body build of the patient characterized. Based on the findings of the general examination, further specific evaluations can be performed. Conditions such as Marfan's syndrome, osteogenesis imperfecta, dwarfism, congenital musculoskeletal deformities are among the more obvious examples of where further detailed examinations will be indicated by the general evaluation.

The patient's gait in the plantigrade fashion, on tiptoes, and on heels quickly demonstrates the presence or absence of leg length discrepancy and of neuromuscular dysfunction of the lower extremities. The cutaneous manifestations of neurofibromatosis (café-au-lait spots and fibroma molluscum) and the presence of hairy patches or dorsal dimples might suggest specific types of scoliosis. The anterior torso should be examined with particular regard to the presence of body hair, including axillary and pubic hair, the state of breast development in girls, and the presence of either congenital or acquired chest wall deformities.

With regard to physical examination of the spinal column, it should first be performed with the patient in the erect position, noting the presence of whatever asymmetries might be determined by means of a plumb level from the spinous process of C7. This permits the determination of how much decompensation is present by the use of various levels to note inequality of shoulder height, rib prominence, and the angle of trunk rotation.

In the Adam's position, with the standing patient bent forward, with his weight evenly distributed and with hands and fingers touching and hanging loosely in front of his fully extended knees, the physician can further characterize the deformity. Moire fringe topography with photographic documentation is now being utilized in many clinics for evaluation and documentation of progression, rather than relying completely upon the x-ray examination. The use of plain photography for documentation is clearly advisable especially in view of the strikingly visual nature of scoliosis deformities.

Radiologic Evaluation

In the normal sequence of a scoliosis work-up, after the history and physical, comes x-ray evaluation. Radiographic studies, in most instances, help define the exact etiology of the scoliosis; in all scoliosis patients they are a major factor in the therapeutic decision-making process. They provide an understanding of the nature of the curvature, its location, its angulation, rotation, and flexibility, as well as defining the patient's skeletal maturation.[18]

The physician ordering films must always consider that radiation exposure should be reduced as much as possible. In the first instance the decision must be made as to whether films are necessary, and in the next instance which views are required. There can be little justification for a "routine scoliosis series," each and every time a patient is examined. Each x-ray request should be completed with consideration to what is to be learned from the film and how it will affect treatment. The films that are requested can be obtained in a manner designed to reduce radiation exposure and still provide diagnostic accuracy. Fast screen-film combinations and the routine use of postero-anterior rather than antero-posterior films reduce breast and thyroid exposure, and leaded shields protect the gonads.[19-21]

All x-ray films should be clearly identified with respect to the patient's name, date on which the films were taken, patient's identification number, and birthdate. The patient's position, whether supine or standing, should be indicated by markers on the x-ray films, and any special circumstances regarding the taking of the film should also be imprinted on the film (such as the patient using a shoe lift on one foot, or the patient being out of the brace for 3 hours, etc). Right side bending, or left side bending, or other markings by means of arrows should define any special types of x-ray films.

Scoliosis films are, by usage and convention, read as if looking at the patient's spine from behind, so due care should be taken that the markings, both permanent and temporary, can be easily read by the physician examining these x-ray films. While special x-ray studies may include such examinations as myelograms, tomograms, and computerized axial tomography, most standard x-ray series for the scoliosis patient consist of an erect postero-anterior view and a lateral view of the erect spine. Supine right and left side bending films are taken to determine spinal column flexibility, and in preoperative evaluations these films determine the amount of de-rotation that takes place at the "end" vertebrae in the side bending view. Bone age can be assessed by means of antero-posterior views of the left hand and wrist. Another indication of skeletal and spinal maturation may be obtained by means of the Risser sign, which is a characterization of the degree of ossification and fusion of the iliac apophysis as it appears to migrate from the anterior superior iliac spine towards the posterior superior iliac spine.[22,23]

Because of the high degree of correlation of congenital scoliosis and genito-urinary anomalies, it is advisable that every congenital scoliosis patient should have an intravenous pyelogram.[24,25] Additional studies that may be warranted by previous studies or by treatment decisions include routine pre-operative lab evaluation of patients scheduled for surgical correction, including complete blood count, urinalysis, basic chemistry profile and coagulation profiles, electrocardiogram. Such studies as pulmonary function evaluation are indicated in those patients who have a history or obvious evidence of pulmonary compromise; they are not warranted in patients with mild to moderate scoliosis.

Treatment of Scoliosis: Strategy and Tactics

The treatment of a scoliotic patient can be broken down into two phases — strategy and tactics. Strategy in scoliosis therapy is quite similar to the strategy that is used in dealing with fractures where, for example, the strategic goals are to reduce the fracture and to maintain the reduction. The same is true for scoliosis; it is necessary to straighten the curve and then to maintain the correction achieved. The tactics of scoliosis treatment are two — nonoperative and operative.

Nonoperative Treatment

Because nonoperative treatment is more effective with milder and more flexible curves, the early detection of scoliosis is important in the nonoperative management of scoliosis. Since one can never be certain whether a curve is of the progressive variety, minor scoliotic deformities that have been documented in skeletally immature individuals periodically should be observed and evaluated intermittently by x-ray examination. Curves that have been identified as progressive in the skeletally immature and that have already reached 20 degrees should be started on brace treatment. Other orthopaedists believe that it is safe to wait until 25 degrees, but there is universal recognition that the decision as to when to commence brace treatment cannot be dependent only upon the Cobb angle measurement. The patient's age, the proximity to skeletal maturation, appearance, general level of intelligence, and cooperativeness of the patient and the family are all factors that must be weighed in the decision to commence orthotic management. The orthoses that have been most widely utilized for mild to moderate scolioses are the Milwaukee brace and the Boston brace. Many others have been devised, such as the DuPont, the Korsair, and the Lyon. A description of all is beyond the scope of this chapter. The Milwaukee brace, devised by Blount and Schmidt, is prescribed for flexible scoliotic curves, having a thoracic component, with an apex above T8 where the prevention of further deterioration is the major goal of treatment. It is also utilized for infantile and juvenile idiopathic scoliotic curves, and for curves of other etiologies as a temporizing and delaying tool in a fashion that will reduce the speed at which a younger curve is progressing. In such instances, the recognition that surgery is quite likely to be necessary is made at the outset of treatment. Rather than fusing the immature spine at an extremely early age (with attendant loss of torso height as a result of cessation of growth in the area fused), the brace is used to limit progression until an age at which spinal fusion may be performed.[26,27]

In general, the interval for application of a Milwaukee brace for progressive adolescent idiopathic scoliosis is between the time it measures 20° and before it progresses to 40° in a skeletally immature child.

Many underarm braces have been devised of which the Boston brace, credited to John E. Hall, is the most prominent. The curves for which they are prescribed are usually less than those requiring the Milwaukee brace. They involve the lower thoracic, the thoraco-lumbar, and the lumbar regions. There has been a noticeably greater patient preference for the underarm braces because they do not have the uprights and throat piece, which affect the patient's appearance and which alter his clothing habits. Yet even they do not have 100% patient compliance and acceptance.[28]

After fabrication and final check by the orthotist, the treating physician should also perform a check-out, not only by physical examination of the pelvic girdle, superstructure, and pad placement, but also by x-ray evaluation of the pad placements which can be assisted by radio-opaque pad markers. It is also essential that the patient be advised on how the brace is to be applied, the schedule of how many hours it is to be worn during the breaking-in period, and what his physical activities may be.

In summary, the use of orthoses for the correction of abnormal spinal curvatures is indicated for an immature and growing spine which is afflicted with mild and flexible curves. The patient's consent must be obtained after having been informed of the goals and likelihood of beneficent results. The physiotherapist should be experienced and enthusiastic in exercise programs for scoliosis and kyphosis, and the orthotist must demonstrate a competence developed through education and experience. The physician's compassionate guidance to the other members of the team is an essential pre-requisite. Although the goals of brace management of scoliotic curves are limited, the achievement of these goals is well worth the efforts made by all concerned.

The use of manipulations, physical therapy, and so-called "therapeutic spinal exercises" alone cannot prevent a progressive deformity. In fact, there are those who believe that specific spinal exercise programs work in a counter-productive fashion by making the spine more flexible than it ordinarily would be and, in so doing, making it more susceptible to progression of the curve.

A new method of treatment for the flexible scoliotic curve that might otherwise be treated in an orthosis involves the use of nocturnal electrical stimulation. The method is still undergoing evaluation so strict guidelines for its utilization have been set up by those who are most familiar with its design and application. The basic concept is to cause contraction of the muscles at the convex apex of the curve by means of an electrical impulse imparted either to the paraspinal muscles subcutaneously or the lateral costal muscles transcutaneously. The stimulation is created only during the sleeping hours, so the obvious attraction of this method is the freedom from the use of the brace during the daytime hours.[29,30]

Operative Treatment

The surgical correction of a spinal curvature is one of the most complex and complicated areas of orthopaedic surgery. The surgical procedure is demanding not only with regard to the need for manual dexterity and precision, particularly in view of the proximity to the spinal cord, but also because the decision-making process in scoliosis care is subject to almost an infinity of variations. The lack of a precise formulation in scoliosis surgical treatment has led to different emphases by different surgeons. While all surgeons stress patient safety, one might emphasize correctability and another prefer speed of convalescence. The availability of many surgical techniques and procedures has also compounded the problems faced by the surgeon, as he attempts to gain familiarity and sufficient experience with each of the techniques.

Usually, the following are considered to be poor prognostic signs: a higher degree of angulation, more severe rotation, shorter curves and more cephalad curves, spinal column, stiffer curves in the immature individual, and looser curves in the mature individual.

I have divided factors that affect the surgical decision into those that may be considered intrinsic to the curve and those extrinsic to the curve. The factors that are intrinsic to the curve include etiology and nature, severity and progression, associated presence of a kyphotic or lordotic component, response of the curve to bracing, mobility and flexibility of the curves with or without vertebral wedging, vertical location of the curves within the spinal column, and the potential for deterioration and production of symptoms such as pain or an unacceptable cosmetic appearance. Factors that are extrinsic to the curve, but that influence the surgical decision, include intelligence and level of cooperation of the patient and family, presence of associated constitutional illnesses, availability of support personnel necessary for a brace team, presence of pain and psychic alterations in the patient, and such factors as the lack of feasibility of a brace program due to the inadequacy of transportation facilities by which means regular monitoring of a brace patient could be achieved.[31]

As noted previously, the strategic goals of any scoliosis treatment are two: (1) curves must be reduced and corrected, and (2) these reductions and corrections must be maintained. Reduction and correction of scoliosis curves can be achieved by means of traction, corrective casts, surgical releases, and surgical instrumentation. The maintenance of the correction is achieved by a solid spinal fusion through arthrodesis of spinal joints using autogenous bone grafting. Surgical instrumentation serves as internal splintage during the postoperative period; casts and braces serve as external splintage during the same period.

The keystone of any surgical treatment program for scoliosis is the achievement of a solid spinal fusion. This is true whether an internal fixation device is utilized or not. While such devices are helpful in achieving correction, in reducing pseudarthrosis rates, and in facilitating the postoperative rehabilitation of scoliosis patients, the most important means to the attainment of a solid spinal fusion is the eradication of intervertebral joints and their replacement with autogenous cortico-cancellous bone graft. Fusion performed on the posterior elements entails eradication of the hyaline cartilage and subchondral cortical bone of the posterior facet joints and the insertion of a cortico-cancellous block of bone into the facet joint; anterior fusion entails removal of the fibrocartilage of the intervertebral disc down to cortico-cancellous bone of the vertebral end-plate, and the insertion of multiple fragments of autogenous bone into the disc space.[32]

The correct fusion level must be selected. To decide which is the correct level, three characteristics of the scoliosis must be identified: (1) the curve pattern, (2) the neutral vertebrae, and (3) the "stable zone" of Harrington. Virtually all idiopathic scoliosis curves will fall into one of five patterns: (1) primary thoracic, (2) primary thoraco-lumbar, (3) primary lumbar, (4) double thoracic, and finally, (5) double primary consisting of one thoracic and one lumbar curve. Neutral vertebrae are those in which the end-plates of adjacent vertebrae are parallel and rotation is neutral. The fusion should always include the cephalad and caudad neutral vertebrae. The third parameter is the so-called "stable zone" of Harrington, which is the area between two perpendiculars erected from the sacral pedicles. The fusion should be extended far enough caudad so that the last fused vertebra falls within this zone. Almost the only exception to these rules is found in the double primary thoracic-lumbar curve, when the fusion should not extend caudally below L4. Because these curves have been found to be stable even when fused only to L4, we should try to preserve as many open lower lumbar joints as possible.[33]

Another area that requires pre-operative planning is the reduction of intra-operative blood loss. While extreme hypotension can cause problems with spinal cord function and renal function, moderate hypotension by means of various anesthetic agents will facilitate surgery by reducing blood loss within the operative field. The use of devices to recover blood lost intra-operatively is routine in many institutions. The use of autologous blood and the use of a "cell saver" intra-operatively is accepted quite enthusiastically by patients undergoing spinal fusion. Obviously, meticulous surgical technique, including careful subperiosteal stripping, cautery of bleeding vessels, and packing with pads or sponges can lead to significant reductions in blood loss.

Another recent addition to the scoliosis surgeon's armamentarium is spinal cord monitoring. It is rare for cord injury to occur, but the consequences of such a calamity are catastrophic. Because it has been shown that the possibility of spinal cord recovery is directly related to the speed with which distraction rods can be removed, it is desirable to know that the spinal cord is functionally intact after the instrumentation system has been installed. The first method used for verifying this was to perform a "wake-up" test: the partially awakened patient demonstrates motor control in his lower extremities. This test, however, requires considerable cooperation from the anesthesiology staff as well as the cooperation of an intelligent patient who has been adequately prepared before surgery.[34] A more recent method of spinal cord monitoring is the use of somatosensory evoked potentials.[35]

Pre-operative, intra-operative, and post-operative antibiotics (for 48 to 72 hours) are routinely prescribed in major scoliosis centers in the United States. The major instrumentation used for correction and reduction of spinal curvatures is Harrington instrumentation, which utilizes both distraction and contraction on the posterior elements to straighten a scoliotic curve effectively. The distracting bar separating two Harrington hooks is positioned along the concavity of the scoliosis and the contracting rod assembly, connecting four or more contracting hooks, half of which face caudally and half of which face cranially, are brought together over the transverse processes of the convexity of the curve. Segmental spinal instrumentation by the Luque method requires two long L-shaped rods which are pre-bent on the basis of pre-operative bending films of the patient so that the congruous and parallel L-rods will be able to straighten the spine when sublaminar wires for each vertebra are attached to the rods. The rods are securely anchored in this fashion to prevent rod migration and each is securely affixed to the other. The two rods complement each other in their function; the concave rod is most highly stressed at the apex of the curve where the convex rod provides greater support. Conversely, the greater stress on the convex rod is at the ends where the concave rod provides greater support. When the wiring process is completed the corrective forces are spread over the length of the curve instead of being concentrated at its extremes. Each vertebra is stabilized by wire to each rod. Recently, Luque has introduced the rectangular bar which has the benefit of much greater strength and rigidity of the construct. Modifications of these two major systems have led to combinations of the two, and the recently available Cotrel–Dubousset system provides more correction and stability.[36-38]

Surgical advances and innovations over the last 30 years have led to corrective forces being applied to the anterior portions of the vertebral column. The work of Hodgson[39] on the anterior spine for tuberculous spondylitis opened the door for such devices as Dwyer instrumentation, which involves the attachment of staples to the convex surfaces of the vertebral bodies. Specially designed screws pass through the staples and snugly attach them to the vertebrae.[40] Through the head of each screw a titanium cable is passed; then, after multiple discectomies, the pulling together of the screw heads along the convexity of the curve effects a sizable correction of the scoliotic deformity. Modifications of the Dwyer system by Hall,[41] and the introduction of the rigid rods of Zielke[42,43] have expanded further the opportunities for anterior correction of scoliotic curves.

Despite the heft and the girth of the surgical implants that have been developed through sophisticated engineering and metallurgic studies, the ultimate maintenance of any reduction or correction of spinal deformity depends upon the achievement of a solid spinal fusion. Otherwise, the continued motion of the multiple vertebral segments will lead to metal fatigue and breakage, or to osseous fatigue and breakage.

The basic procedural components of a spine fusion include the meticulous stripping of the periosteum and soft tissues, the eradication of articular joint surfaces, implantation of autologous iliac crest cancellous bone grafts into the facetectomies, decortication of the posterior elements, and the lavish deposition of large amounts of bone graft (preferably autologous bone although homologous bank bone is useful, particularly in very young and small patients). Anterior fusions are achieved by eradication of the intervertebral discs down to the end-plates of the vertebrae. Similar to posterior fusion, autologous cancellous bone from the iliac crest is inserted into the disc spaces or anterior struts fashioned from the fibula or the resected rib are applied as troughs fashioned into the vertebral bodies.

Subsequent to the fusion, immobilization in a cast or brace is usually warranted, although the proponents of segmental spine instrumentation maintain that the stability is so great that external support is not necessary. Follow-up radiographic examination of spinal fusions is usually performed at 6 and 12 months. It includes oblique x-ray films, which are frequently more helpful in demonstrating the presence of a posterior spinal fusion pseudarthrosis. During the 6 to 12 months of the spinal fusion's maturation, the patient's activities are restricted, limited to sedentary adult activities. Upon solidification and maturation of the fusion, patients are encouraged to resume their normal activity schedule including participation in body contact sports. Female patients who have undergone a spinal fusion for adolescent idiopathic scoliosis are specifically advised in one of their final follow-up appointments that they should not expect to encounter any specific difficulty in bearing children and in raising a family.

Treatment Algorithms

While algorithms have been offered for various medical conditions including scoliosis, it should be recalled that an algorithm is a rule of procedure for solving a mathematical problem. Unfortunately, scoliosis is not a mathematical problem, and, therefore, so-called "algorithms" for scoliosis can only be a personal codification of opinion and experience, not a strict rule applicable in every instance.

In infantile idiopathic scoliosis under 20°, regular observation is satisfactory. Between 20 and 50°, the curve should be braced against progression and attention given to identify such poor prognostic signs as a malignant Mehta angle[44]: if the difference in the rib-vertebral angles measured at the apical vertebra on both the concave and convex sides is greater than 20°, the curve is likely to progress. Over 40 or 50° some are advocating the implantation of subcutaneous Harrington rods according to Moe's method, without a spinal arthrodesis.[45] The subcutaneous rod provides some immediate correction and can be lengthened at intervals as the child grows and the spinal curvature progresses. Luque also claims that segmental spinal instrumentation without arthrodesis achieves the same effect, although there are others who maintain that rigid immobilization afforded by segmental spinal instrumentation leads to autogenous facet joint fusion, a result of the lack of motion necessary to maintain joint function and anatomy. The use of a Milwaukee brace and restricted activities must complement the use of a subcutaneous rod in the unfused spine. At a later age, the patient will require a spinal fusion. The same holds true for Luque procedures which were not originally accompanied by a spinal fusion.

In juvenile idiopathic scoliosis, observation is sufficient for the patient who has a curve under 20°; but, for a progressive juvenile idiopathic curve of over 20°, the patient should be braced (and, possibly, even casted to protect against progression). For patients with curves over 40° to 50°, consideration should be given to the use of internal fixation such as Harrington, Luque, or Cotrel-Dubousset instrumentation, which may or may not be complemented with a spine fusion as described in the preceding paragraph, depending on the patient's age and other factors.

The adolescent with idiopathic scoliosis may be followed if the curve is between 10° and 20°, and braced for progressive curves between 20° and 40°. Between 40° and 50° there is a gray zone where either a brace can be applied or a fusion performed, depending on the curve's location and flexibility, the patient's appearance, attitude, and age. Over 50° in the adolescent idiopathic patient, a fusion is recommended.

Scoliosis progresses after skeletal maturity. It has been demonstrated that this progression is related to the severity of the curve at the time of maturation, as well as its flexibility and pattern.[46] The adult with an idiopathic scoliosis should be observed (between 20° and 40°) no more frequently than once every 4 to 6 years, because the amount of progression is so slight in this group that more frequent examination is not warranted. Between 40° and 60° the patient should, perhaps, be observed at biannual intervals, particularly in women who have had pregnancies during their second and third decades.

Over 60°, spinal fusions should be undertaken according to the signs and symptoms of progression in addition to real or potential neurologic compromise, cardiopulmonary disability, pain, and patient appearance. Because adult spinal columns are much less flexible than those of adolescents, correction is much less and the complications of surgery are noticeably higher in any adult series contrasted with an adolescent series. These complications include pseudarthrosis of the fusion, wound and genito-urinary infection, and various pulmonary complications such as pneumonia, atelectasis, and pulmonary embolus.

For the patient with nonidiopathic scoliosis, bracing should be utilized between 20° and 40°, unless the prognostic indicators are such that there can be little justification for delaying a fusion. Such an instance exists in various types of congenital scoliosis such as a unilateral unsegmented bar which will cause severely progressive scoliosis, or defective formation such as the complete absence of a vertebral body which is certain to cause a progressive kyphotic deformity. In such instances even under 40° a short fusion is warranted because the available experience points to the inevitability of progression of these defects.[47]

Sagittal Deformities

Kyphosis and Lordosis

The spinal deformities primarily affecting sagittal alignment are kyphosis and lordosis. Though spondylolisthesis does affect sagittal alignment, its primary defect is in the horizontal plane. This will be presented in that subsection.

Kapandji states that the curvatures of the vertebral column increase its resistance to axial compression forces, and that the resistance of a curved column is directly proportional to the square of the number of curvatures plus one. For this reason the vertebral column with its three flexible curves — lumbar, thoracic, and cervical — has a resistance of $10 (3^2 + 1 = 10)$, i.e., 10 times that of a straight column.[2]

Because the entire spinal column normally is compensated — or balanced — so that the head is directly over the pelvis both in the sagittal and coronal planes, and since there are four curves (the three flexible curves and the one inflexible, sacral, curve) it follows that the sum total of the angles of the curves will add up to zero. (Because average values vary with age and genetic groupings, I have utilized approximate values in the example. Independent of the specific values, however, is the validity of the concept that the total sum will equal zero — otherwise the spine would be unbalanced or decompensated.)

Curve	Average Value
C3–C7 Cervical	($\pm30°$ concave) = $-30°$
T1–T12 Thoracic	($\pm30°$ convex) = $+30°$
L1–L5 Lumbar	($\pm45°$ concave) = $-45°$
S1–S5 Sacral	($\pm45°$ convex) = $\underline{+45°}$
	Sum 0°

Only when these average values are markedly exceeded will the terms hypo- and hyper-kyphosis or lordosis be applied. It is also clear that there must be a reciprocal increase — or decrease — in the associated curves if the spine is to remain compensated. For example, a hyperkyphosis of 70° in the thoracic spine (40° greater than average) requires 40° of additional lordosis divided usually between the cervical and lumbar spinal curves. The cervical concave curve might become 45° and the lumbar concave curve would become 70° (15° increase in the cervical plus 25° increase in the lumbar equals 40° increase, thereby balancing the 40° thoracic increase). This knowledge is taken advantage of in bracing patients with thoracic kyphosis, as the orthotist purposely will attempt to reduce the compensatory lumbar lordosis, thereby forcing the child to diminish the thoracic kyphosis by attempting to stand straighter. Obviously, other orthotic principles are simultaneously utilized, i.e., the three point pressure principle—posterior pressure over the upper sternum and lower abdomen in conjunction with anterior pressure over the thoracic kyphosis.

Classification of Kyphosis

The classification of kyphosis is diverse (Table 11.2) and its consequences are severe due to progressive deformity, pain, neurologic compromise, and cardio-pulmonary failure. Using the three column concept of Denis,[48] the anterior and the posterior columns can both be involved in the biomechanics of progressive kyphosis; if either the anterior column (which is designed to resist compression), or the posterior column (which is designed to resist tension) fails then a kyphosis results. In a child the factors affecting progression of a kyphosis include: the degree of failure of the anterior and/or posterior columns; the weight of load and duration of the imposition of the load on the failing columns; the amount of angulation present; the amount of growth remaining; and, the consequent effect of the Heuter–Volkman law. (See section on Scoliosis Progression.)

The most common types of kyphosis are postural roundback and Scheuermann's disease. Postural roundback is a milder form of kyphosis; it is more flexible, more correctable actively and passively. It is rare to measure greater than 60° and x-ray films fail to show the vertebral wedging and end-plate changes typical of Scheuermann's disease. Sorenson[49] believed that a Scheuermann's kyphosis should include at least three central vertebrae, each wedged anteriorly more than 5°. The cause of Scheuermann's disease is unknown, opinions vary to include avascular changes of the ring apophyses, intracorporal disc protrusions (Schmorl's nodules, trauma, contractures of muscles or the anterior longitudinal ligament, malnutrition, osteoporosis, and calcium deficiency). It may be that postural roundback is a prelude to a Scheuermann's disease, which has been reported variously as occurring in the general population with a prevalence of 0.5 to 8.0% according to the reporter's criteria.

The presence of pain in association with deformity is also variable, and is more commonly seen the greater the angular severity and the more rigid the curvature. On examination, the dorsal hyperkyphosis will not be totally correctable but the associated compensatory lumbar hyperlordosis will.

Radiologic Evaluation

A lateral x-ray film should be taken in the erect position with the head straight and the arms supported comfortably at shoulder-height in front of the patient. A supine hyperextension film with the kyphos positioned over a radiolucent bolster reveals the correctability of the deformity. The Cobb method of selecting the end vertebrae and angular measurement is used to record the dorsal kyphosis and lumbar lordosis. Vertebral wedging is also recorded, using the angles formed by the superior and inferior end-plates of the involved vertebrae. A coronal radiologic examination reveals whether an associated scoliosis is present. These views

Table 11.2. Classification of kyphosis

I. Postural
II. Scheuermann's disease
III. Congenital
  A. Defect of formation
  B. Defect of segmentation
  C. Mixed
IV. Neuromuscular
V. Meningomyelocele
  A. Developmental (late paralytic)
  B. Congenital (present at birth)
VI. Traumatic
  A. Due to bone and/or ligament damage without cord injury
  B. Due to bone and/or ligament damage with cord injury
VII. Post-surgery
  A. Post-laminectomy
  B. Following excision of vertebral body
VIII. Post-irradiation
IX. Metabolic
  A. Osteoporosis
    1. Senile
    2. Juvenile
  B. Osteomalacia
  C. Osteogenesis imperfecta
  D. Other
X. Skeletal dysplasias
  A. Achondroplasia
  B. Mucopolysaccharidoses
  C. Neurofibromatosis
  D. Other
XI. Collagen disease
  A. Marie–Strumpell
  B. Other
XII. Tumor
  A. Benign
  B. Malignant
    1. Primary
    2. Metastatic
XIII. Inflammatory

From: Bradford DS, Lonstein JE, Moe JH, Ogilvie JW, Winter RB.
In: Moe's Textbook of Scoliosis and Other Spinal Deformities, 2nd
edit. WB Saunders, Philadelphia, 1987, with permission.

also assist in the differential diagnosis of other causes of kyphosis, especially congenital, traumatic compression fractures, infections, tumorous processes, osteochondrodystrophy, and iatrogenic causes such as seen with the post-laminectomy kyphosis or the excision of a vertebral body.

Consequences of Kyphosis

Thoracic kyphosis can become a serious cosmetic problem. The exaggerated compensatory lumbar hyperlordosis is believed responsible for an increased incidence of low back pain in later life, but data are inconsistent. Neurologic complications in Scheuermann's disease are rare, though they may be seen with the earlier appearing, more acutely angular, and more severely progressive forms of kyphosis such as the congenital form and the kyphos of Pott's disease.

Nonoperative Treatment

The treatment of Scheuermann's disease is warranted to correct deformity, alleviate painful symptoms, and to prevent the consequences of the deformity. Effective nonoperative treatment of the skeletally immature can be accomplished by repetitive body casts worn for at least a year, or by the use of the Milwaukee brace which has been reported to improve thoracic kyphosis 40%.[50] In the more rigid curves a preliminary body cast might be used prior to the brace. An exercise program is designed to reduce excess lumbar lordosis by pelvic tilting exercises. Abdominal muscle strengthening reduces thoracic kyphosis by strengthening the thoracic extensor muscle groups and mobilizing the spinal column, making it more susceptible to the corrective forces of the brace. An exercise program by itself has not been shown to be effective in the treatment of Scheuermann's disease.

Operative Treatment

Scheuermann's disease rarely warrants surgical treatment, and never in a skeletally immature patient. The selection of surgical fusion for other types of thoracic hyperkyphosis in the pediatric and adolescent patient is justified when one can document worsening of a kyphotic curve due to the factors enumerated earlier. For example, kyphosis due to congenital anterior bar, noted to be worsening on sequential lateral x-ray films, should be fused promptly upon recognition that the anterior column bar will not grow though the posterior column will. This can only lead to further angulation, deformity and, perhaps, neurologic compromise. A posterior fusion, eradicating the growth potential at the same levels as the anterior bar, will at least effect the maintenance of the status quo. If correction of the deformity is sought, then the posterior fusion in the immature patient can be extended beyond the levels of the anterior bar. The diminution of the potential for growth in the posterior column will exceed the loss of growth potential anteriorly so that the net effect is an anterior column, both normal and abnormal, through the levels covered by the posterior fusion, outgrows the posterior column, thereby reducing the hyperkyphosis in the thoracic spine. This is the same principle that causes the problems following very early fusions of the posterior thoracic spine, for whatever reason. Disproportionate growth rates lead to lordosisation of the thoracic spine. At the minimum it leads to hypokyphosis of the region, i.e., instead of a thoracic kyphosis of 30° the total thoracic kyphosis will be only 5° or 10°.

Because bone heals in compression and dissolves in tension, kyphotic curves over 60° in their maximally corrected condition should be fused both anteriorly and posteriorly. If this rule is not followed, one may anticipate that either the posterior fusion will not heal primarily, or, if it does heal in conjunction with a body cast and prolonged bed rest, delayed pseudarthrosis with attendant loss of correction and, ultimately, instrumentation failure. The spinal column must be fused both on its compressive side (anteriorly in the thoracic region) and its tension side (posteriorly in the thoracic region). My own experience leads me to believe that the preferred course of management for a moderately severe (60° to 90°) kyphotic deformity is the release of the anterior longitudinal ligament, multiple thorough discectomies, packing of the disc spaces with bone chips, and the utilization of autologous strut grafts from the rib, ilium, or fibula (or homologous grafts from the bone bank) which can be positioned to bridge the arms of the angular deformity.

Instrumentation designed to distract the anterior column either temporarily in the operating room (to help attain greater correction in the positioning of the bone struts) or permanently in the very severe (>90°) kyphotic deformities may be useful. It should be noted that following the anterior surgery, traction apparatus (halo-gravity or halo-femoral traction) may be utilized to diminish the kyphotic angle further. A posterior fusion, using Harrington compression rods and hooks with the usual surgical technique for spine fusion (facet joint destruction, facet bone block fusions, autogenous cortico-cancellous bone grafting, and wide decortication) should be performed a week or two later, depending on whether traction is being utilized and is achieving improvement.

These principles of management outlined for spinal kyphotic deformities apply both in the simpler and the more complicated situations, which may, as well, require anterior decompression, e.g., tuberculous abscess with kyphosis, or anterior and posterior resection, e.g. severe kyphosis associated with meningomyelocele where only shortening of the spinal column below the intact neurologic level will allow reasonable correction of the kyphos. Meningomyelocele with its absent posterior elements is an example drawn from nature of the effect that an unstabilized laminectomy has on a growing spine. The deficient posterior column does not prevent progressive kyphosis. Failing to recognize that a neurologically threatening anterior tuberculous abscess must be debrided and drained anteriorly leads to further grief if only a posterior approach is used as this will allow further rapid progression of the angular deformity and neurologic damage due to the deficiencies of both the anterior and posterior columns.

The knuckle of a congenitally fused bone pressing on the anterior cord is resected from an anterior approach, and the taut cord freed to move anteriorly into the area previously occupied by the resected bone. To forestall further angulation a fusion, front and back, is performed in two stages.

Lordosis

Lordosis of the cervical and lumbar regions is a normal condition but hyperlordosis of the regions is abnormal and seen with neurologic states leading to weakened musculature of the anterior neck and abdomen, or spastic extensors of the same regions. Hip flexion contractures cause lumbar hyperlordosis, as do lumbo-peritoneal shunts for hydrocephalus. Rarely, a congenital posterior bar leads to a similar deformity. Commonly, meningomyelocele results in severe lumbar lordosis, as the gluteal paralysis fails to counteract the tight hip flexors. This causes a posture of a forward tilted pelvis, which with growth leads to increase in the thoracic kyphosis and lumbar lordosis. Prompt release of the hip flexion contractures and a spine fusion are indicated as brace treatment is not effective.

If the lordosis is in the lumbar or thoraco-lumbar regions, the use of Dwyer instrumentation placed in the anterior portion of the vertebral bodies will markedly diminish the lordosis which is not fixed. An anterior spine fusion accompanies the instrumentation, and a posterior fusion must also be seriously considered.

Lordosis in the thoracic region, strictly speaking, does not occur until the region becomes concave posteriorly. Usage of the term frequently, however, is associated with what is more correctly a hypokyphosis of the thoracic spine, that is, the kyphosis is less than normal and is approaching 0°. A hypokyphotic thoracic spine is frequently associated with idiopathic scoliosis. It is a factor that complicates treatment as it magnifies the rib hump, intensifies pulmonary compromise, and makes the scoliotic curve refractory to brace treatment: a brace will not correct the scoliosis, but will even exaggerate the lordosis.

Lordosis of the thoracic spine is the result of early posterior fusions, a consequence of the unequal growth of the anterior and posterior columns. The anterior column can grow though the posterior column cannot. The result is to lessen the kyphosis leading ultimately to lordosis.

Horizontal Deformities

The spinal deformities to be considered as arising mainly in the horizontal plane are: spondylolysis and spondylolisthesis, diastematomyelia, and spina bifida. The common denominator in each of these lesions is that the deformity can be appreciated best when the vertebra is viewed in a horizontal fashion, as if a computerized tomogram cut across the involved level of the lesion.

Spondylolysis and Spondylolisthesis

Spondylolysis and spondylolisthesis are terms coined in the 19th century to describe a condition in which there is a discontinuity of the neural arch, usually at the pars interarticularis, which allows the anterior portion of the vertebra to slide forward on the neighboring inferior vertebra, most frequently L5 on S1 (*spondylos*, spine; *lysis*, dissolution or disintegration; *olisthanein*, slip). There are five types of spondylolisthesis according to the 1976 classification of Wiltse, Newman and Macnab.[51] They are: dysplastic or congenital, isthmic (lysis, elongation or acute fracture), degenerative, traumatic, and pathologic. This system of classification is criticized by Marchetti and Bartolozzi[52] as being insufficiently clear, based on mixed criteria as it uses both etiology and topography, and since it excludes iatrogenic forms. Using only etiology as a criterion they "propose a unitary view of developmental spondylolistheses in the sense that the lyses, elongations, the formation defects of the bony hook [i.e., the neural arch which normally precludes forward slippage], the spondylolisthesis, the spondyloptoses, are all morphological expressions, quantitatively different, of the same congenital cause, capable of determining different effects depending on intensity, topography, length of application, moment of occurrence during fetal development." Thus, this view leads to a classification as follows: developmental (with either lysis or elongation) and acquired. The acquired category includes traumatic (acute or fatigue fractures), iatrogenic, pathologic, and degenerative. There are valid reasons for preferring either of these similar classifications, but the former has the advantages of simplicity, priority, and wider usage.

Congenital Spondylolisthesis

This form is more common in females and the degree of slip is likely to be more severe. It is due to a congenital sacral defect with the superior sacral facets oriented so as to allow the inferior facets of L5 to slip anteriorly; the pars is intact but elongated; an S1 spina bifida is common, and the superior facets of the same segment are deficient. The entire L5 segment slides forward and its pars interarticularis, though intact, may be thinned. The S1 nerve root and the lower cauda equina may be compressed from behind by the neural arch of L5 and immediately below by the posterior ridge of the body of S1, thus forming an acute double 90°-curve. In a congenital slip, there are commonly marked rounding of the upper surface of S1 so that it appears as a "sand-pile," and occasionally a buttress of bone from the superior anterior surface of S1 (as if to support the body of L5).

Isthmic Spondylolisthesis

Isthmic spondylolisthesis is possibly the most common type of spondylolisthesis, although a prevalence study in older age groups might demonstrate that degenerative spondylolisthesis is far more common if one accepts minimal slips as the criterion. In the study of Roche and Rowe of 4,200 skeletons, isthmic spondylolisthesis was found in over 4% of the American-European group.[53] Males outnumbered females, and whites outnumbered blacks. Stewart[54] reported a 24% incidence in Eskimos, but with variations of 18.8 to 52.6% depending on geographic location. The lower figure was found south of the Yukon River, and the higher figure north of it. Stewart also found an increasing incidence with increasing age up to 40 years, where the prevalence plateaued at 34%. Aside from this ethnic group study, it is commonly held that slippage rarely increases after age 20.

Though there have been many hypotheses regarding the causation of spondylolisthesis, it has been definitely shown that the etiology is not due to anomalies of ossification of each side of the neural arch, to antenatal or postnatal trauma, or to compression of the L5 pars by the downward pressure of the inferior L4 articular process and superior pressure of the superior process of the sacrum. Others, among them Wiltse,[55] maintain that the deformity is the result of an hereditary predisposition of the involved pars, coupled with specific forces seen in the lordotic and perhaps hyperlordotic posture of the lumbar spine. Thus, repetitive daily micro-trauma leads to stress fractures of the region. Genetic studies suggest a single recessive gene in some family trees, whereas an incomplete dominant gene is seen in other genetic histories. There can be spina bifida at L5, S1, and/or S2. A secondary break of the neural arch may occur.

Isthmic spondylolisthesis is most common at L5–S1, less frequently at L4–L5. It is due to dissolution of the pars interarticularis or, less commonly, to elongation of the pars although the facets are intact. The problem is more commonly seen in males, in the population under 40, and, in the United States, it is less common in the black population. Spina bifida is common (30%), and sacralization rare (1%). The lumbo-sacral angle shows more lordosis according to Rosenberg.[56]

Degenerative Spondylolisthesis

Degenerative spondylolisthesis, also called "pseudospondylolisthesis," may be the most common form of listhesis, depending on the definition criteria. It is due to facet deficiencies secondary to degenerative joint diseases and is seen most frequently at L4–L5 and in females over 40. In contrast to the isthmic type, spina bifida is rare, sacralization is common (20%), and the lumbo-sacral angle is less lordotic.[57]

Traumatic Spondylolisthesis

Traumatic spondylolisthesis is due to an acute fracture of the pars resulting from severe trauma. It is most common in adolescent males. The role of repetitive lesser trauma leading to a stress fracture is not clearly understood.

Pathologic Spondylolisthesis

Pathologic spondylolisthesis occurs with generalized or localized bone disease of the pedicles or the pars regions, allowing the slippage to occur. Wiltse reports an increased incidence of this variety in children with Albers–Schoenberg disease and with osteogenesis imperfecta.[58]

Management of Spondylolisthesis

The forms of spondylolisthesis that affect the pediatric and adolescent age groups more commonly are congenital, isthmic, and traumatic. I shall emphasize these forms of the deformity. Usually, spondylolysis and spondylolisthesis are asymptomatic and may be discovered by incidental x-ray studies. While it is believed that spondylolysis develops between 6 and 10 years of age, the greatest risk of progression occurs thereafter, presumably during the period of the adolescent growth spurt. In the face of increased instability and increased applied forces, i.e., during competitive sports, there is a tendency for increase in symptoms. This explains the increased percentage of patients with complaints as they grow from pediatric to adolescent to adult age groups.

Pain, while uncommon overall in the entire group, is still the most common presenting complaint. Low back pain may be insidious or related to a specific trauma; it is exacerbated by activity and is described as full, constant, and mainly located in the lumbo-sacral midline region. Pain may radiate to the posterior thighs in the more severe degrees of slip. Pain below the knee is rare. Nerve root irritation may be secondary to disc protrusion at L4–L5, compression by the fibrocartilaginous mass at the pars defect, or by stretching over the lack of the body of S1.

There is some correlation between the physical findings and the degree of slip, but it is not strong. A severe slip will cause torso shortening, accentuated sacral prominence, and verticality of the sacrum. Since there is an increased kyphosis at the slippage level, there is an increased lumbar lordosis above to compensate for the deformity. Scoliosis due to rotation and unequal slippage of the involved vertebra is not uncommon. Flexion-extension mobility of the spine is reduced because of paravertebral and hamstring spasm. This also causes gait changes with fully extended hips, flexed knees, some mild equinus of the feet and short, mincing steps. Neurologic findings may include diminished ankle jerk, toe extensor weakness, positive straight leg raising and, rarely, sphincter tone dysfunction or perianal anesthesia.

The defect and the microstructure of the intervening soft tissue in an isthmic spondylolisthesis do not suggest fracture healing. Perhaps this is a reflection of chronicity as the bone ends and the fibrocartilage mass mimic a well-established nonunion or even a neo-arthrosis.

Radiologic Evaluation

Oblique views of L5 show the familiar outline of a Scottish terrier with an elongated or broken neck (at the pars interarticularis): the "broken neck" is the fibrocartilage. Lateral films of the lumbo-sacral junction must be taken in the standing position. Plain tomograms and CT scans help delineate the defect and the deformity of the involved segment. It also defines the status of the associated discs, and the presence of intraspinal tumors. In traumatic lesions the bone scan may delineate the acuteness of a lesion. The body of the involved vertebra tends to be more trapezoidal than rectangular, with the shorter dimension posteriorly in the lytic and listhetic areas. This deformation is called the lumbar index.

$$100 \times \frac{\text{Height of posterior vertebral body}}{\text{Height of anterior vertebral body}} = \text{Lumbar index}$$

The lumbar index averages 89 in the normal spine, 83 in the lytic spine, and 76 in listhetic spines. Meyerding's grading system and that of Taillard use the antero-posterior width of the sacral body as the denominator and the forward translation of L5 as the numerator. The resulting percentage is the percentage slippage. Grade I, 0–25%; II, 26–50%; III, 51–75%; and IV, 76% or more. Marchetti and Bartolozzi, in light of the fact that S1 is often so dysmorphic, prefer to use the width of L5 as the denominator, and the uncovered length of S1 as the numerator. The resulting percentages of the two systems are very similar.[52] The angle of slippage is the angle formed between the superior surface of S1 and the inferior surface of L5.

Spondylolisthesis Treatment

An asymptomatic child with spondylolisthesis should be examined and x-rayed periodically, and encouraged also to avoid impact sports, weight lifting, severe calisthenics, and body mobilization exercises.

Symptomatic children and adolescents should be started on a program of rest, therapeutic exercises, and the use of a total contact low-profile brace. If satisfactory relief is obtained, then they may resume the program charted for the asymptomatic patient. If not, then operative intervention is warranted. Even in the asymptomatic patient with x-ray evidence of either severe (grade III or greater) or progressive slippage, surgery is the treatment of choice: the instability increases with age.

If neurologic symptoms are present, their etiology should be identified and the offending compressive lesion removed. This may require a CT scan and/or a myelogram. Rather than removing the fibrocartilaginous mass at the pars defects, together with the loose posterior neural arch fragment (the so-called "RATTLER" of Crock,[59] as advocated by Gill,[60] there is much to be said for the direct repair of the defect as advocated by Buck,[61] Scott,[62] and Bradford.[63] This is particularly true in the less severe slippages (up to grade II) in the young, since they have an enormous potential for healing. Also, if the activities that accelerated the development of the condition are discontinued, the chances are greater that the combination of the bone graft at the defect and internal fixation of the portions of the deformed segment will "take" and persist. The Gill procedure appears to be contraindicated, certainly in the pediatric and adolescent age groups, but may be useful in the adult where progression is less likely and where nerve root impingement is the major source of pain.

The principal factor in the achievement of pain-free stability is fusion of the lumbo-sacral region from L4 to S1. The elements of successful posterior fusion include facet block grafts, wide decortication from tip of one transverse process to that of the other and, possibly, the use of internal fixation with Harrington, Luque, or pedicle screw instrumentation. Cast immobilization and bed rest do contribute to a higher fusion rate; therefore, if possible, they should be included in the postoperative regimen.

Reduction of the deformity is advocated by some. Using a Risser table, longitudinal traction is applied via pelvic and cephalic casts. Derotation of the pelvis accomplished by using anterior traction straps on the pelvic cast and, finally, localized pressure is applied to the sacrum. This is the method of Marchetti and Bartolozzi.[52] A posterior fusion follows. Others use posterior surgical methods including use of the Harrington distraction rod, and even spinous process traction. A combined anterior-posterior, reduction-fusion, in advanced slippage cases has been advocated by Bradford;[64] more recently, Gaines[65] has presented results of L5 vertebral body resection in instances of severe slippage. Bradford[50] credits MacEwen with the concept. Anterior fusion has had its advocates, but the fear of retrograde ejaculation as a complication of the procedure in males has limited its use.

Diastematomyelia

Diastematomyelia is a congenital deformity of the spinal column. The defect consists of a bony or cartilaginous spicule running from the posterior vertebral body to the neural arch, dividing the neural canal, the spinal cord, and its meninges in two. The pedicles are more widely separated, and the most common site is the area about the thoraco-lumbar junction. A persistent neurenteric canal is thought to be responsible for the defect. The effect on the bifid cord, which is anchored to the spicule, is noted when the spinal cord and the bony spinal column begin to grow at different rates, and the spicule begins to pull the cord distally, leading to neurologic deficits in a child who had been normal earlier.

Clinically the presentation begins with variable, frequently asymmetric and progressive neurologic deficits developing in a previously normal child. Examination of the patient's back may reveal a dimple, hairy patch, or other cutaneous defect in the midline. Plain films may show a bony midline mass in conjunction with a widened interpedicular distance of the involved vertebrae. Myelography shows a bifid dural sac at the stated level; CT scan makes these observations obvious.

The treatment of choice is removal of the deforming spicule and release of the tethered cord.

Spina Bifida Aperta

The entire spectrum of spinal deformity may be seen in association with meningomyelocele, where the problem of spinal deformity is compounded by the associated neurologic defects: paralysis, anesthesia, and bladder and bowel impairment, complicating chronic urinary tract infections, hydromyelia, hydrocephalus, Chiari II malformation, etc. The infections complicate surgical care as well as orthotic management. Another characteristic of meningomyelocele that affects the treatment of the sinal deformity is the dysplasia of the posterior elements, necessary for routine usage of Harrington and Luque instrumentation, and of the bone stock in the skeleton below the lesion—affecting not only the spine but also the iliac crests of the pelvis. These serve as donor sites for autogenous bone grafts and the anchoring points for Luque rods. Lacking the normal stresses seen in weight-bearing, the pelvic bones are thin and fragile.

The basis for spinal deformity in meningomyelocele is paralytic or congenital, according to Raycroft and Curtis.[66] The curves are more common the older the patient and the higher the level of neurologic deficit.[67]

Nonoperative Treatment

Orthotic management is useful in the paralytic variety of spinal deformity to delay curve progression and maintain trunk balance until fusion is feasible. Bracing is contraindicated if the child is obese, or if the parents cannot devote the needed time for a brace therapy program. Cutaneous anesthesia alone is not a contraindication. If progression occurs despite adequate bracing, or if any of the other conditions required for an effective brace program are not met, then the patient should be fused anteriorly and posteriorly as soon as possible. This is particularly true when a kyphotic component is present as well.

Operative Treatment

Operative management of the meningomyelocele patient requires a three-dimensional analysis of the deformity, acute awareness of skin cover and laminal defects, and a detailed analysis of hip flexion contractures and pelvic obliquity. Concomitant problems, such as hydrocephalus and persistent urinary tract infections, should be resolved before spinal surgery is undertaken.

Despite the earlier advocacy[45] of subcutaneous instrumentation without fusion (to avoid excessive spinal growth retardation), it appears that this tactic is not feasible for meningomyelocele patients, nor for certain types of dwarfism or other conditions with diminished capacity for growth. It requires postoperative bracing in any event, and this requirement vitiates its usage in many of the patients described in this section. Usually, these curves necessitate that the fusion extend to the sacrum, that it be sufficiently extended in the cephalad direction, and that it be planned not only for scoliosis, but also for kyphosis and/or lordosis. Because of deficient posterior elements, anterior and posterior fusions are more commonly required in this group of patients.

Conclusion

The management of the spinal deformities in a pediatric population represents a complex challenge that is four-dimensional in scope, and that is frequently changing as newer treatment modalities make themselves available. Nevertheless, there are few challenges as worthy or as satisfying if the results provide a less deformed and more functional spinal column for the patient.

References

1. Andry N: L'Orthopédie, ou l'Art de Prévenir et de Corriger dans les Enfants les Déformités du Corps. Paris, 1741.
2. Kapandji IA: The physiology of the joints. In: The Trunk and the Vertebral Column, 2nd Edit., Vol. 3. Churchill Livingstone, Edinburgh, 1974.
3. White AA III, Panjabi MM: Clinical Biomechanics of the Spine. JB Lippincott, Philadelphia, 1978.
4. Parke WW: Development of the spine. In: Rothman RH, Simeone FA (eds): The Spine, 2nd Edit. WB Saunders, Philadelphia, 1982.
5. Tanner JM: Growth at Adolescence, 2nd Edit. Blackwell, London, 1962.
6. Tanner JM, Whitehouse RH: Clinical longitudinal standards for height, weight, height velocity, weight velocity and stages of puberty. Arch Dis Child 51:170–179, 1976.
7. Tanner JM, Whitehouse RH, Takaisni M: Standards from birth to maturity for height, weight, height velocity and weight velocity: British children, 1965. Arch Dis Child 41:454–471, 613–635, 1966.
8. Duval-Beaupère G: The growth of scoliosis patients. Hypothesis and preliminary study. Acta Orthop Belg 38:365–376, 1972.
9. Winter RB: Scoliosis and spinal growth. Orthop Rev 6:17–20, 1977.
10. Nordwall A: Studies in idiopathic scoliosis. Acta Orthop Scand (Suppl 150), 1973, pp 81–178.
11. Bradford DS, Lonstein JE, Moe JH, Ogilvie JW, Winter RB: Moe's Textbook of Scoliosis and Other Spinal Deformities, 2nd Edit. WB Saunder, Philadelphia, 1987.
12. Scoliosis Research Society, Terminology Committee: a glossary of scoliosis terms. Spine 1:57–58, 1976.
13. Cobb JR: Outline for the Study of Scoliosis in Instructional Course Lectures. The American Academy of Orthopaedic Surgeons, Vol 5. JW Edwards, Ann Arbor, MI, 1948.
14. Nash CL, Moe JH: A study of vertebral rotation. J Bone Joint Surg 51A:223, 1969.
15. Drummond D, Rogala E, Gurr J: Spinal deformity: natural history and the role of school screening. Orthop Clin North Am 10:751–760, 1979.
16. Kane WJ: Editorial: a new challenge in scoliosis care. J Bone Joint Surg 64A:479–480, 1982.
17. Lonstein JE, Bjorkland S, Wanninger MH, Nelson RP: Voluntary school screening for scoliosis in Minnesota. J Bone Joint Surg 64A:481–488, 1982.
18. Young LW, Oestreigh AE, Goldstein LA: Roentgenology in scoliosis: contribution to evaluation and management. Am J Roentgenol 108:778, 1970.
19. Andersen PE Jr, Andersen PE, van der Kooy P: Dose reduction in radiography of the spine in scoliosis. Acta Radiol (Diagn) 23:251–253, 1982.
20. DeSmet A, Fritz SL, Asher MA: A method for minimizing the radiation exposure from scoliosis radiographs. J Bone Joint Surg 63A:156, 1981.
21. Nash CL, Gregg EC, Brown RH, Pillia MS: Risk of exposure to x-rays in patients undergoing long term treatment for scoliosis. J Bone Joint Surg 61A:371–380, 1979.

22. Farren J: Routine radiographic assessment of the scoliotic spine. Radiography 47: 92–96, 1981.
23. Risser JC: The iliac apophysis: an invaluable sign in the management of scoliosis. Clin Orthop 11:111, 1958.
24. MacEwen G, Winter R, Hardy J: Evaluation of kidney anomalies in congenital scoliosis. J Bone Joint Surg 54A:1451, 1972.
25. Vitko R, Cass A, Winter R: Anomalies of the genitourinary tract associated with congenital scoliosis and congenital kyphosis. J Urol 108:655, 1972.
26. Blount WP, Schmidt AC, Keever ED, Leonard ET: Milwaukee brace in the operative treatment of scoliosis. J Bone Joint Surg 40A:511–525, 1958.
27. Blount WP, Moe JH: The Milwaukee Brace. Williams & Wilkins, Baltimore, 1973.
28. Hall JE, Emans JB, Kaelin A, Bancel P: Boston brace system treatment of idiopathic scoliosis. Follow-up in 400 patients finished treatment. Orthop Trans 8:148, 1983.
29. Axelgaard J, Brown JC: Lateral electrode surface stimulation for the treatment of progressive idiopathic scoliosis. Spine 8:242, 1983.
30. Bobechko WP, Herbert MA, Friedman HG: Electrospinal instrumentation for scoliosis: current status. Orthop Clin North Am 10:927–941, 1979.
31. Kane WJ: Basic decision making in management of scoliosis. In: Shannon ES (ed): Instructional Course Lectures, Vol XXXIV. CV Mosby, St. Louis, 1985.
32. Moe, JH: A critical analysis of methods of fusion for scoliosis. J Bone Joint Surg 40A:529, 1958.
33. Bunch WH: Posterior fusion for idiopathic scoliosis. In: Shannon ES (ed): Instructional Course Lectures, Vol XXXIV. CV Mosby, St. Louis, 1985.
34. Hall JE, Levine CR, Sudhir KG: Intraoperative awakening to monitor spinal cord function during Harrington instrumentation and spinal fusion. J Bone Joint Surg 60A:533–536, 1978.
35. Bunch WH, Scarff TB, Trimble J: Current concepts review: spinal cord monitoring. J Bone Joint Surg 65A:707–710, 1983.
36. Harrington PR: Surgical instrumentation for management of scoliosis. J Bone Joint Surg 42A:1448, 1960.
37. Luque ER (ed): Segmental Spinal Instrumentation. Slack, Thorofare, NJ, 1984.
38. Cotrel Y, Dubousset J: New segmental posterior instrumentation of the spine. Orthop Trans 9:118, 1985.
39. Hodgson AR, Stock FE: Anterior spine fusion. Br J Surg 44:266, 1956.
40. Dwyer AF, Newton NC, Sherwood AA: An anterior approach to scoliosis – a preliminary report. Clin Orthop 62:192–202, 1969.
41. Hall JE: The anterior approach to spinal deformities. Orthop Clin North Am 3:81–98, 1972.
42. Zielke K, Pellin B: Neue Instrumente und Implante zur Erganzung des Harrington Systems. Z Orthop Chir 114:534–537, 1976.
43. Zielke K, Stundat R, Beaujean F: Ventrale derotationsspondylodese. Vorlaufiger Ergebnissbericht uber 26 operierte Falle. Arch Orthop Unfallchir 85:257–277, 1976.
44. Mehta MH: The rib-vertebra angle in the early diagnosis between resolving and progressive infantile scoliosis. J Bone Joint Surg 54B:230–243, 1972.
45. Moe JH, Kharrat K, Winter RB, Cummine JL: Harrington instrumentation without fusion plus external orthotic support for the treatment of difficult curvature problems in young children. Clin Orthop Rel Res 185:35–45, 1984.
46. Dawson EG, Moe JH, Caron A: Surgical management of scoliosis in the adult. Scoliosis Research Society, 1972. J Bone Joint Surg 55A:437, 1973.

47. Winter RB: Congenital Deformities of the Spine. Thieme-Stratton, New York, 1983.
48. Denis F: The three column spine and its significance in the classification of acute thoracolumbar spinal injuries. Spine 8:817–831, 1983.
49. Sorenson KH: Scheuermann's Juvenile Kyphosis. Munksgaard, Copenhagen, 1964.
50. Bradford DS, Moe JH, Montalvo FJ, Winter RB: Scheuermann's kyphosis and round-back deformity, results of Milwaukee brace treatment. J Bone Joint Surg 56A:749, 1974.
51. Wiltse LL, Newman PH, Macnab I: Classification of spondylolysis and spon-dylolisthesis. Clin Orthop 117:23–29, 1976.
52. Marchetti PG, Bartolozzi P: Spondylolisthesis. Aulo Gaggi Editore, Bologna, 1986.
53. Roche MB, Rowe GG: The incidence of separate neural arch and coincident bone variations. Anat Rec 109:233, 1951.
54. Stewart TD: The age incidence of neural arch defects in Alaskan natives, considered from the standpoint of etiology. J Bone Joint Surg 35A:937, 1953.
55. Wiltse LL, Widell EH, Jackson DW: Fatigue fracture: the basic lesion in isthmic spondylolisthesis. J Bone Joint Surg 57A:17–20, 1975.
56. Rosenberg NJ, Bargar WL, Freidman B: The incidence of spondylolysis and spon-dylolisthesis in nonambulatory patients. Spine 6:35–38, 1981.
57. Rosenberg NJ: Degenerative spondylolisthesis and surgical treatment. Clin Orthop Rel Res 117:112–120, 1976.
58. Wiltse LL: Spondylolisthesis in children. Clin Ortho 21:156–162, 1961.
59. Crock HV: Practice of Spinal Surgery. Springer-Verlag, New York, 1983.
60. Gill GG, Manning JG, White HL: Surgical treatment of spondylolisthesis without spine fusion. J Bone Joint Surg 37A:493, 1955.
61. Buck JE: Direct repair of the defect in spondylolisthesis. J Bone Joint Surg 61A:479, 1979.
62. Scott JH: Personal communication.
63. Bradford DS: Repair of spondylolysis or minimal degrees of spondylolisthesis by segmental wire fixation and bone grafting. Orthop Trans 6:1–2, 1982.
64. Bradford DS: Treatment of severe spondylolisthesis: a combined approach for reduc-tion and stabilization. Spine 4:423, 1979.
65. Gaines RW, Nichols WK: Treatment of spondyloptosis by two-stage L5 vertebrectomy and reduction of L4 onto S1. Spine 10:680–687, 1985.
66. Raycroft JF, Curtis BH: Spinal curvature in myelominingocele. AAOS Symposium on Myelomeningocele. CV Mosby, St. Louis, 1972.
67. Shurtleff DB, Goiney R, Gordon LH, Livermore N: Myelodysplasia: the natural history of kyphosis and scoliosis. A preliminary report. Dev Med Child Neurol 18:126–133, 1976.

CHAPTER 12

Congenital Malformations of the Spine in Children: Neuro-Imaging

H.S. Chuang

Spinal Dysraphism — Neuro-Imaging

Dysraphism is defined as incomplete or absent fusion of parts that normally unite. The term *spinal dysraphism* was introduced by Lichtenstein in 1940[1] to designate the congenital malformations of the spine that involve defective fusion of the neural tube.

The imaging of these defects in the bony structures is not crucial, but the associated intraspinal abnormality is where the importance of neuro-imaging becomes apparent.[2] With computed tomography (CT), ultrasound (US),[3-6] and magnetic resonance (MR)[7-13] all gaining ground, we must not lose sight of the importance of the plain films which at times provide us with significant information.

The spina bifida spectrum varies from spina bifida occulta (Fig. 12.1A), which is a simple incomplete fusion of the neural arch, to widely spread neural arches (Fig. 12.1B). Associated with spina bifida is meningomyelodysplasia, which is a disorder of the formation of the spinal cord, nerve roots, and thecal sac. These range from the simplest — an isolated tethered cord or tight filum terminale syndrome — to developmental inclusion masses associated with tethered cord such as dermoid, lipoma, epidermoid and teratoma; and all the way to myelocele (meningomyelocele or myelomeningocele), and lipomyelomeningocele, including diastematomyelia.

Though there is no direct correlation between the degree of vertebral abnormality and the underlying neural abnormality,[14] the neural abnormalities are usually associated with a certain type of spinal anomaly.

Spina bifida occulta is associated with isolated tethered cord syndrome. The wide open posterior arches are seen in patients with myelodysplasias such as myelocele and meningo- and lipomyeloceles. The tethered cord may or may not have widened interpediculate distance, but the ones associated with lipoma or dermoid usually do. The diastematomyelia or split cord syndrome always has widened interpediculate distance and the diastematomyelia with bony spurs also has narrowing of the disc space at the level of the diastematomyelias.

The neuroimaging of different dysraphisms will be discussed.

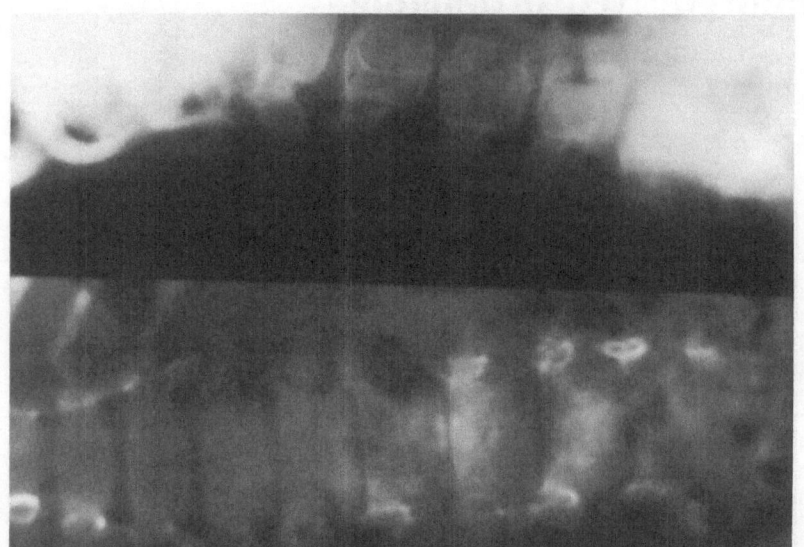

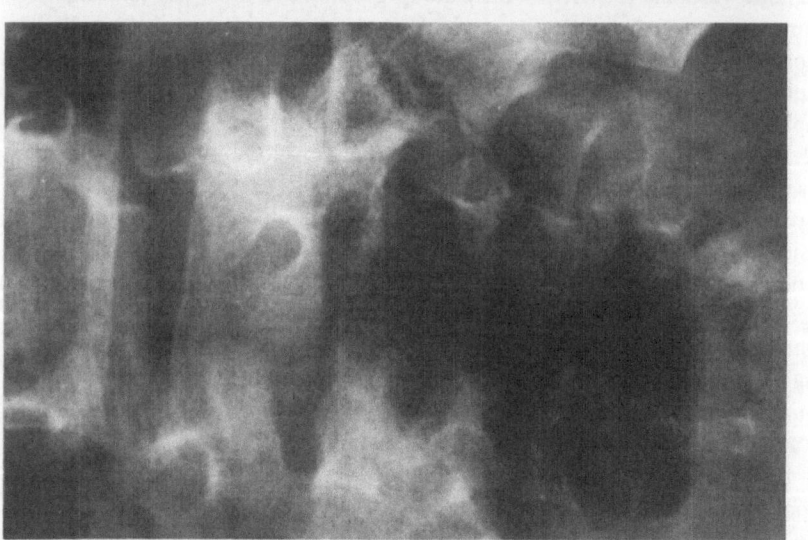

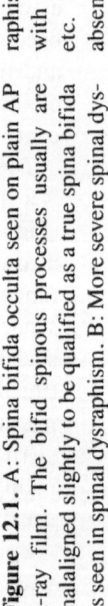

Figure 12.1. A: Spina bifida occulta seen on plain AP x-ray film. The bifid spinous processes usually are malaligned slightly to be qualified as a true spina bifida as seen in spinal dysraphism. B: More severe spinal dys- raphism seen on plain film. This is usually associated with meningomyelocele and lipomeningomyelocele, etc. Note widened interpediculate distances with absence of the posterior elements.

Table 12.1.

	Conus level	Filum size
Type I	≤ L1–2	≤ 1 mm
Type II	< L1–2	> 1 mm
Type III	> L1–2	≤ 1 mm
Type IV	> L1–2	> 1 mm

Isolated Tethered Cord or Tight Filum Terminale Syndrome

The radiologic finding of isolated tethered cord syndrome was first described by Fitz in 1975,[15] using oil-contrast (Ethiodan) for myelography. The criteria at that time were conus level below L1–2 and filum thickness on the supine spine film more than 2 mm. Since the introduction of nonionic contrast medium (metrizamide was the first) and CT for myelography[16] the criteria for tethered cord have not been revised until recently.

By analyzing the radiologic findings and the clinical findings on the post-surgical follow-up examinations in 50 patients, we have now changed the criteria for the tethered cord, which should probably be more correctly named the *tight filum terminale*.

The filum thickness is now being considered as abnormal when it is over 1 mm. The criteria for the filum thickness changed to take into account the difference in surface tension between the oil- and water-soluble contrast media.

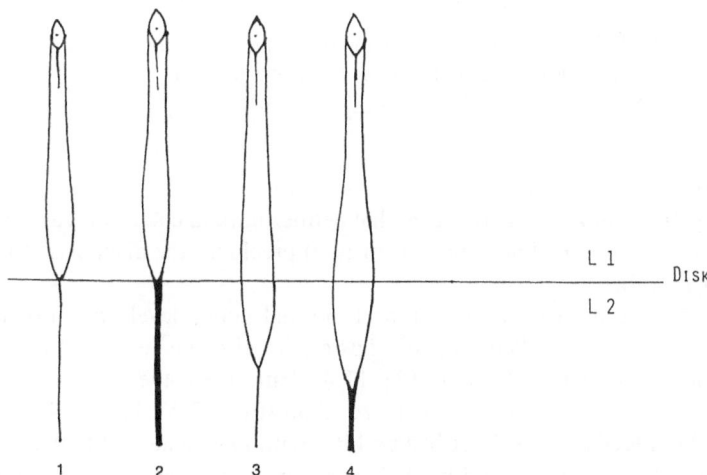

Figure 12.2. Diagram of normal conus level and filum thickness with three patterns of tethered conus. Type 1 is considered as normal — normal conus level and normal filum thickness. Type 2 has normal conus level but thickened filum. Type 3 has low conus level but normal size filum. Type 4 has low conus level and a thickened filum.

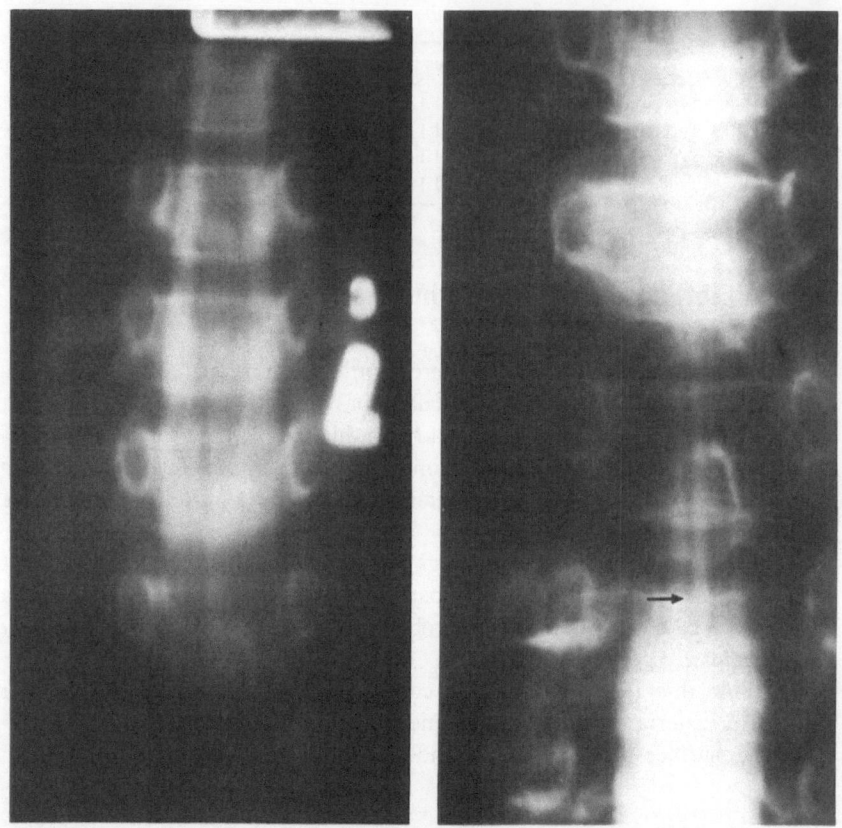

Figure 12.3. A, B: Metrizamide myelography, supine view showing the normal conus level at L1–2 with normal filum thickness of <1 mm (*arrow*).

By categorizing the radiologic findings into four patterns (Table 12.1 and Fig. 12.2), we have come to realize that neither normal conus level alone (L1–2) nor normal filum thickness alone (<1 mm) precludes the diagnosis of tethered cord syndrome.

Pattern 1 is normal, which shows a normal conus level and normal filum thickness (Fig. 12.3). Pattern 2 still has a normal conus level, but the filum is thickened to more than 1.5 mm (Fig. 12.4). Pattern 3 is the reverse of pattern 2 and shows a low conus but normal size filum (Fig. 12.5). Pattern 4 is the full-fledged tethered cord as described by Fitz, with low conus and thickened filum (Fig. 12.6). Patterns 3 and 4 have shown to be associated with intraspinal dermoids. Patterns 2 to 4 all showed significant benefit from surgical treatment, but pattern 1 is doubtful. Therefore, a normal myelographic examination should preclude surgery.

Figure 12.4. Supine projection of metrizamide myelography which shows a filum thickness of 2 mm (*arrow*) but conus is at normal level of L1–2.

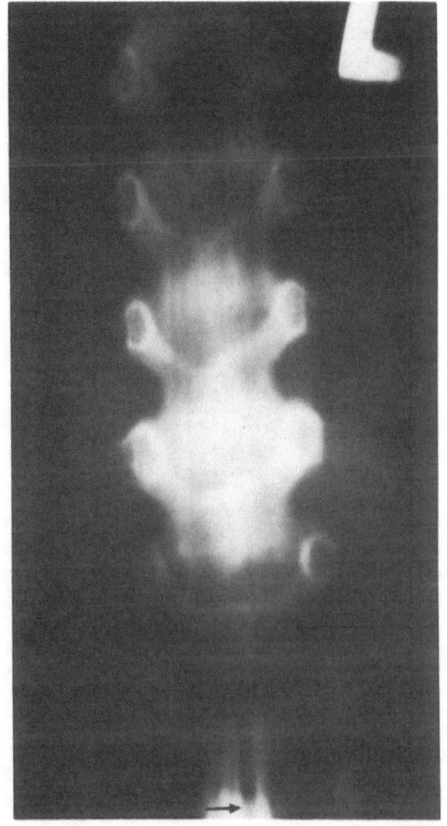

Though US[4,17] (Fig. 12.7) and MR (Fig. 12.8) can give the same diagnosis in pattern 4, pattern 3 is more difficult to diagnose by US and MR, since it is, at times, extremely difficult to note the exact level of the conus on US and MR. In addition, pattern 2 will most likely be missed as it may be difficult to visualize the thickened filum on MR or US. Real-time US does have the advantage of viewing the motion of the cord, and the amount of excursion of the cord is what some people believe determines the tethering.[18]

Therefore, it is the author's opinion that myelography is still the best radiologic tool in the diagnosis of tethered cord. However, it is extremely important to have the diagnosis made on the supine film, since the tethered filum is always posteriorly placed (Fig. 12.9A). CT myelography (CTM) has the added advantage of demonstrating the lipomatous nature of the filum (Fig. 12.9B).

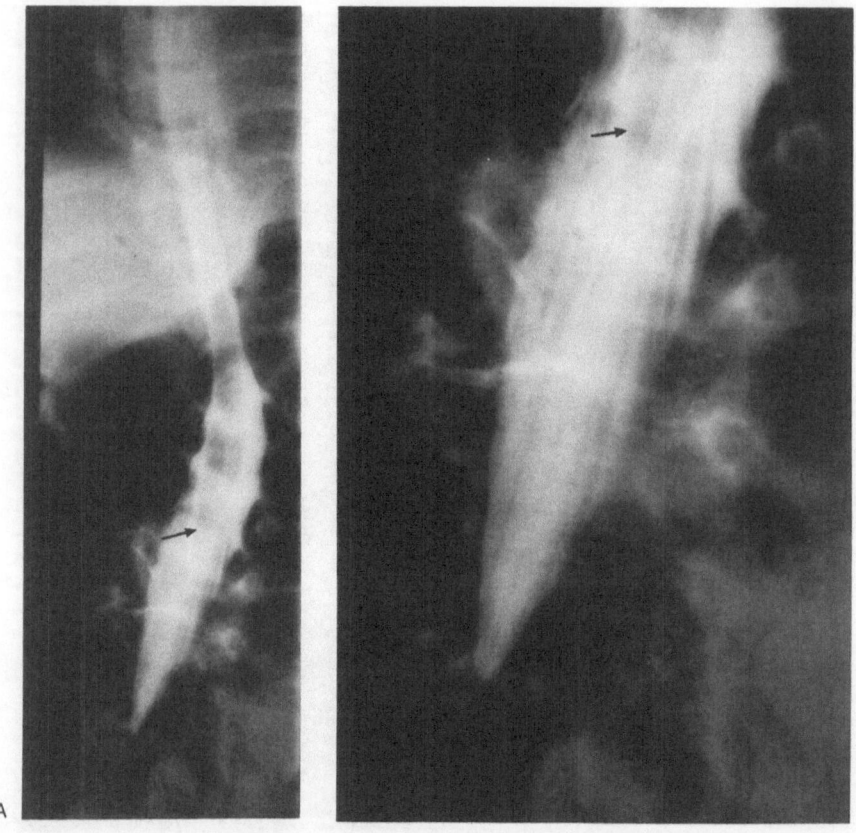

A   B

Figure 12.5. A, B: This is the reverse situation of that seen on Fig. 12.4. In this case, the filum is of normal thickness but the conus (*arrow*) is low, lying below L2.

Figure 12.7. Sagittal ultrasound in a patient with tethered cord and showing the low position conus (*arrow*) and thickened filum (*arrowhead*).

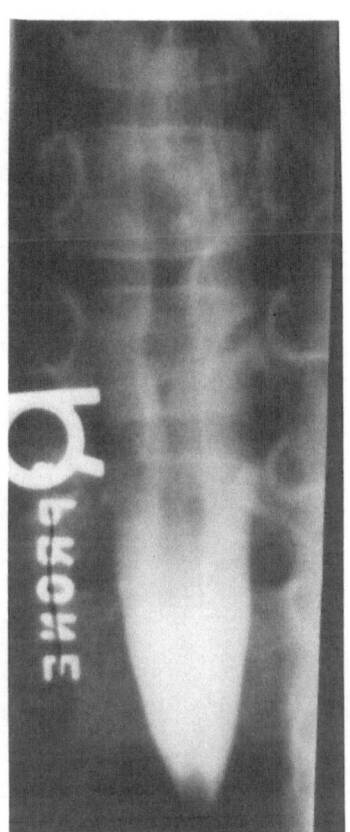

Figure 12.6. Supine metrizamide myelography seen with a low conus and thickened filum. Classical appearance of the tethered cord syndrome.

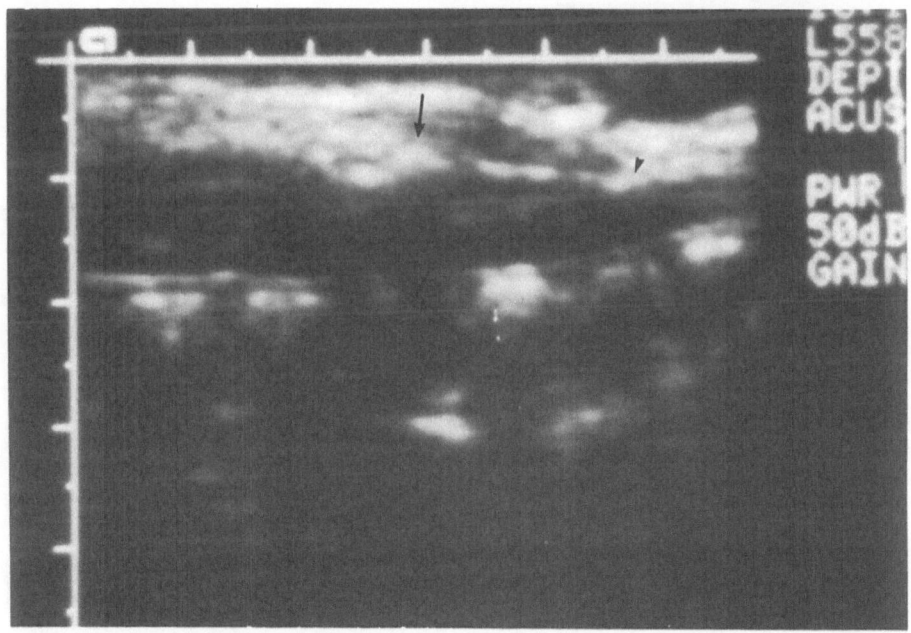

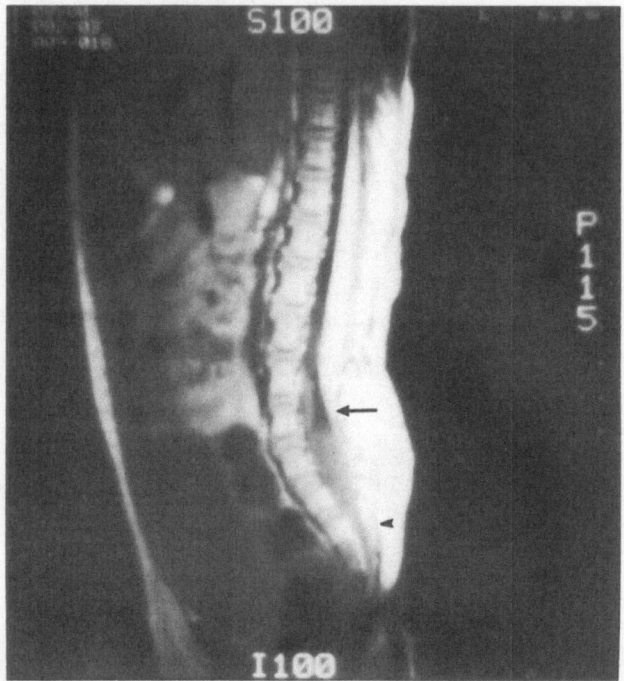

Figure 12.8. Sagittal MR scan showing the classical appearance of low conus (*arrow*) and thickened filum (*arrowheads*). However, this classical appearance is seen only occasionally. The coronal MR scan is more accurate in assessing the position of the conus because the 12th rib is more easily recognized.

Associated Developmental Mass Lesions

Developmental mass lesion is a result of sequestration and overgrowth of normal tissue during embryonic fetal development. These include dermoid and epidermoid. The mass lesions are usually associated with dermal sinus tracts which are epithelial lined dermal tubes connecting the body surface with the central nervous system or its coverings.[19] The inner end of the sinus tract may be expanded to form a dermoid or epidermoid.[19]

The dermoid usually arises from all layers and is derived from epithelium and dermis, and may include hair follicles and sebaceous and sweat glands. The epidermoid is derived from the epithelium alone. However, the lesions are indistinguishable on neuro-imaging but identifiable by histology. However, they are distinguishable on CTM and MR from lipoma, which contains a very high fat content.

The fat content causes a low attenuation value on CT (Fig. 12.10) and an increase in signal on MR (Fig. 12.11). However, the findings are indistinguishable on myelography (Fig. 12.12). The Hounsfield reading on dermoids and

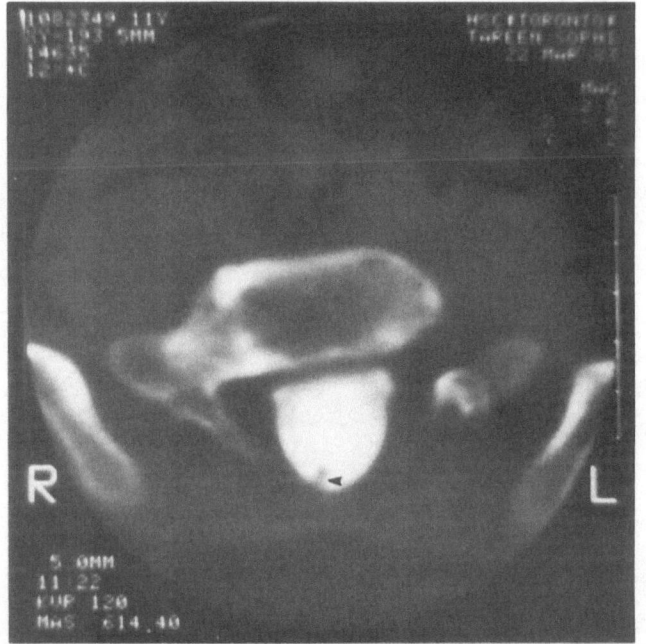

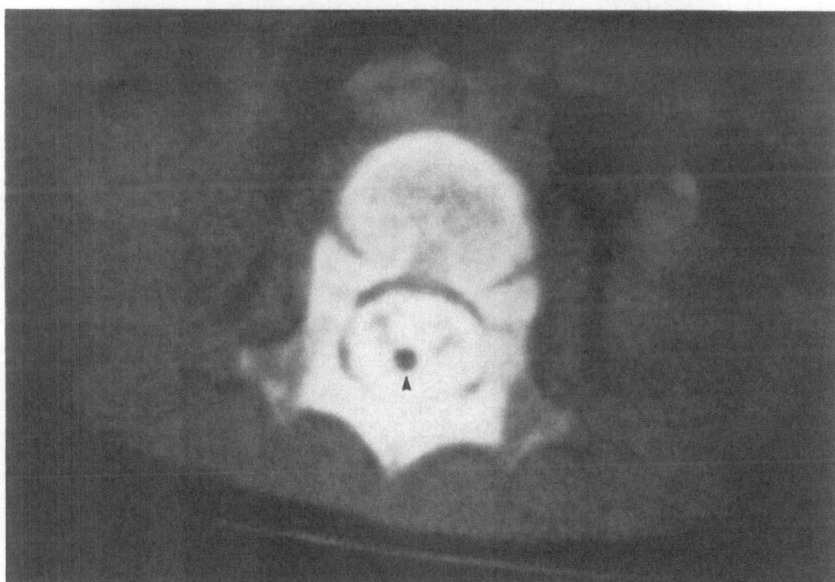

Figure 12.9. A: Axial CT myelography showing the posterior position of the tethered filum (*arrowhead*). B: Axial CT scan with a thickened filum (*arrowhead*). Low attenuation value of the filum suggests fatty infiltration.

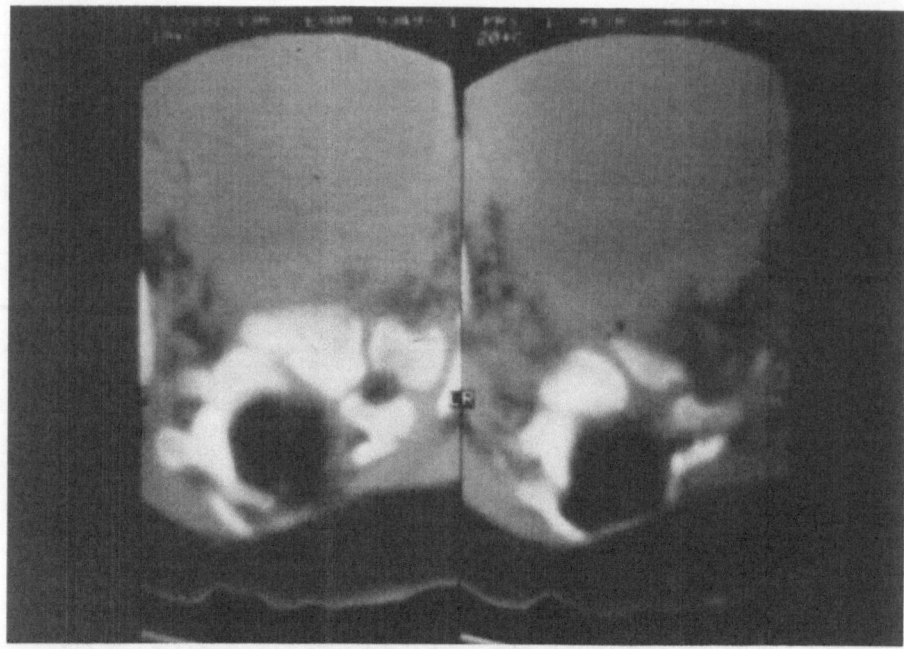

Figure 12.10. Axial CT scan showing spinal dysraphism with intraspinal lipoma seen as low attenuation.

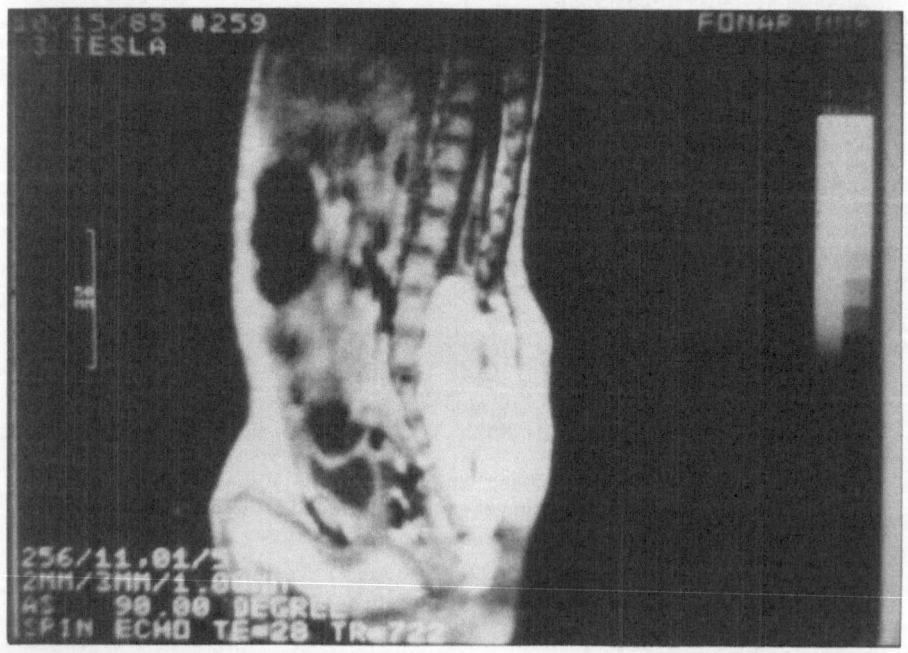

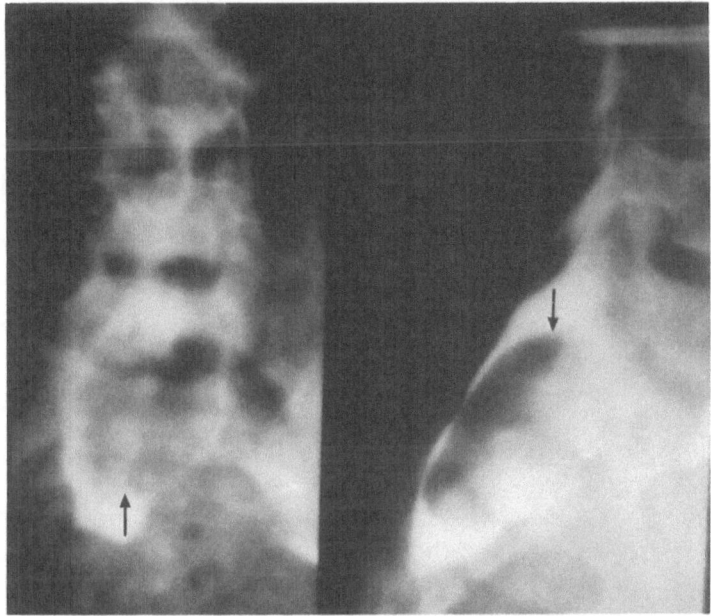

Figure 12.12. Metrizamide myelography, AP and lateral views, showing the same mass lesion (*arrows*) as seen in CT and MR though the myelogram does not differentiate with lipoma and dermoid.

epidermoids varies between $+30$ and -30 units, whereas the lipoma is in the range of -50 to -60 units.[14]

CTM may also show the dermal sinus tract as a filling defect placed posteriorly leading from the dura to the mass lesion in cases of dermoids (Fig. 12.13). The dermoids may vary from 4 to 5 mm to 15 cm in size, in which case there will be a spinal block.

The dermoids have a preselection for the lumbo-sacral region ($\sim 60\%$)[20] with decreasing frequency through the thoracic to cervical region.[21] In contrast, the distinction of epidermoid is more or less equal.[22] There is also an association of dermoid with nonsurgical diastematomyelia in the lower thoracic region.

The dermal sinus at the skin may be several levels below the dermal sinus seen entering the subarachnoid space; therefore, it is important that CTM or MR should cover a wide area of the spine.

◄

Figure 12.11. Sagittal MR of a lipoma. Increased signal with the T1 weighted image indicates lipomatous tissue. Incidental finding is a small syrinx adjacent to the lipoma at the conus.

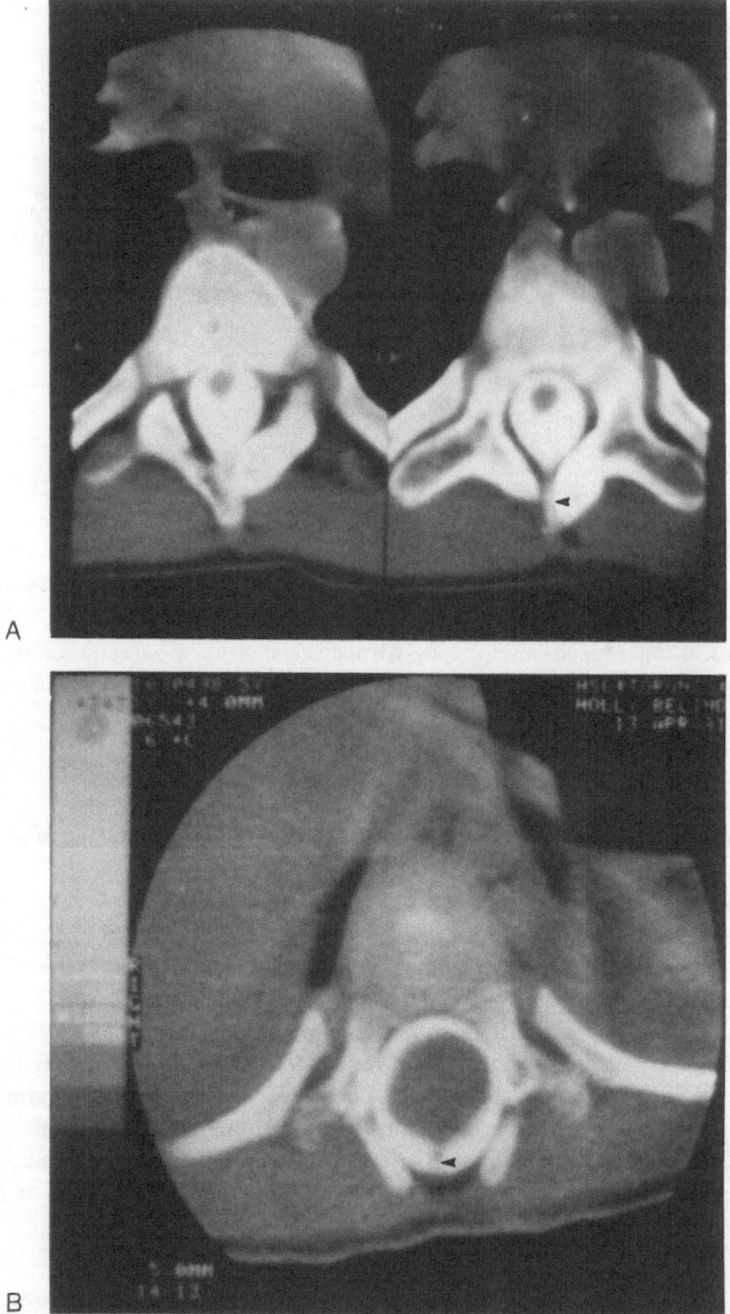

Figure 12.13. A: Dermal sinus tract (*arrowhead*) seen on axial CT scan with intrathecal metrizamide. B: Dermoid within spinal cord seen on axial CT scan as an enlargement of the cord. Note the posterior dermal sinus attachment (*arrowhead*).

In cases of lipoma, occasionally the lesion may be large enough to be studied by CT alone without contrast; otherwise MR may be the examination of choice. When present in the lumbo-sacral region, it is usually associated with tethered cord in which case spina bifida occulta is a finding.

The last of the mass lesions seen is teratoma, which is a neoplasm derived from all three layers, namely mesoderm, endoderm, and ectoderm, but occur at a site where they do not usually exist. They may be confined to the sacro-coccygeal region in which they will have the appearance of a dermoid or they may involve the entire spinal cord.

Lipomeningomyelocele

Lipomeningomyeloceles (LMMC) are meningoceles with lipomatous tissue connecting the subcutaneous fat to the intraspinal contents.[23] They constitute 20% of the skin-covered lumbo-sacral masses.[24] The condition is predominant in females.[25-27]

X-ray films of the lumbo-sacral spine reveal widened interpediculate distance with absence of the posterior elements to a varying degree (Fig. 12.14). The

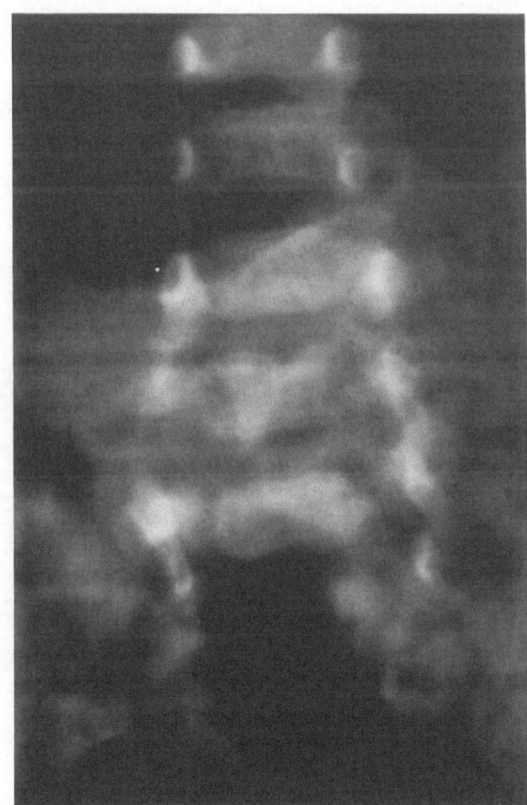

Figure 12.14. AP view of the lumbo-sacral spine shows the widened interpediculate distance with varying degrees of absence of the posterior elements.

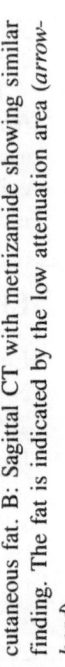

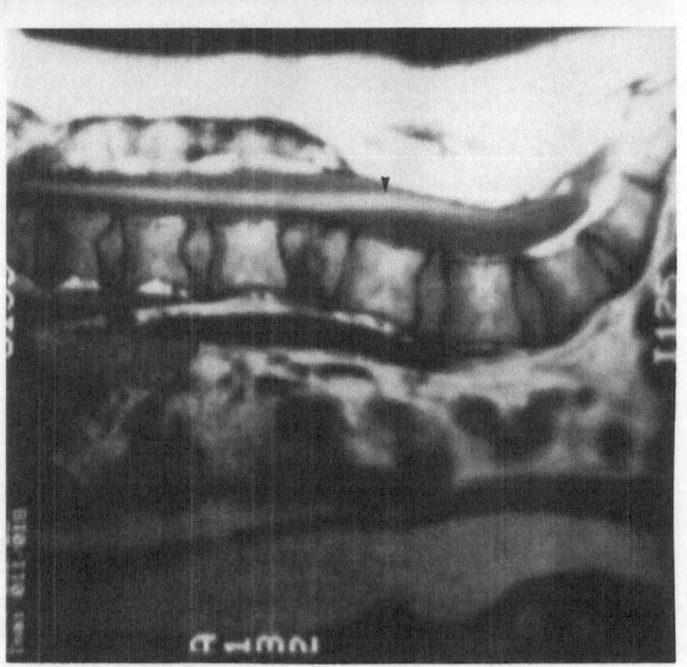

Figure 12.15. Lipomeningomyelocele. A: T1 weighted sagittal MR of lumbo-sacral region with increased signal caused by lipomatous tissue blending the cord (*arrowhead*) with the sub- cutaneous fat. B: Sagittal CT with metrizamide showing similar finding. The fat is indicated by the low attenuation area (*arrow- head*).

spina bifida which consists of absence of laminae extends through multiple levels. Butterfly vertebrae[28] and segmentation anomalies of the vertebral bodies have been reported in up to 43%[29]; and sacral asymmetry, confluent sacral foramina, and partial sacral agenesis up to 50%.[30,31]

The position of the conus is usually low and blends in with the subcutaneous fat which has penetrated into the subarachnoid space. This is best appreciated on sagittal MR images (Fig. 12.15A) where the fatty components appear as areas of increased signal on T1 weighted images blending into the spinal cord. CTM will demonstrate a similar finding with its low attenuation values of fat. If the patient is small enough, direct sagittal scanning,[32] similar to MR, can also be performed (Fig. 12.15B). Otherwise reformatted thin slice axial images will offer similar results though not as esthetically pleasing (Fig. 12.16). In newborns and neonates, US has also been helpful (Fig. 12.17).[3,4]

Though myelography alone does not offer the differentiation between cord and lipomatous tissue or masses, it does show the abnormal presence of the mass and the position of the conus (Fig. 12.18).

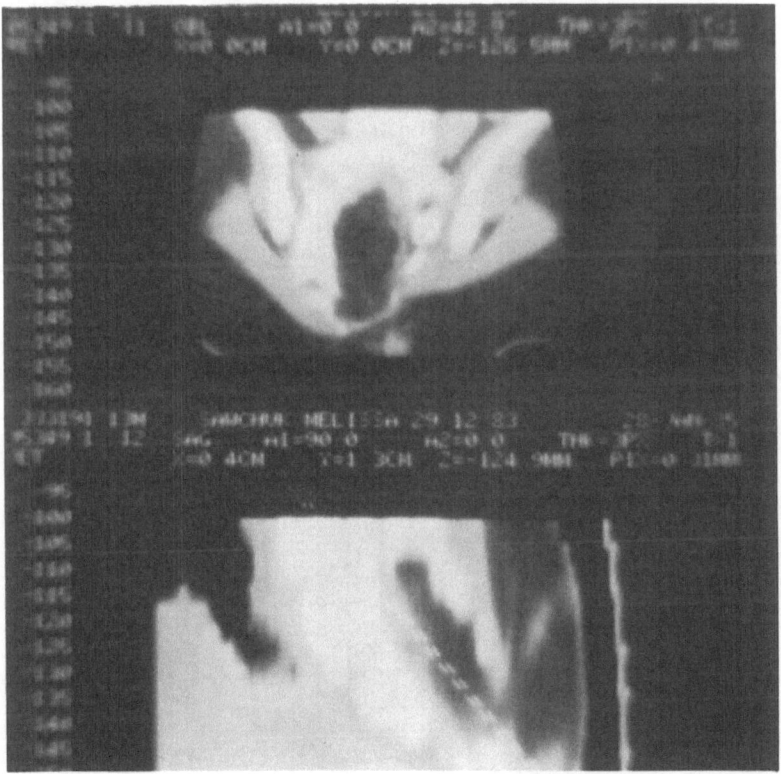

Figure 12.16. Reformatted sagittal CT from axial images showing the same finding of lipomeningomyelocele.

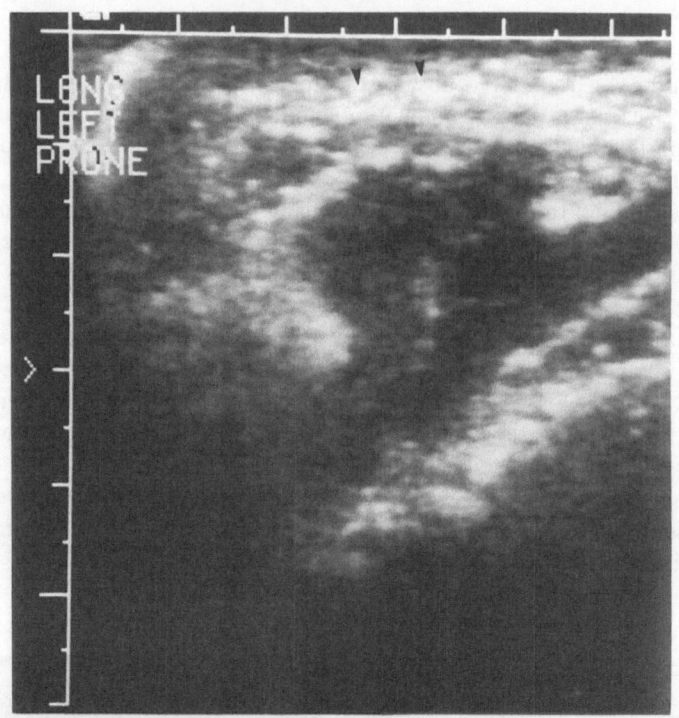

▲
Figure 12.17. Ultrasound appearance of lipomeningomyelocele showing the increased echogenicity of fat and the low conus (*arrowheads*).

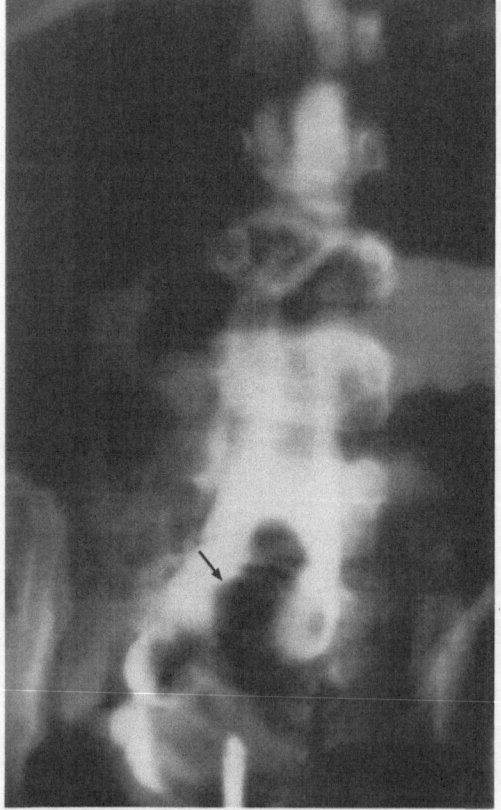

◄
Figure 12.18. AP view of metrizamide myelography in a patient with lipomeningomyelocele. Note the lobulated mass lesion (*arrow*) blending into the spinal cord.

Meningocele and Myelocele

Meningocele is an extension of the meninges outside the spinal cord through a spinal defect. By definition, it should contain no neural tissue.[33,34] A meningocele does not have to be protruding posteriorly or dorsally only; it can be anterior (Fig. 12.19) or lateral (Fig. 12.20), or even intraspinal.[21]

Any of the modalities will be good and useful in demonstrating the anomaly though CT has the added advantage of demonstrating the associated bony anomaly better with less contrast required than regular myelography.

When neural tissue or elements are found in the meningocele, it becomes a myelocele (synonyms are myelomeningocele or meningomyelocele).

Plain film again shows the grossly widened posterior elements which on CT scan shows the pedicles to be pointing postero-laterally rather than postero-

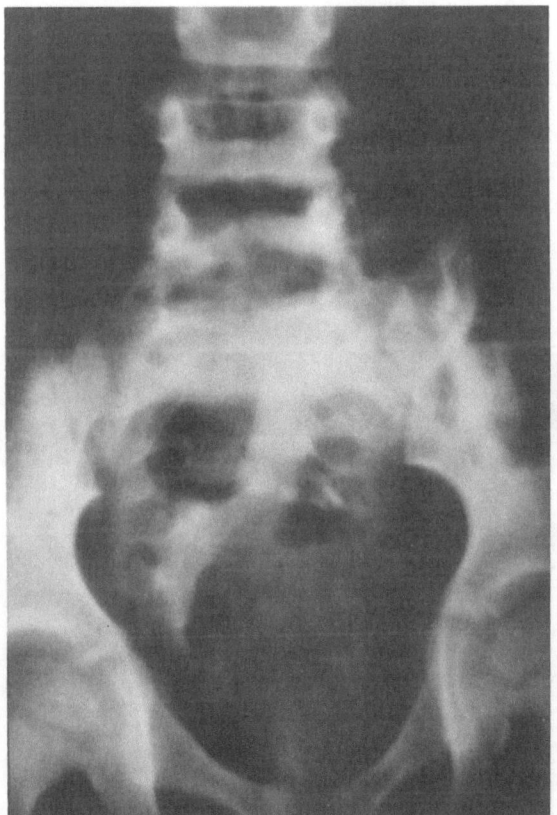

A

Figure 12.19. Anterior meningocele. A: AP x-ray film of anterior meningocele with a defect seen on the left side of the sacrum. B: AP and lateral metrizamide myelogram; meningocele is indicated by *arrows*. C: Axial CT scan without intrathecal metrizamide. Anterior meningocele (*arrow*) displaces bladder to the left.   *(Continued)*

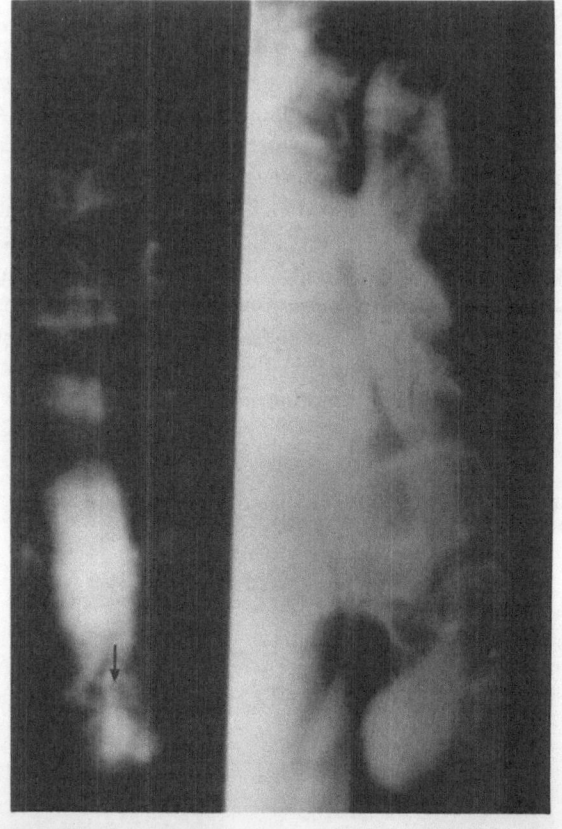

B

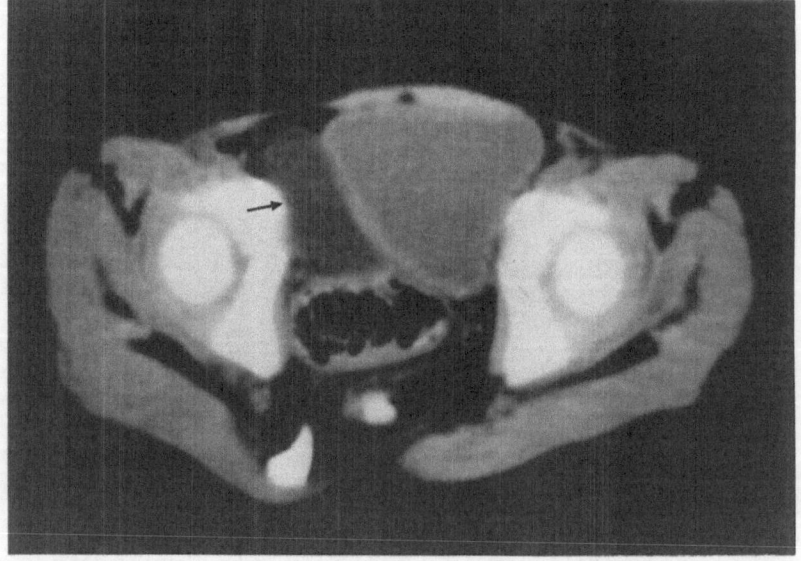

C

Figure 12.19. *Continued.*

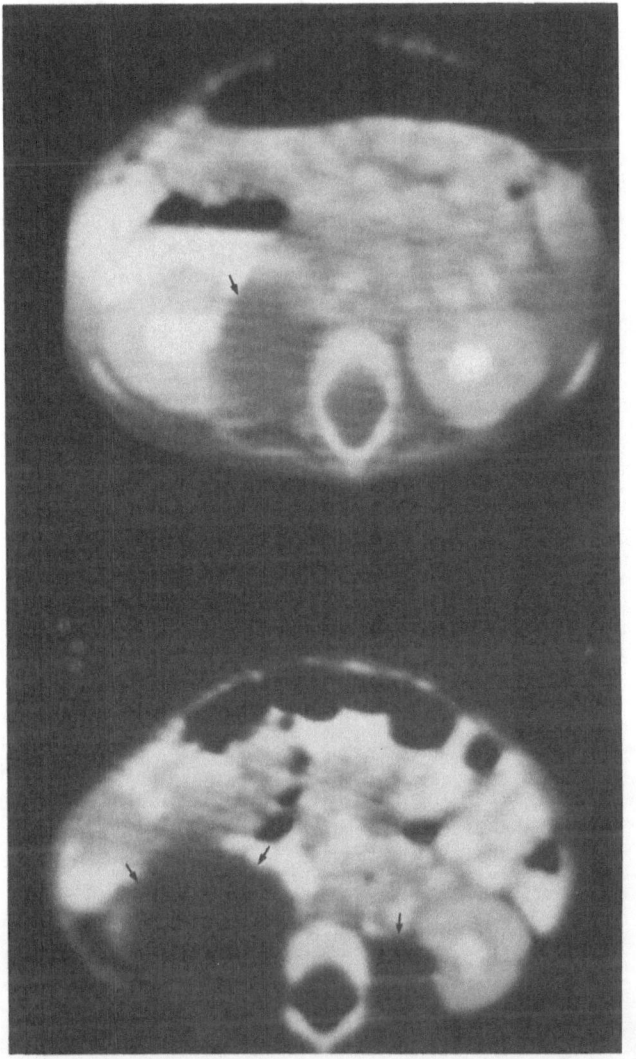

A

Figure 12.20. A: Axial CT scan without intrathecal metrizamide. Lateral meningoceles (*arrows*) seen at lumbar level. B: Same patient's CT scan with intrathecal metrizamide with meningoceles (*arrows*) filled with contrast.   *(Continued)*

medially (Fig. 12.21). The laminae also point postero-laterally as well (Fig. 12.21).

Scoliosis of the spine is often associated with the dysraphism. There may be associated kyphosis as well. Other associated bony abnormalities include hemivertebrae, vertebral fusion, and so forth. The scoliosis and kyphosis may be developmental as a result of muscle imbalance. Depending on the level of the

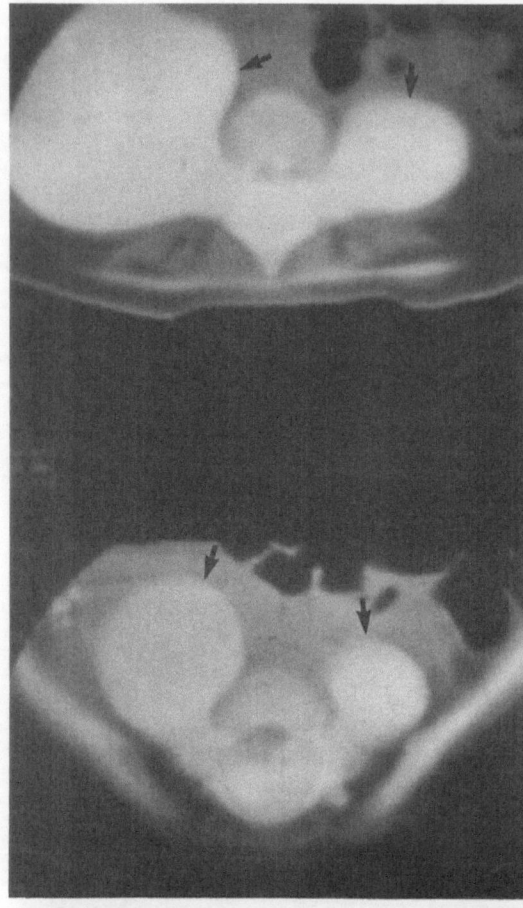

Figure 12.20. *Continued*

B

Figure 12.21. Axial CT scan in a patient with meningomyelocele. Portions of the laminae and spinal processes are missing. The remaining laminae are pointed postero-laterally. ▼

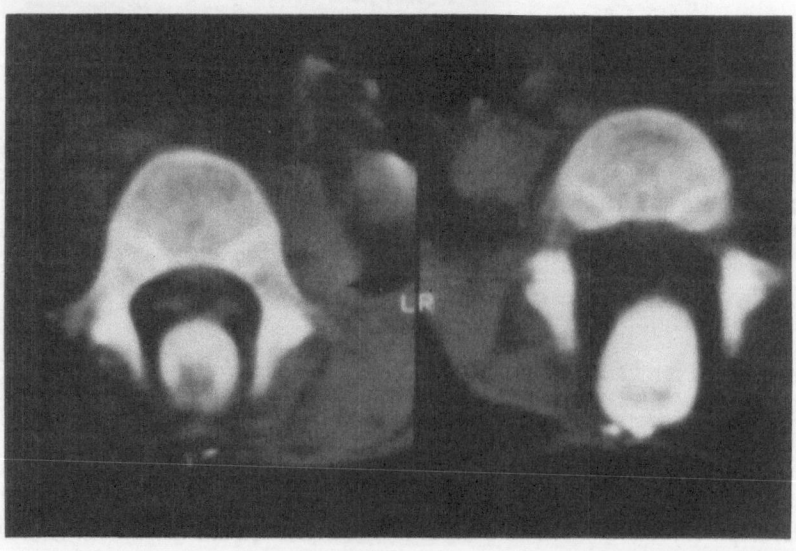

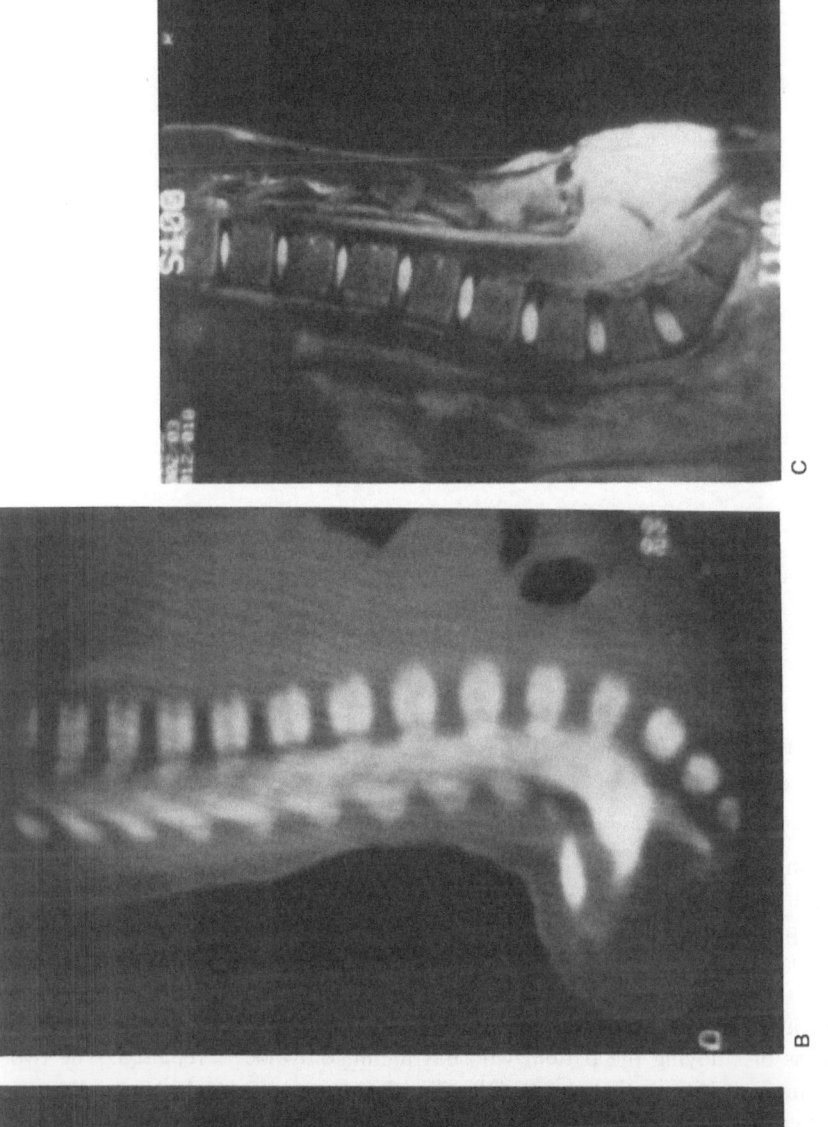

Figure 12.22. Sagittal scans and lateral view of meningomyelocele showing the tethering of the cord to the placode. A: Lateral view of metrizamide myelogram. B: Direct sagittal CT scan. C: Sagittal MR best demonstrating the abnormality.

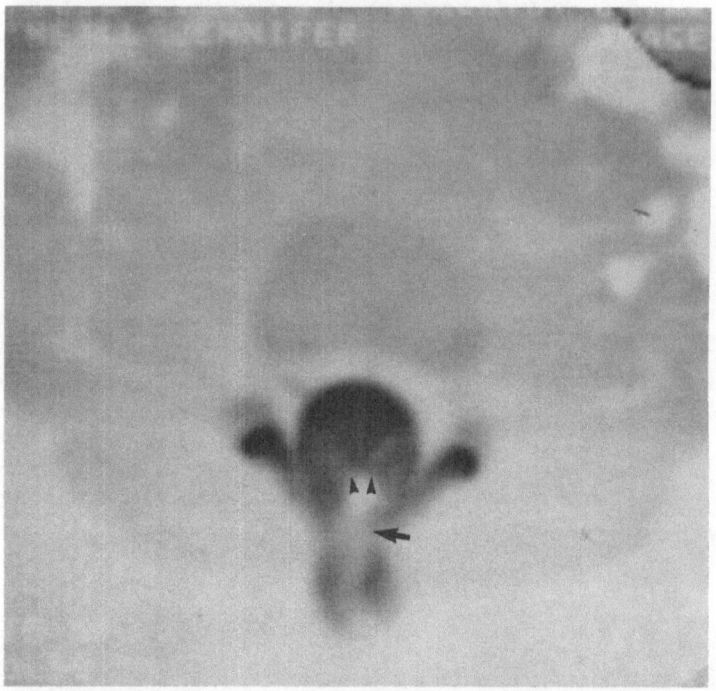

Figure 12.23. Axial CT scan of a tethered placode (*arrow*) with the dorsal nerve roots travelling ventrally (*arrowheads*).

meningomyelocele, the development of the scoliosis varies from 25 to 80%; the higher the level of myelocele the more likely is scoliosis to develop.

Kyphoscoliosis is a significant concern in the neuro-imaging of the spine because it is extremely difficult to image on MR in regard to positioning. In addition, the use of rods for correction of the scoliosis poses difficulty in resolution with artefacts. Before the time of MR, myelography and CTM have been the only means of studying the patient who has meningomyelocele repaired. The two common conditions that are associated with meningomyelocele are retethering of the cord to the placode and development or syringohydromyelia.

Myelography is usually difficult to perform in these cases because of the low position of the cord, and in some cases a grossly dysraphic spine associated with multiple other bony anomalies, making direct puncture impossible. However, a typical myelographic finding will be that of a low cord to the level of the previous meningomyelocele with, at times, nerve roots seen to be traversing cephalad rather than caudal. The tethering of the cord to the placode of the repaired meningomyelocele is best demonstrated by CTMM (Fig. 12.22). With the posteriorly placed cord, the dorsal nerve roots at the conus level will be traversing ventrally rather than dorsally (Fig. 12.23).[14]

CT is also much better than myelography in demonstrating the low position of the tonsils and vermis seen in Chiari II malformation – a condition associated with meningomyelocele (Fig. 12.24). In this respect, sagittal MR[16,17] is even better in demonstrating the position of the tonsils and vermis in addition to the cervico-medullary kink (Fig. 12.25) which is another classic finding in Chiari II malformation.[36,37]

MR is also much more superior than CT scan in diagnosing syringohydromyelia or, in short, syrinx.[38-42] These are mostly, if not all, true hydromyelia (Fig. 12.26). Hydromyelia, the dilatation of the central canal which is filled with

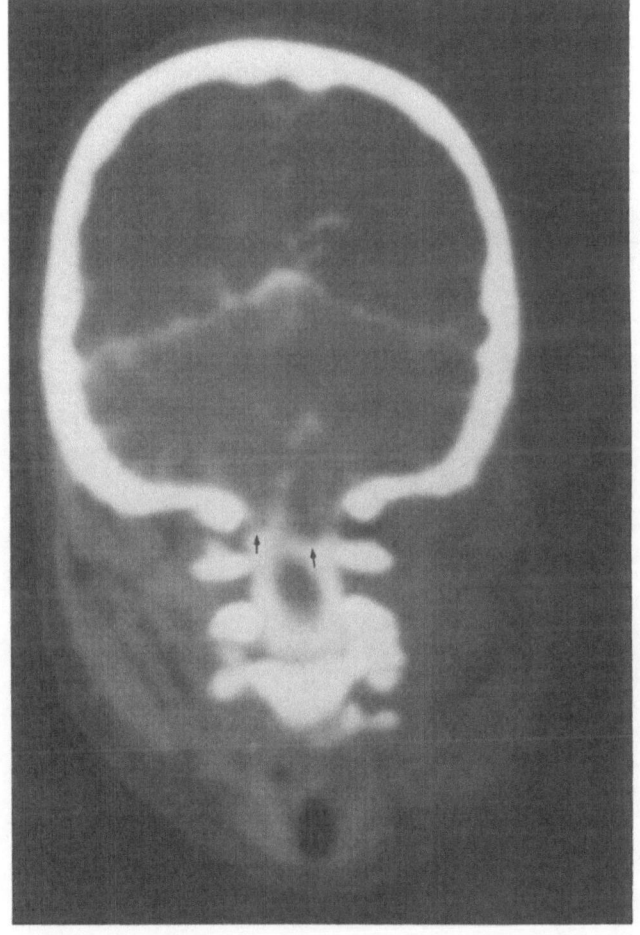

A

Figure 12.24. Chiari II malformation seen on metrizamide CT scan. A: Coronal view showing the low tonsils (*arrows*). B: Axial view showing the low tonsils (*arrows*). C: Axial CT scan with metrizamide showing the low vermis (*arrow*).

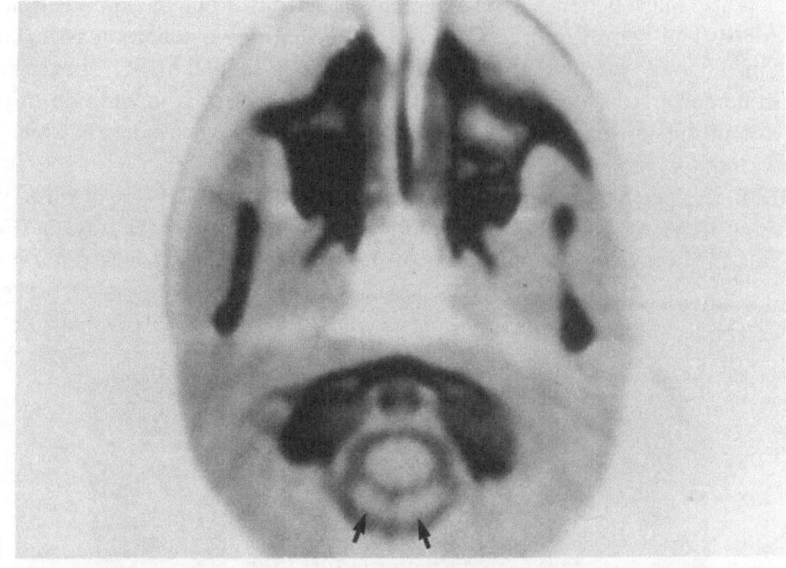

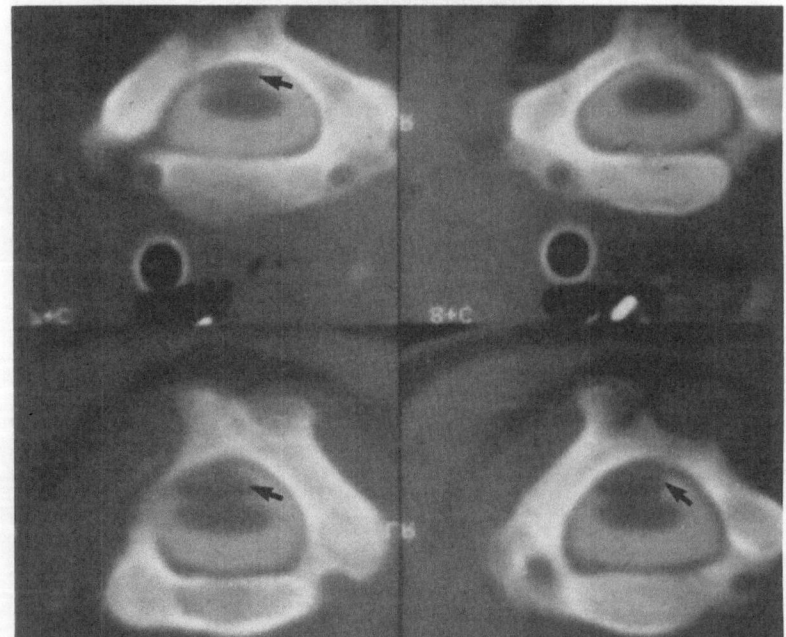

Figure 12.24. *Continued*

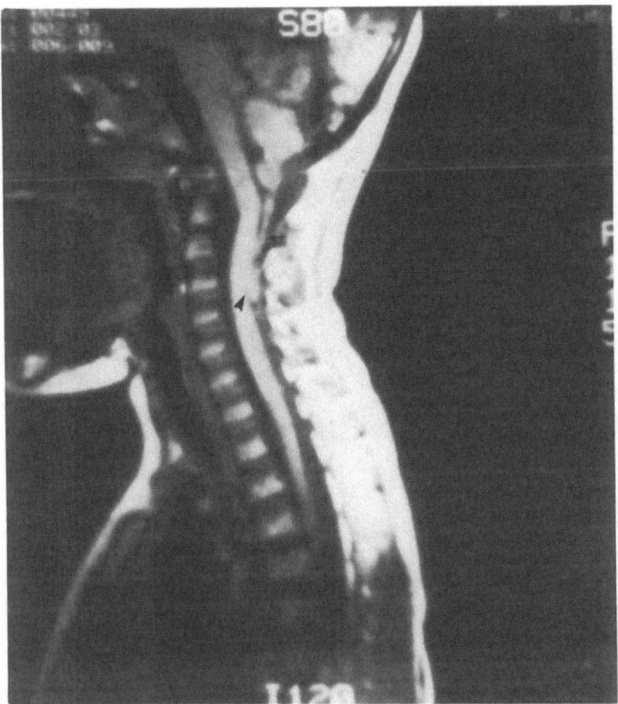

Figure 12.25. Sagittal MR scan demonstrating the low vermis (*arrow*) and the cervico-medullary kink (*arrowhead*).

cerebrospinal fluid is always distended as seen on the MRI, whether it is loculated or not. In contrast, on CTM, the cord can be seen as enlarged (Fig. 12.27) or flattened (Fig. 12.28).[14,43,44] If one is lucky enough, one may fill the dilated central canal through the obex (Fig. 12.28).[43] The diffusion of the contrast through the cord to be concentrated in the central canal on the delayed CT scan is not always successful or reliable in children.

An interesting finding, however, is that we have never observed a collapsed syrinx on MR scan. This suggests that collapsed syrinx is seen only after lumbar puncture and injection of contrast for myelography. Possibly, the disturbed CSF dynamics after lumbar puncture causes the shift of fluid compartments in hydromyelia through the obex.[45] The percentage of flattened cord versus enlarged cord seen on CT scan is approximately 50/50.

Myelography of Chiari II malformation associated with meningomyelocele is one of the most difficult to perform since there are pathology at both ends. Inadvertent puncture of the hydromyelia sac is not uncommon either at the lumbar or cervical level, though patients had no untoward results or discomfort (Fig. 12.29). Purposeful direct puncture of the syrinx has also been performed (Fig. 12.30) before the time of MR to estimate the size and extent of the sac in order to facilitate treatment.

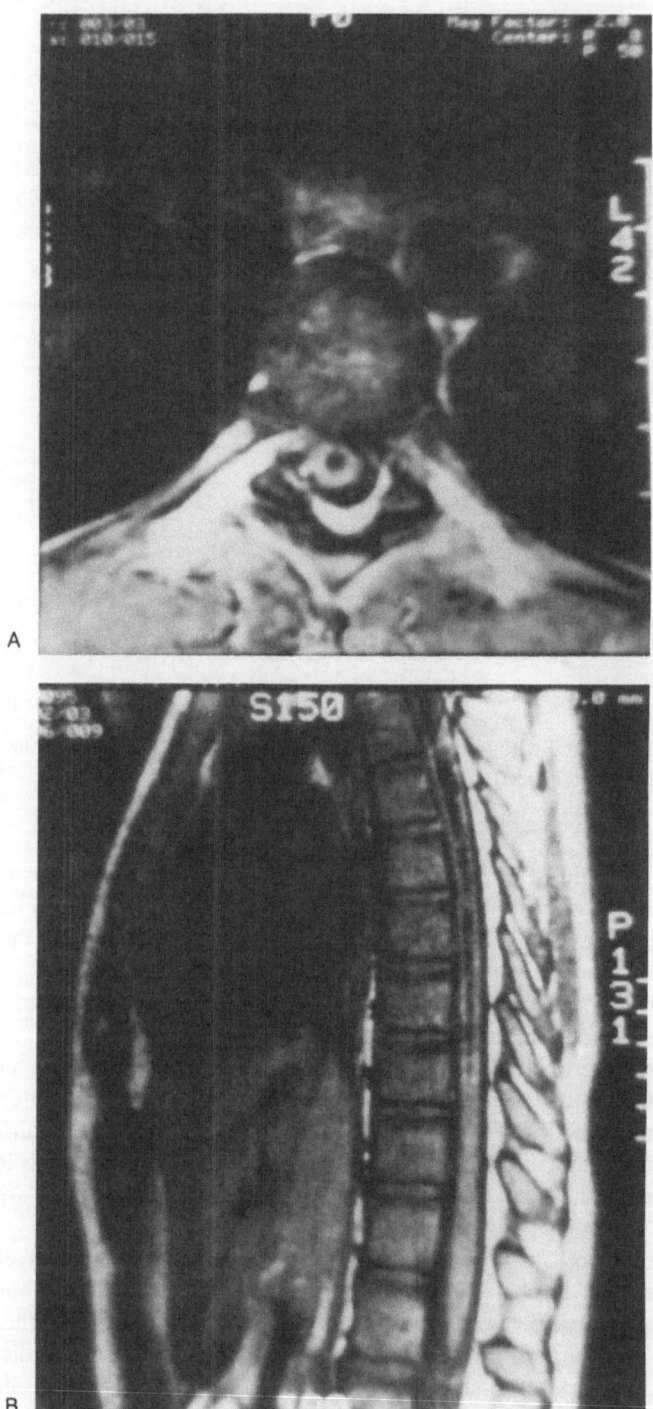

Figure 12.26. Hydromyelia seen on MR scans as decreased signal attenuation within the cord. A: Axial. B: Sagittal. C: Sagittal with loculated hydromyelic sac.

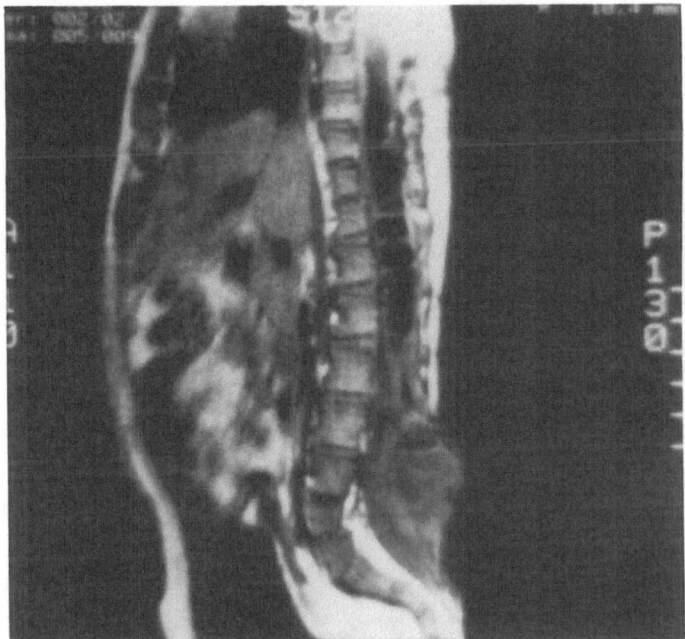

C

Figure 12.26. *Continued.*

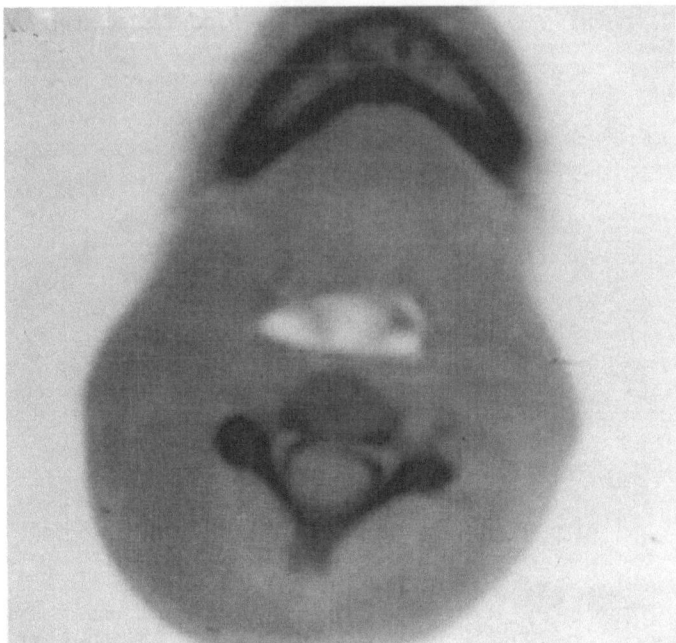

Figure 12.27. Axial CT scan with metrizamide demonstrating the enlarged cord from hydromyelia.

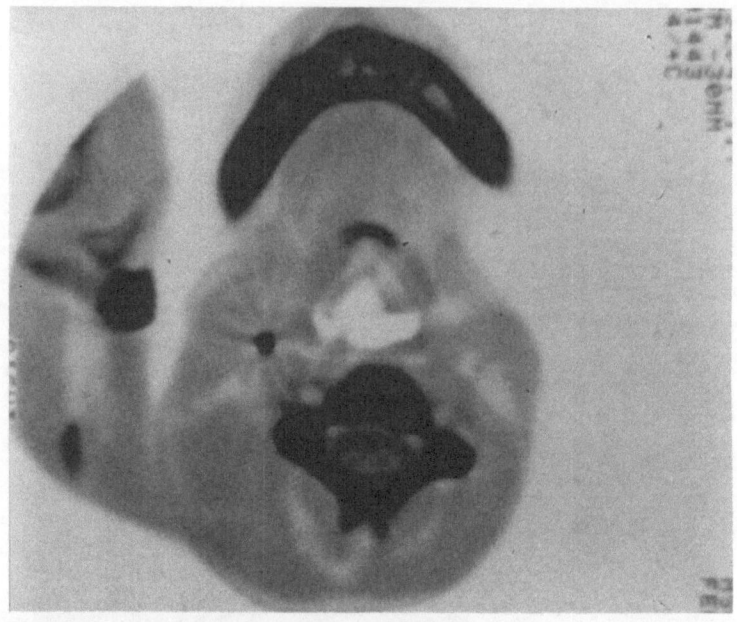

▲
Figure 12.28. Hydromyelia. The dilated central canal is filled with metrizamide secondary to a wide open obex. The cord is flattened.

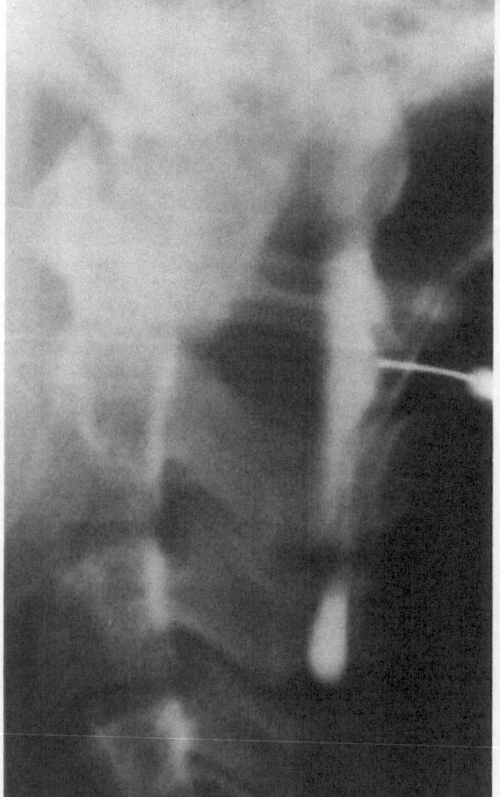

Figure 12.29. Lateral view of metrizamide myelogram performed on a patient with Chiari II. C1–2 puncture performed and metrizamide was injected into syringobulbia and syringohydromyelia.

Figure 12.30. Direct injection of metrizamide and hydromyelia cavity to determine the extent and size of the cavity before time of MR scan.

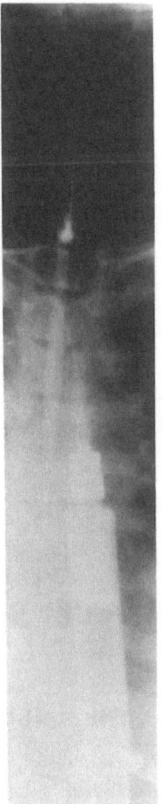

However, the availability of MR has eliminated the use of myelography except in very selective cases such as the presence of metallic rods. In these cases myelography is still helpful, though examinations may be extremely difficult in regard to puncturing the subarachnoid space. In cases where lumbar puncture is impossible, we have punctured the subarachnoid spaces at C1–C2 in 12 patients. We have no complications or complaints in all 12 patients and the examinations were satisfactory. However, it is not recommended for normal usage and the person performing the procedure should be properly trained. A potential complication is puncturing the posterior inferior cerebellar artery with the low tonsils. Puncturing the tonsils or vermis is generally not a concern. Visualization of the syrinx on US is difficult though not impossible (Fig. 12.31) mainly because of the bony acoustic shadows from the neural arches. In neonates and in intra-operative ultrasound, it is very useful.

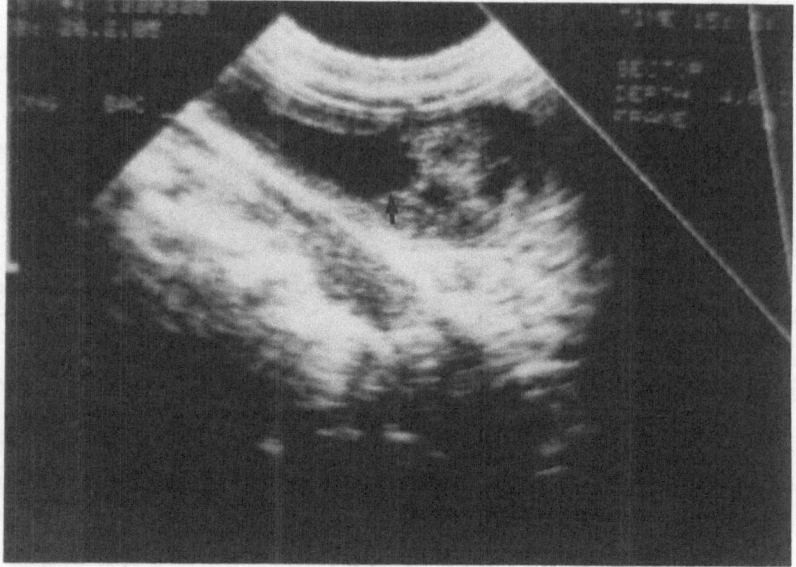

Figure 12.31. Longitudinal ultrasound showing the terminal syrinx (*arrow*) in the conus.

Diastematomyelia

Diastematomyelia means clefting or splitting of the cord. However, until recently, it has been used to mean "surgical diastematomyelia" where there is the presence of a fibrous cartilage or bony spur splitting the dural sac and the cord in the sagittal plane (Fig. 12.32).[47] In this type, surgical removal of the spur is the treatment of choice. In contrast, the "split cord syndrome" shows only splitting of the cord with no splitting of the dural sac and is not related to any spurs[16,47,48] (Fig. 12.32B). The split cord without spur was previously considered rare,[49] but has been observed more and more commonly since CTM.[16,48] Only 34% of the "diastematomyelia" seen have true bony spur and 67% are split cords without spurs.

In surgical diastematomyelia, the plain film often reveals the diagnosis. Typical findings include widening of the interpediculate distance with narrowing of the disc spaces at the level of the spurs. The bony spur can sometimes be seen on the plain film though, at times, this can be extremely difficult in view of the dysraphic state. Myelography demonstrates the surgical diastematomyelia well (Fig. 12.33A), but is not ideal for the split cord which is much more to visualize (Fig. 12.33B). MR and CTM are the methods of choice, since they demonstrate both types of diastematomyelia very clearly in the axial images (Fig. 12.34).[43,48,50-52] CTM has the added advantage in being able to show the bony component and nerve roots distinctly and allow reformatting in the oblique plane (Fig. 12.35).

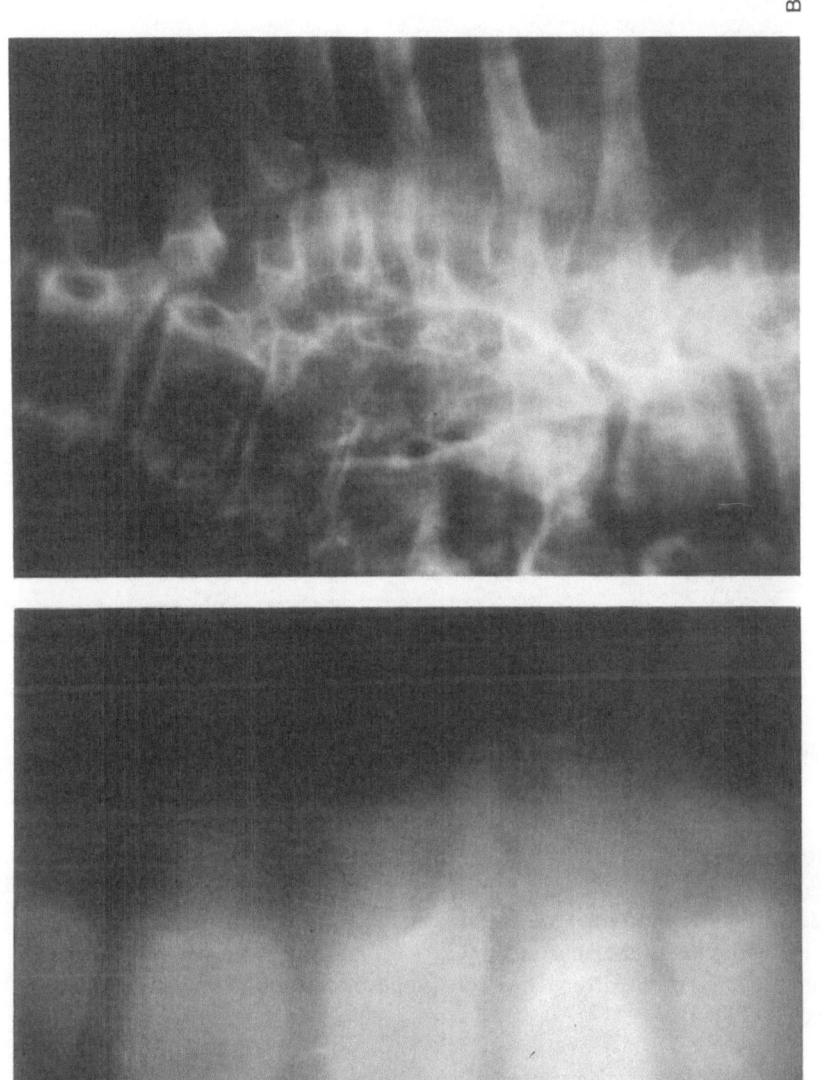

Figure 12.32. A: Lateral tomogram of bony spur in a patient with diastematomyelia. B: AP view of thoracic spine showing the classical appearance of diastemato-myelia. Note the increase in interpediculate distance and narrowing of the disc spaces.

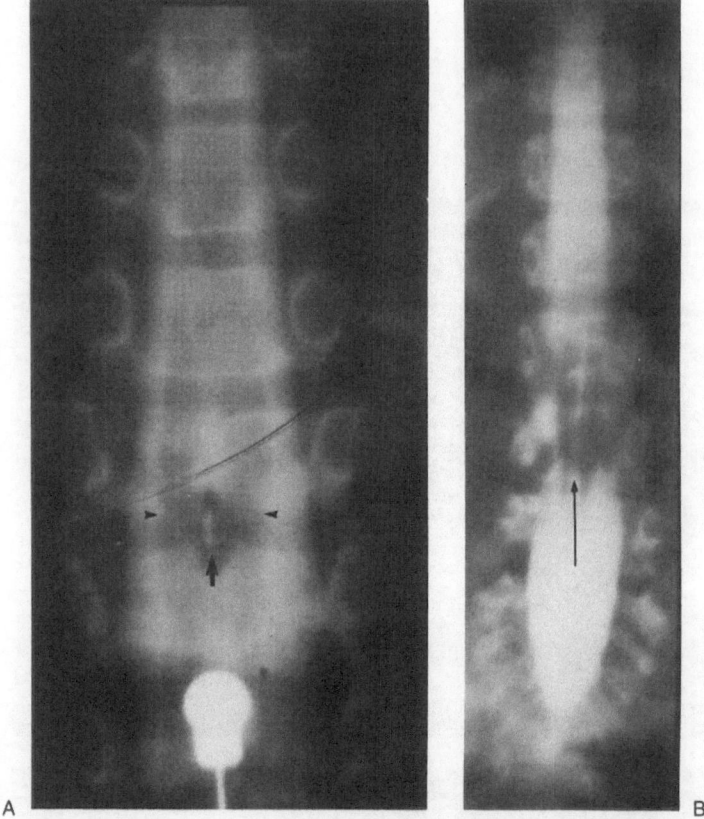

Figure 12.33. A: Metrizamide myelogram of surgical diastematomyelia with the bony spur (*arrow*) and splitting of the cord (*arrowheads*). B: Tethered cord and split cord without spur. Metrizamide (*arrow*) seen between the split cord.

Rarely, in infants, US or intravenous enhanced CT can also demonstrate the anomaly (Fig. 12.36) of the split cord.

The "split cord syndrome" has a high frequency of tethering (~68%).[14] The cords may reunite at the conus or they may remain separated with one or both coni tethered. Syringohydromyelia may also develop in either one or both of the split cords (Fig. 12.37).[53]

Neurenteric Cysts

This is a form of split notochord syndrome, the most common being the neurenteric cyst. Other names for this condition include foregut duplications or dorsal enteric cyst. It represents a persistence of the transient open passage (the

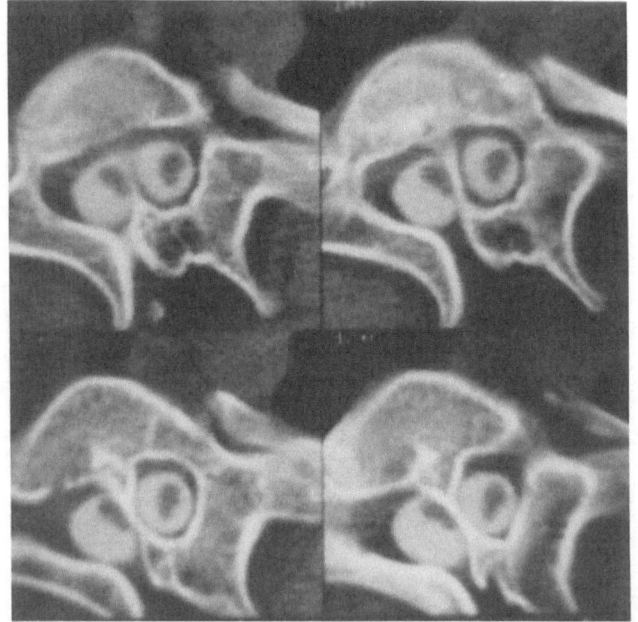

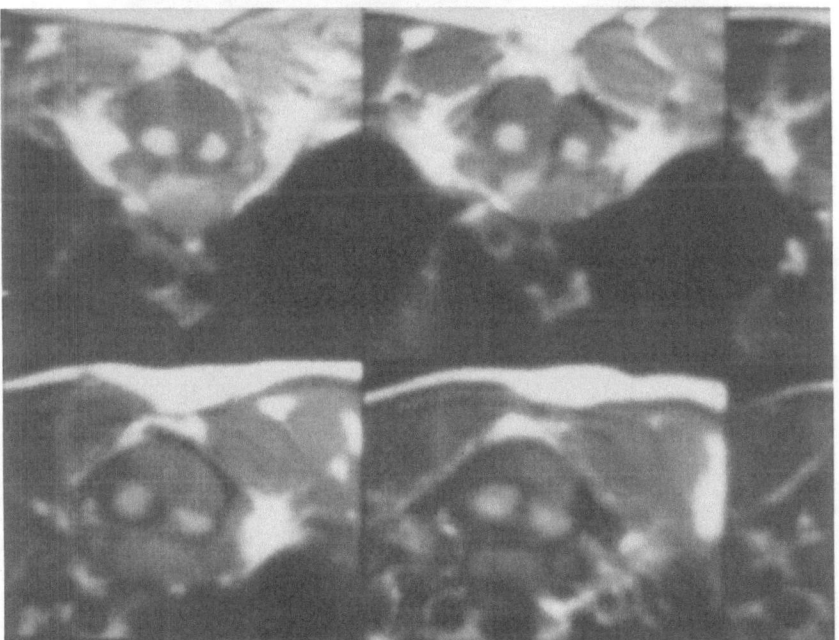

Figure 12.34. A, B: Surgical diastematomyelia with bony spur seen on CTMM (*A*) and MR (B). C, D: Split cords without spurs seen on CTMM (C) and MR (D). *(Continued).*

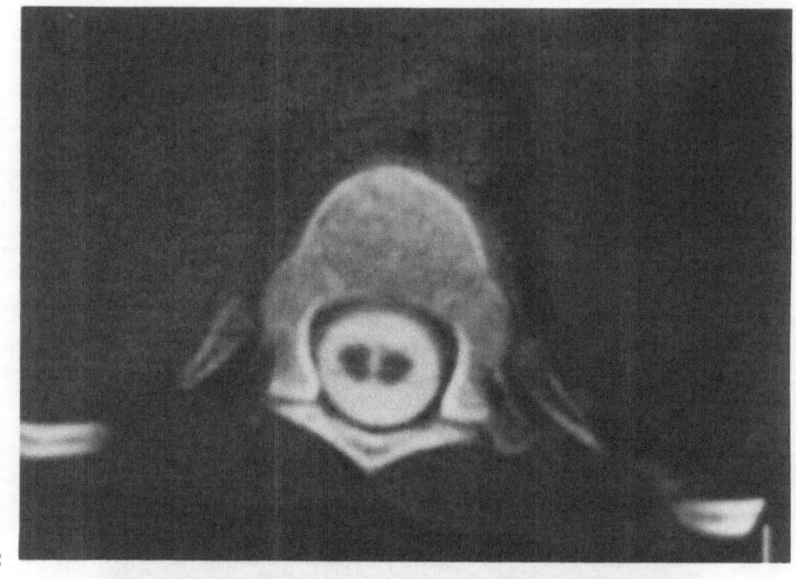

C

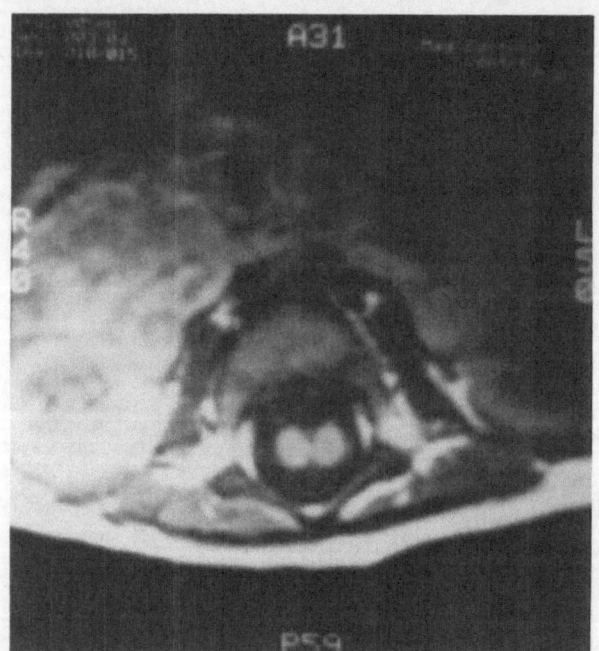

D

Figure 12.34. *Continued.*

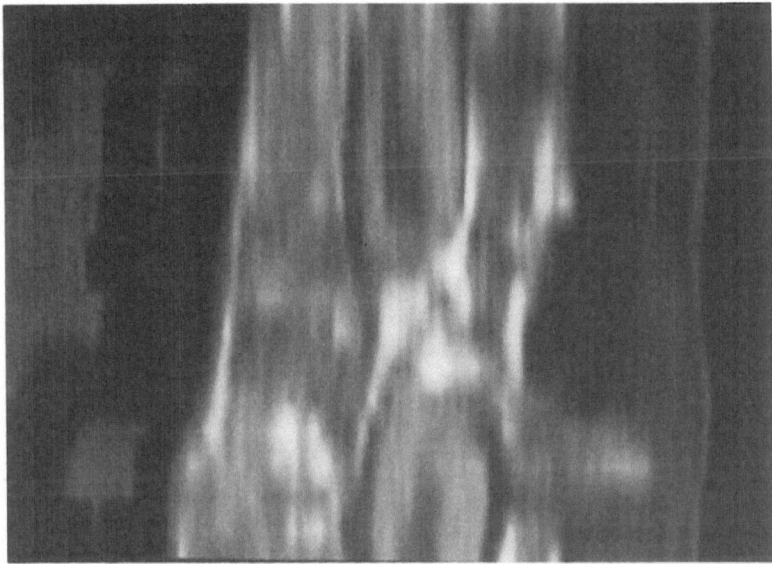

Figure 12.35. Reformatted CTM of diastematomyelia with bony spur. Reformation performed at the plane of the bony spur.

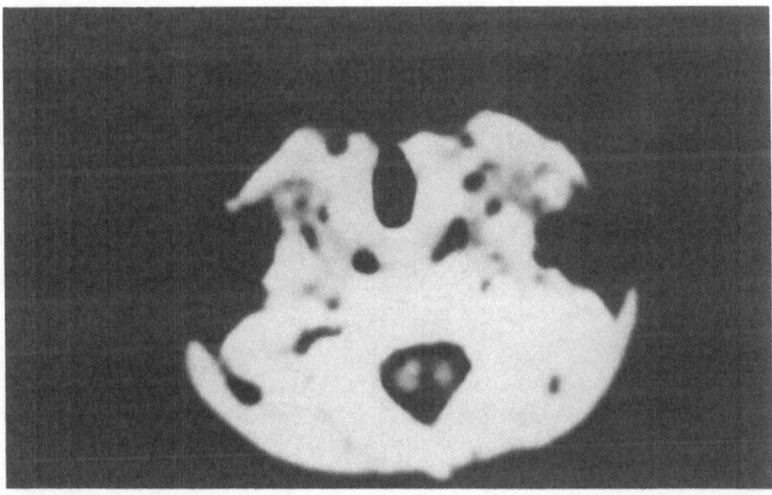

A

Figure 12.36. A: IV enhanced axial CT demonstrating the split cord at the cervical level. B: Transverse ultrasound demonstrating the same finding (*arrows* indicate the separate cords). *(Continued.)*

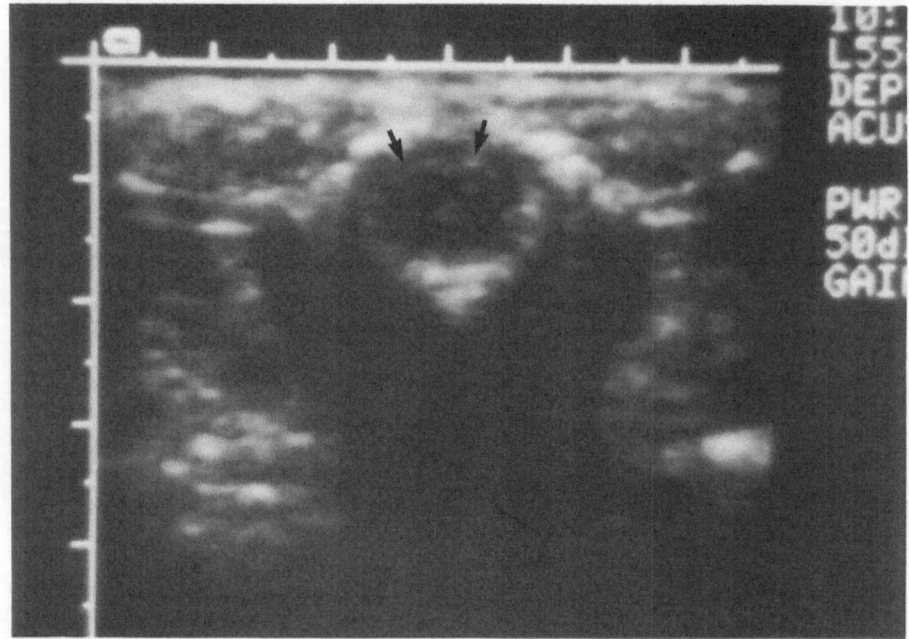

Figure 12.36. *(Continued).*

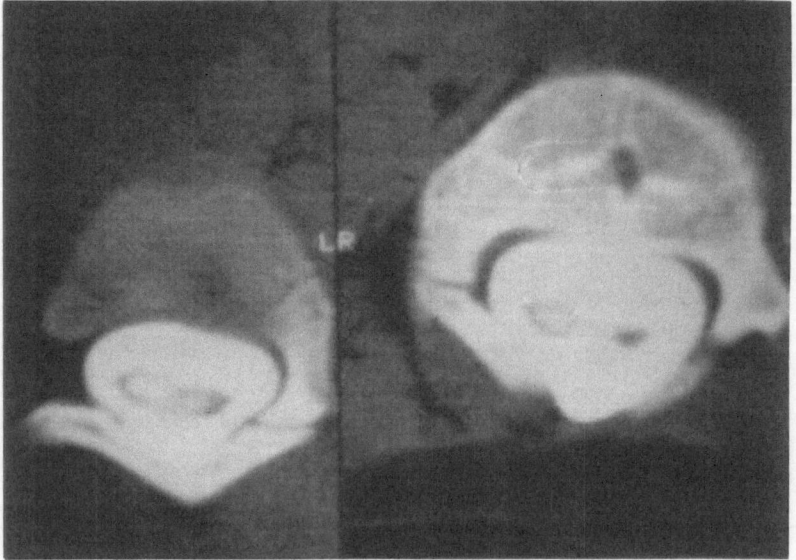

Figure 12.37. Split cord with syrinx seen on CTM (axial view). The syrinx continues on the right half of the hemicord viewed as metrizamide in the syrinx cavity.

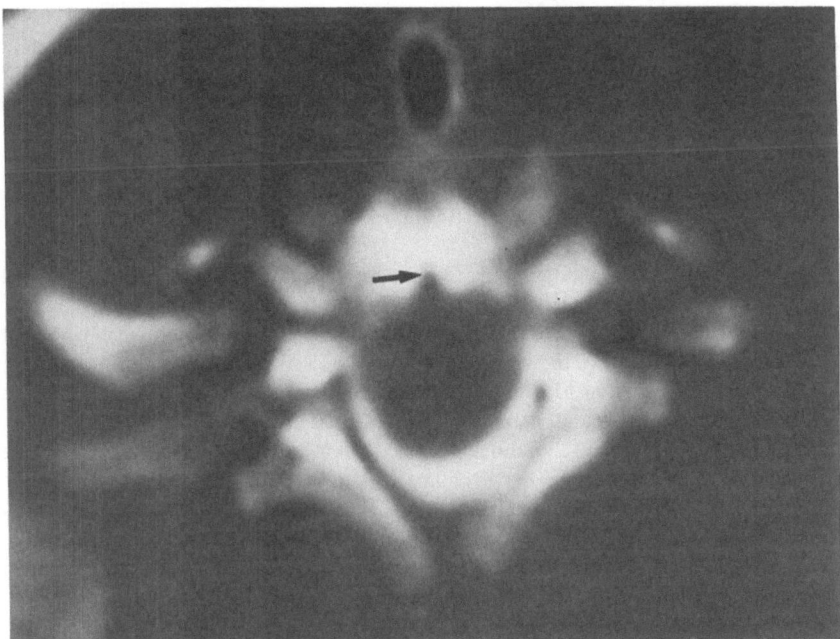

Figure 12.38. Neurenteric cyst causing enlargement of the cord. Note canal of Kovalevsky (*arrow*) anteriorly splitting the vertebral body.

neurenteric canal of Kovalevsky) or the third embryonic week between the yolk sac and the notochord canal. The persistence of the canal of Kovalevsky is always accompanied by some form of anterior vertebral dysraphism as well as abnormalities of neural elements and of tissue derived from the endoderm.[54]

The neurenteric cyst is most often situated in the upper thoracic region but may occur at any level.

The lesion is more common than previously thought[14] and CTM with axial spurs is definitely the method of choice[54] (Fig. 12.38).

Though not very many cases have been reported on MR, its use in neurenteric cyst detection and diagnosis is undoubtedly excellent.

Summary

Different radiologic techniques have been discussed for diagnosis of the spectrum of spinal dysraphism and the associated anomalies. Though MR appears superior in most aspects, it is the least available and the most expensive. If it is readily available, it should be the first method of choice except in cases for simple or isolated tethered cord syndrome.

US can be used instead of MR in all neonates as a screening procedure because it is relatively inexpensive and readily available. CTM is a good and solid diagnostic tool except in cases of syringohydromyelia where MR is definitely superior and should be the method of choice.

References

1. Lichtenstein JE: "Spinal dysraphism," spina bifida and myelodysplasia. Arch Neurol Psychiatry 44:792–810, 1940.
2. Tadmor R, Ravid M, Findler G, Sahar A: Importance of early radiologic diagnosis of congenital anomalies of the spine. Surg Neurol 23:493–501, 1985.
3. Hobbins JC, Grannum PAT, Berkowitz RL, Silverman R, Mahoney MJ: Ultrasound in the diagnosis of congenital anomalies. Am J Obstet Gynecol 134:331–345, 1979.
4. Naidich TP, Fernbach SK, McLone DG, Shkolnik A: Sonography of the caudal spine and back: congenital anomalies in children. AJR 142:1229–1242, 1984.
5. Naidich TP, McLone DG, Shkolnik A, Fernbach SK: Sonographic evaluation of caudal spine anomalies in children. AJNR 4:661–664, 1983.
6. Scheible W, James HE, Leopold GR, Hilton SVW: Occult spinal dysraphism in infants: screening with high-resolution real-time ultrasound. Radiology 146:743–746, 1983.
7. Zimmerman R, Bilaniuk L: Applications of magnetic resonance imaging in diseases of the pediatric central nervous system. Magnet Reson Imaging 4:11–24, 1986.
8. Packer RJ, Zimmerman R, Sutton LN, Bilaniuk L, Bruce DA, Schut L: Magnetic resonance imaging of spinal cord disease of childhood. Pediatrics 78:251–256, 1986.
9. Han JS, Kaufman B, El Yousef SJ, Benson JE, Bonstelle CT, Alfidi RJ, Haaga JR, Yeung H, Huss RG: NMR imaging of the spine. AJR 141:1137–1145, 1983.
10. Modic MT, Weinstein MA, Pavlicek W, Starnes DL, Duchesneau PM, Boumphrey F, Hardy RJ: Nuclear magnetic resonance imaging of the spine. Radiology 148:757–762, 1983.
11. Altman NR, Altman DH: MR imaging of spinal dysraphism. AJNR 8:533–538, 1987.
12. Roos RAC, Vielvoye GJ, Voormolen JHC, Peters ACB: Magnetic resonance imaging in occult spinal dysraphism. Pediatr Radiol 16:412–416, 1986.
13. Barnes PD, Lester PD, Yamanashi WS, Prince JR: Magnetic resonance imaging in infants and children with spinal dysraphism. AJNR 7:465–472, 1986.
14. Pettersson H: Spinal dysraphism. In: CT and Myelography of the Spine and Cord. Springer-Verlag, Berlin, 1982, pp 39–57.
15. Fitz CR, Harwood-Nash DC: The tethered conus. AJR 125:515–523, 1975.
16. Resjo IM, Harwood-Nash DC, Fitz CR, Chuang SC: Computed tomographic metrizamide myelography in spinal dysraphism in infants and children. J Comput Assit Tomogr 2:549–558, 1978.
17. Raghavendra BN, Epstein FJ, Pinto RS, Subramanyam BR, Greenberg J, Mitnick JS: The tethered spinal cord: diagnosis by high-resolution real-time ultrasound. Radiology 149:123–128, 1983.
18. Sarwar M, Crelin ES, Kier EL, Virapongse C: Experimental cord stretchability and the tethered cord syndrome. AJNR 4:641–643, 1983.
19. Mount LA: Congenital dermal sinuses as a cause of meningitis, intraspinal abscess and intracranial abscess. JAMA 139:1263–1268, 1949.

20. Naidich TP, McLone DG, Harwood-Nash DC: Spinal dysraphism. CT of the spine and spinal cord. In: H. Newton and G. Potts (eds): Modern Neuroradiology, Vol. 1. Clavadel Press, San Anselmo, 1983, pp 299–354.

21. Harwood-Nash DC, Fitz CR: Neuroradiology in Infants and Children, Vol. 3. CV Mosby, St. Louis, 1976, pp 1072–1227.

22. List CF: Intraspinal epidermoids, dermoids and dermal sinuses. Surg Gynecol Obstet 73:525–538, 1941.

23. Naidich TP, McLone DG, Mutluer S: A new understanding of dorsal dysraphism with lipoma (lipomyeloschisis): radiologic evaluation and surgical correction. AJR 140: 1065–1078, 1983.

24. Lemire RJ, Graham CB, Beckwith JB: Skin-covered sacrococcygeal masses in infants and children. J Pediatr 78:478–954, 1971.

25. Bruce DA, Schut L: Spinal lipomas in infancy and childhood. Childs Brain 5:192–203, 1979.

26. Chapman PH: Congenital intraspinal lipomas: anatomical considerations and surgical treatment. Childs Brain 9:37–47, 1982.

27. McLone DG, Mutluer S, Naidich TP: Lipomeningoceles of the conus medullaris. Concepts in Pediatric Neurosurgery, Vol. 3, ASPN. S. Karger, Basel, 1982.

28. Swanson HS, Barnett JC Jr: Intradural lipomas in children. Pediatrics 29:911–926, 1962.

29. Gold LHA, Kieffer SA, Peterson HO: Lipomatous invasion of the spinal cord associated with spinal dysraphism: myelographic evaluation. AJR 107:479–485, 1969.

30. Dubowitz V, Lorber J, Zachary RB: Lipoma of the cauda equina. Arch Dis Child 40:207–213, 1965.

31. Roller GJ, Pribaum HFW: Lumbosacral intradural lipoma and sacral agenesis. Radiology 84:507–511, 1965.

32. Altman N, Rusztyn A, Harwood-Nash DC, Fitz CR, Chuang S: Direct sagittal CT of infants for evaluation of the spine. GE CT Clinical Symposium, Vol. 7, No. 3, 1984.

33. Northfield DWC: The Surgery of the Central Nervous System: A Textbook for Postgraduate Students. Blackwell Scientific Publications, 1973, pp 467–536.

34. Lemire RJ, Loeser JD, Leech RW, Alvord EC Jr: Normal and Abnormal Development of the Human Nervous System. Harper & Row, Baltimore, 1975.

35. Shurtleff DB, Goiney R, Gordon LH, Livermore N: Myelodysplasia: the natural history of kyphosis and scoliosis: a preliminary report. Dev Med Child Neurol 18 (Suppl 37):126–133, 1976.

36. Lee BCP, Deck MDF, Kneeland JB, Cahill PT: MR imaging of the craniocervical junction. AJNR 6:209–213, 1985.

37. Han JS, Benson JE, Yoon YS: Magnetic resonance imaging in the spinal column and craniovertebral junction. Radiol Clin N Am 22:805–827, 1984.

38. Samuelson L, Bergstrom K, Thomas KA, Hemmingsson A, Wallensten R: MR imaging of syringomydromyelia and Chiari malformations in myelomeningocele patients with scoliosis. AJNR 8:539–546, 1987.

39. Pojunas K, Williams AL, Daniels DL, Haughton VM: Syringomyelia and hydromyelia: magnetic resonance evaluation. Radiology 153:679–683, 1984.

40. Yeates A, Brant-Zawadzki M, Norman D, Kaufman L, Crooks L, Newton TH: Nuclear magnetic resonance imaging of syringomyelia. AJNR 4:234–237, 1983.

41. Sherman JL, Barkovich AJ, Citrin CM: The MR appearance of syringomyelia: new observations. AJNR 7:985–995, 1986.

42. Lee BCP, Zimmerman R, Manning JJ, Deck MDF: MR imaging of syringomyelia and hydromyelia. AJNR 6:221–228, 1985.
43. Resjo IM, Harwood-Nash DC, Fitz CR, Chuang S: CT metrizamide myelography in syringohydromyelia. Radiology 131:405–407, 1979.
44. Aubin ML, Vignaud J, Jardin C, Bar D: Computed tomography in 75 clinical cases of syringomyelia. AJNR 2:199–204, 1981.
45. Kan S, Fox AJ, Vinuela F, Debrun G: Spinal cord size in syringomyelia: change with position on metrizamide myelography. Radiology 146:409–414, 1983.
46. Miller JH, Reid BS, Kemberling CR: Utilization of ultrasound in the evaluation of spinal dysraphism in children. Radiology 143:737–740, 1982.
47. Naidich TP, Harwood-Nash DC: Diastematomyelia: hemicord and meningeal sheaths: single and double arachnoid and dural tubes. AJNR 4:633–636, 1983.
48. Scotti G, Musgrave M, Harwood-Nash DC, Fitz CR, Chuang SH: Diastematomyelia in children: metrizamide and CT myelography metrizamide myelography. AJR 135:1225–1232, 1980.
49. Dale AJD: Diastematomyelia. Arch Neurol 20:309–317, 1969.
50. Arredondo F, Haughton VM, Hemmy DC, Zelaya B, Williams AL: The computed tomographic appearance of the spinal cord in diastematomyelia. Radiology 136:685–688, 1980.
51. Han JS, Benson JE, Kaufman B, Rekate HL, Alfidi RJ, Bohlman HH, Kaufman B: Demonstration of diastematomyelia and associated abnormalities with MR imaging. AJNR 6:215–219, 1985.
52. Thron A, Schroth G: Magnetic resonance imaging (MRI) of diastematomyelia. Neuroradiology 28:371–372, 1986.
53. Schlesinger AE, Naidich TP, Quencer RM: Concurrent hydromyelia and diastematomyelial. AJNR 7:473–477, 1986.
54. Harwood-Nash DC, Fitz CR: CT and the pediatric spine. CT metrizamide myelography in children. In: Post MJD (ed): Radiologic Evaluation of the Spine. Masson, New York, 1980, pp 4–33.

Index

Adam's position, 228
Alar sacral hooks, 214–215
"Anisocoria, vertebral," 123, 126
Anterior fusion, 246
Apical segment, agenesis of, 5
"Apical vertebra," 226
Archenteric cysts, 134
Arnold–Chiari malformation, 45, 46, 60; see also Chiari malformations
Arthrodesis, 129–130
  following reduction of listhesis, 130
  postero-lateral, 129–130
Arthrogryposis multiplex congenita, 192
"Arthrogrypotic-like" deformity, 144
Atlas, 21–23
  arch defect of, 3–4
  dysplasia of, 4
  fusion of, 4
  malformations of, 3–5
  occipitalization of, 36, 39
  split, 41
Axis, 22, 23
  fusion of, 12
  malformations of 4, 5–13

Back pain, 121, 244
Basilar invagination, 23, 30–35
Basilar line, 30–31
"Basilar impression," 33
Basi-occipit, 31, 32
  hypoplasia of, 35–36
  transitory supplementary fissure of, 33–35

Basi-oticum, 31, 32
"Bayonet deformity," 120
Bidigastric line, 23, 30
Bimastoid line, 30
Bladder, neurogenic, dysfunction, 156, 158
Blood loss, intraoperative, 232
Blood scavenging system, 207
Boston brace, 230
Braces, 205, 247
Bronchiogenic cysts, 134
Butterfly vertebra, 265

C1–C2 dislocation, 41, 43–44
C2 pedicle, absence of, 10–11
Canal of Kovalevsky, 287
Cauda equina syndrome, 121
Caudal abortion, 153–154
Caudal malformations, 95
"Caudal regression syndrome," 144, 153–154
Cervico-occipital area, ossification centers in, 22
Cervico-occipital canal, stenosis of, 44
Charcot–Marie–Tooth disease, 193
Chiari malformations, 45, 46, 57–86
  clinical features, 68–80
  historical background and definitions, 57–60
  "hydrodynamic" theories, 61–63
  "maldevelopmental" theories, 65–68
  mechanical theories, 63–65
  neuro-imaging of, 72–80, 273–274, 275, 278

Chiari malformations (*cont.*)
  physiopathogenic interpretations,
    60–68
  posterior fossa decompression in,
    82–86
  treatment of, 80–86
  type I malformation, 57, 58, 68, 70
  type II malformation, 58, 68–72
  type III malformation, 58
  type IV malformation, 58, 59
Chondrification, 1
Chordoma, 50
Cobb measurement, 215, 224, 226
Colloid cysts, 139
Computed tomographic metrizamide
  myelography (CTMM), 182–183,
  271, 272, 283–284
Computed tomography (CT), 251, 253,
  259–274, 277–278
Conus medullaris, 177
Coronal deformities, 223–236
Cotrel-Dubousset system, 233
Coupling phenomenon, 222
Cranialization, 20
Craniolacuniae, 72–73
Cranio-vertebral junction, 19
  embryology of, 20, 21
  infections of, 48–49
  injuries of, 49
  malformation of bones in, 23–44
  normal and abnormal aspects of, 19–50
  ossification of, 30
  pathologic anatomy of, 92–96
  tumors of, 50
Crede maneuver, 158
CT (computed tomography), 251, 253,
  259–274, 277–278
CT myelography (CTM), 255, 280, 288
CTMM (computed tomographic metrizamide myelography), 182–183, 271,
  272, 283–284
Cysts
  archenteric, 134
  bronchiogenic, 134
  colloid, 139
  Dandy-Walker, 61
  dorsal enteric, 282
  enteric, 134
  enterogenous, 134

  foregut, 134
  intraspinal, 137
  neurenteric, *see* Neurenteric cysts
  posterior fossa neuroepithelial, 139
  prevertebral, 137, 139
  teratomatous, 134, 135

Dandy–Walker cyst, 61
Dandy–Walker syndrome, 46, 47
Deformed spine, long-term care of,
  221–248
Dermoid, 258–262
Developmental mass lesions, 258–263
Diabetes, maternal, 149–150
Diastematomyelia, 91–107, 246
  CT scan in, 103, 105
  cutaneous anomalies in, 99
  dorsal, 94
  double, 92
  embryology of, 96–97
  frontal, 92
  incomplete, 92
  mechanical factors in, 97–98
  MRI in, 103
  myelography in, 102–103, 104
  neuro-imaging of, 100–104, 280–286
  "non-mechanical" factors in, 98
  physiopathology of, 97
  review of literature on, 91–92
  signs and symptoms of, 98–103
  surgery in, 104–107
  surgical, 280
  surgical indications in, 106–107
  tethered spinal cord and, 178
  treatment of, 104–107
  x-ray findings in, 101–102
Diplomyelia, 91, 95–96; *see also*
  Diastematomyelia
Dorsal enteric cyst, 282
Duchenne's muscular dystrophy, 192
Duhamel syndrome, 153
Dwyer system, 197, 214, 233
Dysautonomia, familial, 191
Dysraphism, 147
  defined, 251
  spinal, neuro-imaging of, 251–288
"Dystrophie cruro-vésico-fessière," 144,
  145

Electrical stimulation, nocturnal, 231
Embryo, human, sagittal section of, 29
Embryonic cells, 167
Enteric cysts, 134
  dorsal, 282
Enteric diverticulum, posterior,
    140–141
Enteric fistula, dorsal, 139–140
Enterogenous cysts, 134
Epidermoid, 258, 261
Epiduritis, 19
Examination, physical, 227
"Exercises, spinal therapeutic," 230

Falx fenestration, 75
Familial dysautonomia, 191
Femoral agenesis, 156, 157
Filum, thickened, 183, 185–187
Flexion pain, 19
Foregut cysts, 134
Foregut duplications, 282
Froriep's occipitoblast, 20
Fusion, spinal, 235
  anterior, 246
  solid, 232
Fusion levels
  correct, 232
  selection of, 211

Galveston technique, 215, 216
Gastrocystomas, 134
Gill procedure, 245
Grisel's syndrome, 48–49
"Growing Luque" procedure, 216

Halo-wheelchair traction, 196–197
Harrington, "stable zone" of, 232
Harrington instrumentation, 195–199,
    214–215, 233
Hemisacrum, 158
Hemivertebra, 13–14, 15, 145
  lumbo-sacral, 16
Heuter-Volkman Law, 226
Hip dislocation, 162, 195
Horizontal deformities, 241–247
Hounsfield reading, 258, 261

Hydrocephalus
  primary, 61–62
  secondary, 62–63
Hydromyelia, 45–46, 50, 273, 275–279
Hyperkyphosis, 236
Hyperlordosis, 117, 241

Idiopathic scoliosis (IS), 189, 194, 224
  adolescent with, 235
  infantile, 234
  juvenile, 235
Infantile idiopathic scoliosis, 234
Intestinoma, 135
Intracranial neurenteric cysts, 139
Intraoperative blood loss, 232
Intrasphenoidal synchondrosis, 33
Intraspinal cyst, 137
Intraspinal neurenteric cysts, 135–139
Intravenous pyelogram, 229
"Inverted Napoleon's cap," 123, 124
IS, see Idiopathic scoliosis

Jejunal diverticulum, 137
Junghann's pseudospondylolisthesis, 116
Juvenile idiopathic scoliosis, 235

Klippel–Feil syndrome, 12, 60
Knee disarticulation, 161
Kovalevsky, canal of, 287
Kyphoscoliosis, 100, 272
Kyphosis, 236–237
  classification of, 237, 238
  consequences of, 239

Lachapelle's dog, 127
Laminectomy, 107
Lipoma of cord, 158, 160
  neuro-imaging of, 260–262
Lipomeningocele, 174
Lipomeningomyelocele (LMMC), 177,
    179
  dorsal, 182
  neuro-imaging of, 263–266
  untethering, 185, 187
LMMC, see Lipomeningomyelocele

Long-term care of deformed spine, 221–248

Lordosis, 236, 241
exaggerated, 122

Lumbo-sacral agenesis, sacral agenesis and, *see* Sacral and lumbo-sacral agenesis

Lumbo-sacral hemivertebra, 16

Lumbo-sacral vertebra, malformations of, 16–17

Luque instrumentation, 208, 213, 214, 215, 233

Magnetic resonance (MR), 251, 279, 288

Marique–Taillard classification, 125, 245

Mass lesions, developmental, 255–263

Maternal diabetes, 149–150

Meningoceles
neuro-imaging of, 267–272
presacral, 174

Meningomyelocele, 46, 70–71, 267
incidence of, 158
neuromuscular scoliosis and, 191–192
operative management of, 247
repaired, 178–180

Meningomyelodysplasia, 251

Meyerding's classification, 124, 125, 245

Micturition reflex, spinal, 156

Milwaukee brace, 201, 203, 230

Moire fringe topography, 228

Morquio's disease, 49

Motion segment, 221–222

MR (magnetic resonance), 251, 279, 288

Mulholland chair, 203, 204

Muscular dystrophy, Duchenne's, 192

Myelocele, 251
neuro-imaging of, 267–272

Myelodysplasia, 59

Myelography
computed tomographic metrizamide (CTMM), 182–183, 271, 272, 283–284
computed tomography (CTM), 256, 280, 288

Myelomeningocele, 267; *see also* Meningomyelocele

"Napoleon's cap, inverted," 123, 124

Neurenteric cysts, 134–141
defined, 134
development of, 139–141
intracranial, 139
intraspinal, 135–139
neuro-imaging of, 282, 287
pathogenesis of, 140, 141
pathology of, 134–135
radiologic features of, 138
treatment of, 138–139

Neurofibromatosis of von Reckling-hausen, 50

Neurogenic bladder dysfunction, 156, 158

Neurolysis and posterior arch removal, 129

Neuromuscular scoliosis (NMS), 186–216
classification and incidence of, 189–192
current treatment of, 200–215
etiology and pathogenesis of, 192–193
known causes of, 190
literature review of treatment of, 195–199
meningomyelocele and, 191–192
myopathy in, 192
natural history of, 194–195
neuropathic, lower motor neuron, 191
neuropathic, upper motor neuron, 190–191
operative treatment of, 206–215
orthotics with, 201–205
syringomyelia and, 191

NMS, *see* Neuromuscular scoliosis

Nocturnal electrical stimulation, 231

Nonidiopathic scoliosis, 235

Occipital condyles, vertebralization of, 37–40

Occipitalization of atlas, 36, 39

Occiput, 20–21, 22

Odontoid base, agenesis of, 5

Odontoid process
agenesis of, 5, 49
dysplasia-dysgenesis of, 5–10
mobile, 39, 41

"OEIS complex," 144–145
Orthopaedic syndrome, 92, 99–100
Orthopaedics, term, 221
Orthoses
    in neuromuscular scoliosis, 201–205
    thoracic suspension, 202, 203
Os odontoideum, 5, 6
Ossiculum terminale, 5, 7–10
Ossification, 1
    from birth to age of 8 years, 24–28
    of cranio-vertebral junction, 30
    secondary, 23
Ossification centers in cervico-occipital
    area, 22

Pain, back, 121, 244
PFT (pulmonary function testing), 206
Physical examination, 227
Pneumonia, 200, 201
Poliomyelitis, 189, 191
Polyarthritis, 46–48
Posterior arch removal, neurolysis and,
    129
Posterior fossa decompression, 82–86
Posterior fossa neuroepithelial cysts, 139
Postural roundback, 237
Presacral meningoceles, 174
Prevertebral cyst, 137, 139
Prosthesis for lumbo-sacral agenesis, 161,
    162
Pseudospondylolisthesis, 120, 243
    Junghann's, 116
Pulmonary function testing (PFT), 206
Pyelogram, intravenous, 229

Reduplicated ileum, 137
Rostral malformations, 94–95
Roundback, postural, 237

Sacral and lumbo-sacral agenesis,
    144–163
    associated malformation in, 159
    autopsy case reports of, 154–155
    classification of, 145–148
    clinical characteristics of, 156
    defined, 144–145

    with duplication of ureter, 157, 158
    embryology of, 153–154
    etiology of, 148–153
    with femoral agenesis, 156, 157
    neurologic complications with,
        158–160
    orthopedic management of, 160–162
    pedigree of families with, 151
    urologic complications of, 156–158
    visceral malformation in, 160
Sacralization, 15, 16–17
Sacro-coccygeal teratomas, see Teratomas
Sagittal deformities, 236–241
Scheuermann's disease, 237
    treatment of, 239–241
Schmitt–Fischer angle, 30
Sciatica, 121
Scoliosis, 189, 223
    bracing for, 162
    classification of structural, 224, 225
    evaluation of, 227–229
    idiopathic, see Idiopathic scoliosis
    incidence of, 193
    management of, 226
    measurement of, 224, 226
    neuromuscular, see Neuromuscular
        scoliosis
    nonidiopathic, 235
    nonoperative treatment of, 229–231
    operative treatment of, 231–234
    progression of, 226
    radiologic evaluation of, 228–229
    structural versus nonstructural, 224
    treatment algorithms for, 234–236
    treatment of, 229–236
Segmental spinal instrumentation (SSI),
    198–200
Solid spinal fusion, 232
Somatosensory evoked cortical potential
    (SSEP), 216
Spheno-occipital synchondrosis, 33, 35
Spina bifida, 41
Spina bifida aperta, 246–247
Spina bifida occulta, 94, 251, 252
Spinal cord
    lipoma of, see Lipoma of cord
    monitoring, 232–233
    tethered, see Tethered spinal cord
"Spinal deformity," concept of, 223

Spinal dysraphism, neuro-imaging of,
    251–288
"Spinal exercises, therapeutic," 230
Spinal flexibility, determination of, 207
Spinal fusion, see Fusion entries
Spinal instrumentation, 180
    segmental (SSI), 198–200
Spinal micturition reflex, 156
Spinal-pelvic fusion, 162
Spine
    coronal deformities of, 223–236
    deformed, long-term care of,
        221–248
    growth over time, 222–223
    horizontal deformities of, 241–247
    normal curves for, 221
    sagittal deformities of, 236–241
Spine straightening procedure, 180
Split atlas, 41
"Split cord syndrome," 251, 280, 282; see
    also Diastematomyelia
"Split notochord syndrome," 139
"Spondylo-centers," 32
Spondylolisthesis, 113–130, 242
    classification of, 113–116
    clinical manifestations of, 121–122
    congenital, 242
    congenital theory of, 116
    degenerative, 116, 243
    dysplastic, 113–114, 115
    dysplastic theory of, 117
    grade I asymptomatic, 124, 129
    grade II, 129
    hereditability of, 117
    history of, 113
    incidence of, 117
    isthmic, 114, 116, 242–243
    management of, 244
    pathogenesis and natural history of,
        116–119
    pathologic, 116, 243–244
    pathologic features of, 119–120
    radiographic features of, 122–128
    radiologic evaluation of, 244–245
    term, 116
    therapeutic approaches in, 128–130
    traumatic, 116, 117–118, 243
    traumatic theory of, 116
    treatment of, 245–246

trophostatic theory of, 117
    true, 116
Spondylolysis, 113, 114, 119, 242; see
    also Spondylolisthesis
    asymptomatic, 128
Spondyloptosis, 122, 127
Spondylothoracic dysplasia, 14
SSEP (somatosensory evoked cortical
    potential), 216
"Stable zone" of Harrington, 232
Still's disease, 19, 43, 46–48
Suboccipito-palatine line, 30
Subtrochanteric amputation, 161
Syringohydromyelia, 272, 273, 282
Syringomyelia, 45–46, 50
    scoliosis and, 191
Syrinx, terminal, 280

Taillard classification, 125, 245
"Teratoid tumor," 134
Teratomas, 169–175, 263
    diagnosis of, 170–174
    literature review of, 167–170
    origin of, 167
    pathology of, 170
    presacral or postsacral, 170
    technique for excision of, 172–173,
        174–175
    term, 167
    treatment of, 172–173, 174–175
Teratomatous cysts, 134, 135
Terminal syrinx, 280
Tethered spinal cord, 177–187
    clinical manifestations of, 179–182
    conditions associated with,
        177–179
    diastematomyelia and, 178
    investigation of, 182–184
    neuro-imaging of, 253–259
    treatment of, 184–187
"Therapeutic spinal exercises," 230
Thickened filum, 183, 185–187
Thoracic suspension orthosis, 202, 203
Thoracic vertebrae, malformations
    affecting, 12, 13–15
Tight filum terminale syndrome, 253–259
TLSO (underarm body jacket), 194, 202,
    203, 205

Torticollis, 19
Traction, 207–208
Tuberculosis, 48
Tuberculous osteoarthritis, 19

Ultrasound (US), 251, 265, 288
Underarm body jacket (TLSO), 194, 202, 203, 205
Ureter, duplication of, 157, 158
US (ultrasound), 251, 265, 288

"Vater" association, 144
Vertebra(ae)
  "apical," 226
  block, 41, 42
  butterfly, 265
  classification of congenital anomalies, 1–3
  cranio-vertebral junction, see Cranio-vertebral junction

development of, 1
hemivertebra, see Hemivertebra
lumbo-sacral, malformations of, 16–17
major anomalies of, 3–17
malformations of, 1–17
thoracic, malformations affecting, 12, 13–15
wedged, 13
"Vertebral anisocoria," 123, 126
Vertebral bodies, fusion of, 130
Vertebralization of occipital condyles, 39–40
Von Recklinghausen, neurofibromatosis of, 50

Wedged vertebra, 13

Zielke rod, 214, 233